೪ ೪ ೪

Counseling in Speech-Language Pathology and Audiology

JANE SCHEUERLE
University of South Florida

Merrill, an imprint of
Macmillan Publishing Company
New York

Maxwell Macmillan Canada
Toronto

Maxwell Macmillan International
New York Oxford Singapore Sydney

Cover photos: Copyright © Richard Hutchings (Info Edit); David Young-Wolff, Alan Oddie, Myrleen Ferguson, Tony Freeman (PhotoEdit); and Larry Hamill
Editor: Ann Castel
Production Editor: Mona M. Bunner
Art Coordinator: Raydelle M. Clement
Text Designer: Anne Flanagan
Production Buyer: Pamela D. Bennett
Electronic Publishing Coordinator: Marilyn Wilson Phelps

This book was set in New Century Schoolbook and was printed and bound by Book Press, Inc., a Quebecor America Book Group Company. The cover was printed by New England Book Components.

Macmillan Publishing Company
866 Third Avenue
New York, NY 10022

Macmillan Publishing Company is part of the
Maxwell Communication Group of Companies.

Maxwell Macmillan Canada, Inc.
1200 Eglinton Avenue East, Suite 200
Don Mills, Ontario M3C 3N1

Library of Congress Cataloging-in-Publication Data
Scheuerle, Jane.
    Counseling in speech-language pathology and audiology / Jane
Scheuerle.
        p. cm.
    Includes bibliographical references and index.
    ISBN 0-675-21157-3
    1. Communicative disorders—Patients—Counseling of.
2. Communicative disorders—Psychological aspects. 3. Speech
therapist and patient. 4. Audiologist and patient. I. Title.
RC428.8.S34   1992
616.85'506—dc20   91-19173
                                                                            CIP

Printing: 1 2 3 4 5 6 7 8 9   Year: 2 3 4 5

❦ ❦ ❦

Preface

*T*he goal of this book is to describe and present *counseling* as an essential role of the speech-language pathologist and audiologist. The content is generated around four considerations of professional training and delivery of services to communicatively disordered clients and their families. Those considerations are bridging the gap between classroom learning and clinical performance; de-mystifying the counseling process; identifying the therapist as the primary tool for therapeutic intervention; and discovering natural and learned elements of social-interactive communication that the counselor brings to bear in care management of clients and their families.

Issues associated with counseling in communication disorders are separated into seven clusters. Each cluster of issues is the focus of a chapter. Each chapter contains exercises designed to emphasize to the reader that use of counseling skills demands active, objective involvement of the therapist with each individual being served. Chapters 1 through 5 discuss counseling in service to clients and caregivers. Chapter 6 looks at some applications of counseling skills and practices to career choices. Chapter 7 suggests needs and methods for ongoing evaluation of counseling in treatment of communication disorders.

Now, as this volume goes to press, I want to thank the many contributors. Teachers, students, clients, and colleagues helped me explore the ideas contained here. Kelmie Hollahan carefully read drafts of early chapters, Jerry B. Crittenden encouraged me to achieve what sometimes seemed impossible, and Mary Pannbacker analyzed the current status of counseling in the literature of communication disorders. Finally, I acknowledge the enormous contribution of my family—Bill, Angela, and Ramsey. Not only did they tolerate my immersion in this project for several years, but they generously contributed information and resources from their respective fields of expertise.

ℰ ℰ ℰ

Contents

CHAPTER 1

Common Ground Between Communication Disorders and Counseling 1

CHAPTER 2

Hidden Talents: Ordinary Interactive Behaviors as Helping Skills 29

CHAPTER 3

Serving Clients Across Ages   79

CHAPTER 4

Serving Clients Across Disorders   141

CHAPTER 6

Helping—Throughout a Career 243

CHAPTER 7

Evaluating Counseling Skills of Clinicians 267

APPENDIX A

Counseling in Communication Disorders as Addressed in the Literature 287

APPENDIX B

Suggested Interactive Stimulus Materials by Age 294

APPENDIX C

Supplementary Reading 295

❦ ❦ ❦

Common Ground Between Communication Disorders and Counseling

Issues

❦ *Communication disorders and counseling emerged as two significant human services disciplines of the 20th century resulting from social evolution.*

❦ *Change in individual and socio-cultural human values focused interest on communication disorders and their treatment.*

❦ *The clinician is the single most significant therapeutic tool available in the treatment of communication disorders.*

❦ ❦ ❦

THE CHALLENGE OF THE COMMUNICATIONS DISORDERS DISCIPLINE

The field of Speech-Language Pathology and Audiology, like other human service occupations that have gained prominence in the last century, continues to generate more subject matter than any individual can address authoritatively. Still, speech-language pathologists and audiologists face the challenge of serving clients responsibly across the spectrum of human communicative disorders.

The successful practitioner in the treatment of communication disorders must respond appropriately to diverse requests for help from clients and their families. Consider for a moment the wide variety of clients who seek the help of the speech-language pathologist or audiologist. The clinician works with babies and their families, aging men and women, executive officers of multimillion dollar corporations, the rural poor, school children, international opera and film stars, and migrant workers. Additionally, speech, language, and hearing clinicians are typically well-educated, technically skilled, nurturing, caring people who value linguistic communication as a unique human behavior. Attempting to serve the needs of all clients can be overwhelming; however, the process does not require that professionals who treat or manage communication disorders furnish immediate answers to all questions or solutions to all problems. Instead, clinicians learn a variety of non-invasive techniques to induce positive behavioral and/or attitudinal changes in clients and their families. Table 1.1 lists the clinical techniques used most frequently in treatment of communication disorders.

No academic program can fully prepare students for every possible communication disorder and treatment situation they may encounter throughout their careers. Proficient clinicians acquire a bank of knowledge and skills from which they select an appropriate scientific assessment or intervention technique for each client. In practice they adapt what they have learned and apply it as needed.

Importance of Personal Traits in the Interactive Process

In addition to acquiring the knowledge and skills of the discipline, clinicians internalize, interpret, and adapt that knowledge according to individual strengths and preferences. That is, each clinician takes to the treatment setting, to the client, and to the family a unique blend of personal characteristics. Roles of clinicians vary then, not only according to what they learn in university training programs, but according to individual characteristics, their perspectives on life, their grasp of reality, and their hopes and fears. The client and the client's family or care-givers perceive these attributes as degrees of competency, interest, support, caring, understanding, and/or acceptance.

Table 1.1
Common clinical techniques in the treatment of communicative disorders

Technique	Description
Observation	Watching and listening
Assessment	Evaluating responses to stimuli and spontaneous behaviors to determine level of severity and limits of ability
Demonstration	Modeling; showing desired behavior
Elicitation	Stimulating spontaneous responses
Instruction	Telling or describing
Reinforcement	Using social or material stimuli
Diagnosis	Analyzing spontaneous and elicited behaviors to identify disorder or category of disorder
Planning	Arranging strategic steps for change
Referral	Introducing client to a timely, preferred resource
Discussion	Sharing information with client and family
Recommendation	Prioritizing procedural steps
Summarization	Recapitulating experiences concisely
Dismissal	Giving ultimate approval, agreed to by client and family

Just as the clinician is an integral part of the treatment paradigm, so is the client with the communication disorder (Backus & Beasley, 1951). Over the last half century it has become increasingly clear that communication disorders cannot be successfully treated as single entities, separable from other traits of the person with the communicative impairment. Communication disorders that impede normal participation in routines of family and community are critical handicaps. Communicatively impaired individuals and their families seek help as they work toward maximizing communication abilities in everyday life. They require opportunities to learn to cope with aspects of disordered communication that cannot be normalized. The client and the family, like the clinician, influence treatment progress by their unique combination of traits that have evolved from the experience of daily living within their culture. The blend of clinician, client, and family traits significantly influences the initial interview session and therapeutic process thereafter.

Tables 1.2 and 1.3 indicate a variety of significant experiential aspects that influence the interaction of individuals in prevention, diagnosis, and treatment of speech, language, and hearing disorders. Review of clinician, client, and family traits shows that each of the three parties displays many characteristics that fall into common behavioral categories. Differences will occur within each trait category on an individual basis related to the context of the moment. Even identical twins, the most similar of human beings, display differences in behaviors within these trait categories.

Management of the blend of individual traits in interpersonal relationships of clinician and clients is basic to prevention and intervention in communication disorders. The clinician must facilitate mutual respect and trust and utilize client abilities to foster positive change in communicative abilities (Flower, 1984; Cornett & Chabon, 1988). The term *counseling* encompasses the skills and techniques involved in treatment activities such as achieving and maintaining compatibility, alleviating stress, empathizing with joy or sorrow, or addressing reality.

Table 1.2
Aspects of experience affecting interpersonal relationships common to clinicians and clients/families

Aspect	Components
Culture	Beliefs, values, ethics, ethnic group
Environment	Urban, surburban, rural
Family	Responsibility, tolerance, acceptance, expectations
Age	Young, middle age, old
Gender	Male, female
Personality	Feelings, attitude, behavior
Communication style	Formal, restrained, standard, assertive
Personal goals	Plans, hopes, needs, expectations

Table 1.3
Aspects of experience affecting interpersonal relationships differing for clinicians and clients/families

For the Clinician

Aspect	Components
Socioeconomic status	Childhood, current, and expectations
Education	General, professional
Experience	Personal, professional
Reputation	Community, professional
Clinical Style	Structured, non-directive, client-oriented
Professional strengths	Experience, training
Professional goals	Treatment, supervision, administration

For the Client/Family

Aspect	Components
Socioeconomic status	Secure, independent, dependent
Education	Highest level for each family member
Experience	History, motivation
Communication needs	Environmental influences
Communication disorder	Onset, type etiology, history, status, prognosis, coping style and skill

Counseling is formally defined as advising, directing, and exchanging opinions and ideas. However, this much-used term has a history of misinterpretation. In the mid-1900s the term counseling became associated with the practice of clinical psychology and, in that context, denoted a mysterious relationship with hidden workings of the mind and emotions. Because of this negative connotation, the terms *counselor* and *counseling* were not commonly used in other human service professions until much later.

As the discipline of psychology developed through the first half of the 20th century, scholarly research on aspects of human behavior produced definitive information concerning human thoughts, feelings, and behavior; norms and differences; and assessment and treatment. Also, incorporation of case study techniques that had been productive in social work drew aspects of psychology into the applied sciences. Thus the single discipline of psychology diversified into a host of specialized fields, including physiological psychology, perception and cognition, human and animal learning, developmental psychology, personality/clinical psychology, and social psychology.

Increased knowledge gradually eradicated superstitions about unexplained deviant human behavior. The mental illness-wellness dichotomy, inherited from earlier medical approaches to unusual behavior, gave way to a recognition that a broad range of human behavior may occur without indicating mental illness. Among these behaviors were the communication disorders of deafness, loss of language, and impaired speech.

Theories formulated in psychology have been applied to treatment of communication disorders. Twentieth-century learning theory, linguistic theory, existential and humanistic psychology, as well as medical discoveries, profoundly altered medical-physical perspectives found in pre-1900 records of diagnosis and treatment of speech, language, and hearing impairments.

Counseling, defined as giving direction for management of current and future events, now forms an integral part of many well-established and respected occupations. People now commonly seek counseling from lawyers, clergy, physicians, teachers, psychologists, social workers, speech-language pathologists, and audiologists, as well as family members and friends.

Counseling as Helping

The introduction of the concept of *helping* into the treatment of deviant human behavior as a primary characteristic of therapeutic interaction reflects the 19th-century thinking of philosopher Soren Kierkegaard. According to Kierkegaard (1962), the clinician as a person is the most powerful ingredient in the therapeutic process. The values and expectations of the clinician and the ability to communicate those characteristics to the client are essential for effective therapy (Beutler, 1979; Spielberg, 1980; Strupp, 1980). This leads to consideration of the meaning of therapy. Therapy is an interactive process with the intended outcome of producing positive change in the client. Yet, assuming the absence of physical force, drugs, hypnotism, or brainwashing, clients are free to change according to their abilities and designs. Therefore, for the purposes of this book, therapy is defined as a process by which the clinician establishes an environment in which the client and family can and will change.

Carl Rogers (1958) first described helping relationships as the essence of counseling. Rogers defined helping relationships as interpersonal relationships in which one person has the intent to promote another's growth, development, maturity, improved function, and/or improved coping with life. That description ideally applies to all disciplines in the field of human services. In communication disorders, treatment involves the three critical components of any helping relationship: (a) the teacher, counselor, therapist, or helper; (b) the student, client, patient, or helpee; and (c) what they do together, that is, the lesson, guidance, therapeutic process, or interaction (Ellis, 1973; Glasser, 1965; Schwartz, 1978).

Rogers's contribution of this view of counseling as helping formed a major span in the bridge between psychology and other disciplines that deal with human psychosocial conditions. Yet, practical understanding of the concept and specific applications of helping and subsequent training for its use in other disciplines remain largely undeveloped. Without specific training in helping skills, speech-language pathologists and audiologists tend to think of the term *counseling* as simply instructing and advising. In practice, clinicians generally develop high levels of helping relationships as natural functions of their personalities, communication styles, and clinical roles rather than from skills they have learned.

This situation reflects the need to identify abilities and skills that actualize helping relationships to facilitate treatment of communication disorders. From this process, the reader can develop a selected reservoir of helping skills to apply in the practice of speech, language, and hearing therapy. Many of the values, expectations, and skills needed for helping in communication disorders originated from the socio-cultural milieu out of which the discipline grew.

❦ ❦ ❦

ORIGINS OF THE COMMUNICATION DISORDERS DISCIPLINE

Communication is a unique human behavior. Dr. Charles Van Riper (1972) defined communication as *disordered* when it calls attention to itself, interferes with the transmission of ideas, or causes maladjustment in the communicator.

In general, the discipline of communication disorders, like earlier interest in speech correction, evolved from culturally supported ideas and principles (Eldridge, 1968). First is recognition of the unique features of human communication. That is, among all known animals, only humans use symbolic language to express and comprehend cognitive information, use propositional language to deal with abstractions, and use language to create poetry, state scientific principles, or elicit pathos and laughter. A second principle upon which the field of communication disorders is based recognizes that all human beings have the right to realize their individual potentials. Neither of these ideas was new in 1927 when Robert West and his colleagues formalized their commitment to helping the communicatively impaired by establishing The American Academy of Speech Correction (Padden, 1970). Since then other influences have led to the evolution of a widely recognized discipline for prevention and intervention in handicapping conditions related to disorders of speech, language, and hearing.

Factors Identified for Success

The success of any sociocultural endeavor to provide services for handicapped individuals requires the convergence of three factors. The first factor is that the need, or the market, must exist and be identified in sufficiently large numbers to warrant the provision of more than incidental services. By the last decade of the 20th century, it has generally become accepted that 10 to 20 percent of the population experiences communication disorders. Expected increases in both the elderly population and the incidence of birth defects predict continued growth of the consumer market for services dealing with communication disorders. Certainly the need for services has been established.

The second factor is the availability of (re)habilitative services. The need for skilled practitioners led to a demand for university programs to train qualified researchers, teachers, and practitioners in the many subspecialties of communication sciences and disorders. The establishment of these educational programs necessitated regulatory bodies and liaison personnel with other sociocultural agencies. Local, state, and national regulators and professional associations monitor personnel training and provision of services.

The third requirement for the successful provision of services to communicatively handicapped individuals is adequate funding and community support. The identification of the market and the availability of rehabilitative services is meaningless without a reliable source of economic support for these services within the local community and government. Achievement of that type of support demands extensive popular commitment to the value of such services for the betterment of society through betterment of the individual.

Since 1927, dedicated communication specialists and clients and their families have sought to demonstrate the needs and rights of citizens with communication disorders. Convergence of these two elements—needs and rights—implies an obligation for society at large to assume responsibility to rehabilitate communicatively handicapped individuals so that they can fulfill their unique promise. As evidence of some success in these efforts, the United States Department of Defense has instituted speech and hearing services in veterans' hospitals; federal and state agencies spend vast sums on special education; some health insurance programs cover payment for communication therapies; the National Institute for Deafness and Communication Disorders has been established; and most recently, in July, 1990, legislators passed the Americans With Disabilities Act. These and other measures reflect the strides made in swaying public opinion toward the value of (re)habilitation of speech, language, and hearing during this century.

These changes in public and individual attention to human communication have influenced the student of communication disorders. The writing of this book is an example of the effect of those changes. To understand their full significance, it is important to examine the historical ramifications of precedents of modern communication sciences and disorders.

❧ ❧ ❧

EMERGENCE OF THE COMMUNICATION DISORDERS AND COUNSELING FIELDS

The beliefs underlying the communication disorders discipline evolved from the philosophies and perceptions of the human condition that began to emerge during the 18th century. Values and beliefs held throughout the western world at that time were primarily based on Judeo-Christian theologies and practices. Those doctrines viewed people as beloved creatures of a just but loving deity, recognized good and evil, and justified reward and/or punishment in life on earth or in an afterworld. Belief in equality, freedom, and the pursuit of individual fulfillment formed the foundation of the United States, evident in the Declaration of Independence, the Constitution, and the Bill of Rights. The belief in the rights of all citizens to achieve their best echoes the thoughts of John Locke (1632–1704), Soren Kierkegaard (1813–1855), and John Stuart Mill (1806–1873).

A Middle Class Emerges

Prior to the Industrial Revolution (ca. 1750–1860) the population was largely divided into two classes: wealthy landowners and laborers. The latter, peasants and serfs, had no recognized individual rights except as relegated to them by their masters. Health and welfare were a matter of birthright, usually reserved for the wealthy. There was medical treatment of physical illness, but only theological explanations for disturbances in human behavior such as stuttering and mutism.

When industrialization changed the roles of men, women, and children, a new socio-economic class emerged. That new stratum of society, the middle class, exceeded subsistence economy in their daily lives and found time for and interest in identifying and addressing needs, rights, and inequities among all three social classes: upper, middle, and lower. For the first time, a large segment of the population owned real property and chattel, worked for a living wage in respectable and respected positions, and could hope for a better life (Churchill, 1964).

The new middle class became demanding consumers of manufactured products, participants in government, and crusaders for realistic political philosophies. In these new roles, this group called for compulsory elementary education, literacy for the masses, and equal rights under the law for all citizens. Volunteers and private associations provided charity for limited numbers of the ill, homeless, and hungry. These latter efforts were the forerunners of professional social work.

Literacy and Access to Information

Another factor affecting social values came with the rise of capitalism and private enterprise. Newspapers and weekly journals became available, providing commentary on current events and recording speeches and discussions. These print media disseminated information, influenced thinking, and shaped behavior. Access to information previously limited to the wealthy class stirred appreciation of reading in the common citizen.

Access to information increased the perceived value of education. Reading increased social awareness among the new, upwardly mobile middle class readers, as they learned about people and events beyond the scope of their day-to-day experience. The 19th-century works of Charles Dickens are particularly credited with focusing popular attention on rampant poverty, social injustice, and the plight of powerless and homeless urban children.

Independence and Value of the Individual

The American and French Revolutions and their aftermath in the late 18th century had occupied much of the energies of the United States and the European populations during the early years of the Industrial Revolution. Largely because of its insular nature, England was in the forefront of recognizing opportunities for fostering social change during the next 100 years (Churchill, 1964). During this time, capitalism fostered private enterprise and gained prominence in the old, new, and colonial worlds. Urbanization intensified as people sought prosperity and social mobility. In both England and the United States, an individual's financial resources largely determined social mobility, but other factors became important: education, manner of dress, language usage, and manner of speaking.

❦ ❦ ❦

CHANGE IN HUMAN VALUES

Stirred by rapid economic growth and migratory patterns in the population, political and social leaders, scholars, and philosophers recognized the unprecedented evolution of society, its dreams and expectations. They saw achievements in science and technology and their negative and positive side effects, at all levels of human endeavor. Local, national, and international laws regulated boundaries, trade, exploration, and colonization.

Literacy and the Social Conscience

Nationalism, like liberalism, gained a strong foothold in England and Europe. John Stuart Mill's treatise on political theory, *On Liberty* (1859), is considered the most significant statement of the liberal position on the importance of freedom for discovery of truth and for the full development of the individual. Mill raised dual questions: What more or better can be said of any condition of human affairs than that it brings human beings themselves nearer to the best they can be, or what worse can be said of any obstruction to good than that it prevents this? Such ponderance of humanity by a public spokesperson suited people who had experienced the influences of industrialization and who had also read *Oliver Twist* (Dickens, 1838), *Jane Eyre* (Bronte, 1847), and *Wuthering Heights* (Bronte, 1848). These works, like others of that time, challenged the literate, economically and socially secure public to consider as problems of society the conditions of children, women, the poor and uneducated, the insane and their families, and the needs, rights, and ultimately the nature of human beings.

Although Victorian class structure was rigidly controlled, contemporary literature, art, and music gave evidence of discontent with blindness to social injustices (Hughes, 1980). The popularity of novels and essays espousing liberalism demonstrates the readiness of newly literate segments of society to acknowledge social conditions reflected in their literature. In such a climate it is little wonder that the 1859 publication of John Stuart Mill's *On Liberty* generated immediate and long-term private and public discussion, analysis, criticism, and rebuttal. It is interesting to note that the *Communist Manifesto,* which Marx and Engels wrote in 1848 and which excluded the balancing effect of the new middle class, met little acclaim until much later in history and in another culture.

Among the power struggles of the time was the initiation of political unification of Italy. By 1861, the Pope had lost considerable amounts of land, wealth, and power, significantly reducing the position and power of the Roman Catholic Church and its teachings in world politics. In America, economic, expansionist, and constitutional arguments erupted into the War Between the States, leading to the emancipation of slaves and the acknowledged constitutional equality of all people (Boorstin, 1987; Commanger, 1950).

❦ ❦ ❦

SCIENTIFIC INFLUENCES

Biology and Medical Technology

Another powerful influence on social evolution was Charles Darwin's *The Origin of Species,* published in 1859. That biological treatise, as well as his later *Descent of Man* (1871), presented evidence that change in species is more probable than had been ascribed to living things on the planet. Darwin's works challenged perceptions of the self and long-held beliefs.

As if to emphasize society's changing perception of life and the human condition, scientific advances in the 1900s helped to remove much of the mystery long surrounding health, illness, epidemics, and curative agents. Louis Pasteur discovered germs and initiated the field of microbiology. Other breakthroughs include the development of a smallpox vaccination and the identification of bacteria that cause tuberculosis and Asiatic cholera. The introduction of sanitation and anesthetic and antiseptic procedures for surgery saved lives and reduced pain. Nursing, established and popularized as a merciful helping profession, created new roles for women. Perception of human significance in the universe changed again with Antoine Lavoisier's proof that matter can neither be created nor destroyed, but only changed in form.

Behavior-Observations and Treatment

Along with increased efforts to solve perplexing health problems and prolong life, medical records show documentation of certain illnesses and injuries that were accompanied by loss of the ability to speak and to understand language among their patients. Records reveal health-related speech disturbances of articulation, stammering, deafness, aphasia, and ways to occlude palatal clefts. Physicians trained assistants to work with speech-handicapped patients (Boome, Baines, & Harris, 1950). Recognition of deafness as a problem of communication rather than one of mental deficiency gave rise to the development of ways to communicate with and educate deaf children. Such endeavors were precursors of the field of speech-language pathology and audiology.

❦ ❦ ❦

APPLICATION OF SCIENTIFIC ADVANCES TO SOCIAL CHANGE

New knowledge and technology bombarded every field of endeavor. Market demands stimulated industry, which in turn demanded longer hours and more effort from poorly paid, unskilled laborers. Individual creativity and productivity initiated demands for patents and copyrights. To accommodate those demands, legislators created public agencies and passed laws through national and international agreements. Thus, bureaucracy vastly increased to implement and monitor the laws.

Development of Social Work

Many factors focused the attention of influential men and women toward defining human values in the late 1800s and early 1900s (Beutler, 1979). Altruism inherent in social philosophy, accidents of time and place, and recognition of power, rights, and responsibilities of individual citizens converged to create this focus. People found creative ways to solve perplexing social problems. For example, in New York, in the absence of child protection laws, social workers used animal cruelty laws to argue for the removal of abused children from dangerous parents. In London, the need to fight and control the crime that accompanied urbanization led to the creation of The Peelers, an organized police force that later became Scotland Yard.

Development of Case Study Techniques

Social workers developed case management techniques and case studies as ways to define practical and timely solutions to daily problems (Armitage, 1975; Fischer, 1978). For example, in the late 19th and early 20th centuries, urban social problems were so extreme in large cities such as New York and Boston that groups of children roamed the streets searching for food and shelter. By using case study techniques, thousands of abandoned children were identified and alternative ways of life offered them using private and public support. Remedies applied to this unprecedented social problem included orphan trains and urban hostels.

Development of Psychology as a Discipline

In Vienna, dramatic changes in traditional approaches to human behavior occurred as a result of the treatment of Anna O., a woman in a famous case in the annals of psychiatry. Joseph Breuer, a physiologist at the University of Vienna, had been unable to treat Anna O.'s hysteria with hypnosis, the preferred treatment at the time. Instead, he encouraged Anna O. to talk about her past and the circumstances of her current problem. Breuer discovered the talking treatment was as effective as hypnosis had been on similar patients. Sigmund Freud later used Breuer's talking technique to develop his Psychoanalytic Theory between 1882 and 1900 (Bernstein, 1965). The discovery that mental disturbances can be independent of and separate from physical illness provided a major break from psychiatry, the medical specialty in treatment of mental illnesses. Whereas psychiatry utilized sedatives and restraints to control patients who were diagnosed as agitated or dangerous, psychology introduced the notion that behavior is related to life experience, of which the physical aspects are only a part. Thus, the discipline of psychology was born. Interestingly, social work and psychiatry were practical applied fields that identified and remediated problems of daily living and of health, respectively. By contrast, psychology developed as the empirical study of observable human behavior, particularly learning, mental and emotional illness, and perception.

❧ ❧ ❧

APPROACHES TO THE STUDY OF HUMAN BEHAVIOR

As the field of psychology developed during the next 100 years, many theories emerged to explain human behavior. Although in actual chronology the theories overlapped one another, a review of their development shows a critical transition in perception of human nature through study of human behavior. It is convenient to consider the major approaches to study of human behavior under five categorical headings: psychology of learning, Freudian psychology, Gestalt psychology, organismic psychology, and existential-humanistic psychology.

Psychology of Learning

The psychology of learning includes behaviorism and conditioning and is based on rigorous empiricism. Research concentrated on overt, observable behaviors of subjects, both humans and lower animals. Past experience and physical condition of the subject's body were considered to influence current and predictable behavior under given circumstances. The leading proponents of this theory were Ivan Pavlov, John Watson, Clark Hull, and B. F. Skinner. Three behavior therapies have evolved from their work since the 1950s: behavior modification, reciprocal inhibition therapy, and implosive therapy.

Behavior modification refers to use of stimuli to reinforce behavior in a subject or client who is free to act in any way. That is, upon performance of a desired behavior, the subject receives a meaningful reward. Such reinforcement generates an increase in the incidence of the desired behavior. The opposite is true if the reward-stimulus is negative. That is, one expects to observe a decrease in the incidence of the undesired behavior (Skinner, 1957).

Reciprocal inhibition therapy (RIT) was designed to reduce anxiety by eliciting a response to inhibit the anxiety. Examples of techniques applied in this therapeutic model are assertiveness and relaxation training. Preceded by desensitization training, application of assertion or relaxation skills inhibits anxiety reactions in circumstances known to evoke anxiety in a given individual (Wolpe, 1958).

Implosive therapy (IT) is a procedure in which the therapist applies the principle of extinction of a conditioned response to a conditioned stimulus. The therapist elicits extreme anxiety in the neurotic client through visualization of circumstances that evoke negative emotions and symptomatic behavior. In this way the patient can experience the extreme of emotional response without reinforcement by presence of the object which normally elicits the response (Shipley, 1979).

Freudian Psychology

Freudian psychology is both a philosophy of human nature and a theory of human behavior. Three basic principles underlie the theory. These principles are that (a) human behavior expresses the need to reduce psychological tensions and maintain psychological homeostasis; (b) the individual attempts to accommodate behavior to context, that is, to reality; and (c) earlier behaviors are repeated as attempts to control stimuli (Ford & Urban, 1964).

Personality theory based on Freudian psychology introduced the concepts of id, ego, and superego, and later added an explanation of preconsciousness to consciousness and unconsciousness. According to this theory, current behavior is linked to past experiences. Freud's contributions to knowledge about child development, human sexuality, and neuroses have led to understanding of normal human behavior and the development of therapies to help change deviant behavior, particularly anxiety-related behavior. Responses to anxiety or fear of the unknown are called *defense mechanisms* and include fixation, regression, repression, denial, reaction formation, projection, and displacement. These internal responses are manifested through behavior and can vary along a continuum from mild involvement to profound illness, such as psychoses and neuroses. Treatment of such illnesses may require physical therapy, psychotherapy, and/or behavior therapy.

Gestalt Psychology

German psychologists developed Gestalt psychology after World War I, based on the belief that behavior cannot be separated from the whole being. Thus, the total configuration or the context of an event is essentially a contributing component to behavior. Additionally, Gestaltists dealt with perception as psychological closure or completion of integrated relationships among phenomena. Therefore, awareness of reality and one's reactions to it are paramount considerations in normal maturation as well as in therapeutic treatment of psychological problems.

Perls (1969) defined anxiety as the gap between now (the known present) and then (the unknown future). Abnormal behavior reflects holes or discontinuities in the gestalt. Gestalt therapy undertakes to supply what is missing so that the patient has a unified physical, psychological, and symbolic configuration. To achieve wholeness, the patient must become aware of self and other. This awareness, involving internal behaviors of knowing, sensing, valuing, and choosing, results in maturation, self-integration, and self-regulating growth.

Organismic Psychology

Organismic psychology is much like Gestalt psychology. The originator of this theory was Kurt Goldstein, a German neurologist who worked with brain-injured soldiers from World War I. He introduced the idea that the organism must be seen as a unit, not a combination of parts. When one aspect of the nervous system is affected the total system is affected. Evidence that overall neurological efficiency is altered following a single lesion is noted in an acquired sensory deficit. When a prior stimulus is repeated, the impaired nervous system reacts in a different but integrated way.

This theory created distinct definitions of fear and anxiety. Fear is the emotion that impels the organism to "fight or flight," while anxiety is fear of the unknown. Reactions to anticipated fearful situations lead the patient to maintain rigid controls to avoid the feared situation. When the patient encounters those feared situations, fear increases along with the anxiety, and the patient makes adjustments to avoid a recurrence of situations that cause fear.

Every normal person, as described by Goldstein (1959), operates on a single-drive principle, that of self-actualization (SA). The normal person is more than pathology-free; he seeks new experiences, enjoys spontaneity, and is creative in pursuing the total fulfillment of his potential. Thus, self-actualization differs from self-preservation, which is maintenance of *status quo*. Organismic psychology also presented the essential principle of communion, which was described as active participation and cooperation in mutually shared interpersonal relationships.

Existential-Humanistic Psychology

Existential-humanistic psychology evolved from existential philosophy. Existentialism is concerned with reality and the relationship between reality and the individual's awareness of reality (May, Angel, & Ellenberger, 1958). Early existentialists believed that urbanization and impersonalization of industrialized western society led to alienation of individuals from nature, from other human beings, and from themselves. Because of that alienation or aloneness, individuals experience a unique awareness of reality, both internal and external, and of their relation to that complex reality.

The existential perspective delineates and specifies six human characteristics:

1. Being is becoming, a dynamic emerging of potential.
2. Death is inevitable.
3. Individual freedom and responsibility for making choices carry with them risks of anxiety over change as fulfillment is sought, and guilt for refusal to seek fulfillment.
4. The individual exists in and shares in the design of his world and is aware of himself in that world where human relationships bring about change in both participating parties.
5. Past, present, and future are interrelated through the emerging of potential. That is, the future of the individual is influenced by past and present being.

6. Imagination allows the individual to remove himself from immediate experience and to use propositional language to evaluate and compare himself with expectations and memories.

These six characteristics help determine the course of therapy, which is based on the patient's intrinsic value system. In the therapeutic relationship, the helper attempts to understand the patient with the goal of helping develop the patient's potential, encouraging development within the context of the patient's existence and a commitment to discover the self.

Among the significant contributions to humanistic psychology since 1950 is Victor Frankl's *Man's Search for Meaning* (1965). Frankl introduced the premise that, without value or meaning, people stop growing or becoming, begin to decline, atrophy, and die. Abraham Maslow (1968) created the concept of a "hierarchy of needs," which prioritizes behaviors of individuals. The hierarchy is composed of physiological needs (food and shelter), safety and security, belongingness (affection and identification), self-esteem (self-respect), and self-actualization (fulfillment of potential).

Rogerian psychology demonstrated that the psycho-therapeutic process is not the singular province of psychiatrists. Rogers used the terms *interviewing, counseling,* and *helping* to describe his relationships with clients, students, family, and others. Thus, psychology, no longer limited to the *study* of human behavior, includes *treatment* of deviant human behavior as well. Through use of the same skills, helping can be applied to daily problems of the normal individual. Figure 1.1 suggests the emergence and interrelationships of current human services and the application of concepts of counseling and helping.

Rogers (1958, 1961) also initiated intensive study of the influence of the therapist's behavior on that of the client. His principles of helping supplanted traditional therapist behaviors of interrogation and advising with intensive interpersonal communication between clinician and client. The goals of such treatment were to understand and empathize with the client. To achieve the desired relationship, certain conditions are required: (a) two persons must be in contact (the client has a need for help, while the helper has knowledge and skills to provide help); (b) the helper values the client as a person (unconditional positive regard) and is empathic with the client; and (c) the client perceives the helper's positive regard and empathy.

To meet the demands of the helper's role, according to Rogers, therapists must possess qualities of genuineness, respect, empathy, concreteness, self-disclosure, immediacy, confrontation, warmth, and self-actualization (Spielberg, 1980). Rogers (1961) presented a hypothesis of helping relations of all kinds, including family, children, friends, colleagues, students, and clients.

Figure 1.1
Human services emerge to meet perceived human needs.

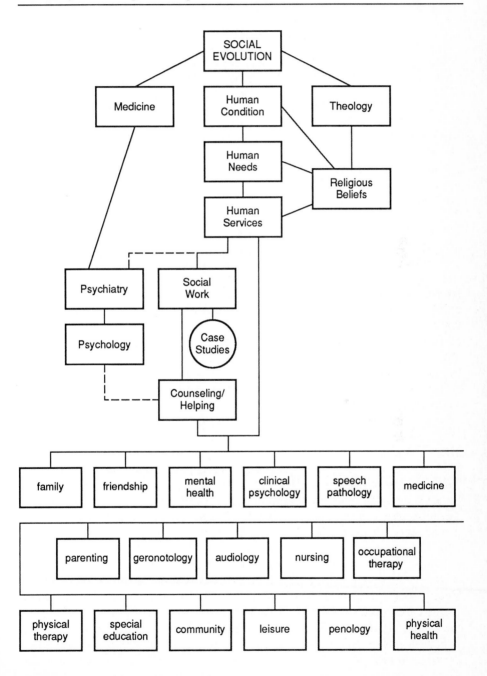

If I create a relationship characterized on my part: by genuineness and transparency, in which I am my real feelings; by a warm acceptance of and prizing of the other person as a separate individual; by sensitive ability to see his world and himself as he sees them; then the other individual in the relationship will experience and understand aspects of himself which previously he has repressed; will find himself becoming better integrated, more able to function effectively; will become more similar to the person he would like to be; will be unique and more self-expressive; will be more understanding, more accepting of others; will be able to cope with the problems of life more adequately and more comfortably. (Rogers, 1961: 37–38)

This hypothesis applies not only to the practice of psychology or psychotherapy but to all disciplines seeking to develop creative, adaptive, and autonomous individuals (Arkof, 1974).

❦ ❦ ❦

APPROACHES TO TREATMENT OF COMMUNICATION DISORDERS

Importance of (re)habilitation of communication disorders grew naturally from emerging concerns for individual fulfillment. Although the ability to speak and hear normally are still largely taken for granted, by 1980 awareness of communication disorders, their onset, severity, duration, and amelioration began to permeate allied health care fields and education settings. Because linguistic oral-aural communication has long been recognized and labeled "a unique human behavior," it was quite natural that approaches to communication disorders should have initially followed behavioristic trends (Scheuerle, 1979). Some early therapies that grew out of the need for speech correction in schools tended to follow popular principles of learning theory. Techniques of behavior modification continue to lend themselves well to treatment of some clients who exhibit deviant communication behavior. However, the nature of that treatment relies upon external sources of control for reinforcement.

Treatment procedures that evolved in university settings, often housed in medical colleges and hospital clinics, varied according to several factors. These factors include the background of practitioners, the needs of patients, the policies of the institution, and the disciplines of professional colleagues available to work on treatment teams. These university settings engendered application of the medical model of diagnosis, assessment, treatment, and dismissal to care management of patients with communication disorders (Scheuerle, 1979).

Furthermore, many early speech-language pathologists had extensive training in psychology (Boome, Baines, & Harris, 1950). Influences of psychotherapy are evident especially in theories and treatment of stuttering and in management of functional voice disorders. Some treatment settings involved clients who exhibited complex psychological and behavioral disorders, at least one of which was a communication disorder (Rousey, 1974; Shadden, 1987). From these experiences, humanistic influences on therapy for communication disorders are readily noted.

The broad knowledge base and complexity of therapeutic skills needed in professional treatment of communication disorders demanded increased emphasis on counseling by practitioners in the discipline (Durieux-Smith, Manion, & Finkelstein, 1988; Eisenstadt, 1972; Goldberg, 1979; Ling-Phillips, 1981; McWilliams & Smith, 1973; Pannbacker, 1977). The status of counseling expertise varies among professionals, and research on the effectiveness of counseling practices between 1975 and 1990 is scarce. (See Appendix A, Part 1.)

William H. Perkins (1982) edited *General Principles of Therapy,* the first of a planned series of reference volumes on therapy for any problem of speech, language, or hearing. The series, to be composed of eighty-seven chapters, was designed to depict unique forms of therapy that apply to specific aspects of language, articulation, voice, fluency, and hearing disorders in children and adults. In this first volume, contributors address the theories and principles on which therapies are based. Five chapters are devoted to behavioral management; three deal with counseling and psychotherapeutic intervention. The implication here, as in other literature on communication disorders, is that successful treatment of individuals with a wide variety of speech, language, and hearing problems requires understanding and skill in a broad spectrum of therapeutic and counseling techniques. (See Appendix A, Part 2.) In fact, clinician responsibilities cited in literature of the discipline under the name of counseling are so numerous that they are overwhelming. Viewed in this way it is understandable that the teaching of counseling in training programs is not readily embraced.

In his book on counseling in communication disorders, Luterman (1984) traced the interaction of behaviorism and humanism in that discipline up to the mid-1900s. Lee Edward Travis (1957), like Charles Van Riper (1939), clearly believed that speech therapy was closely akin to psychotherapy. Yet Luterman explains that even in the 1980s, few practitioners in the field of communication disorders are comfortable in both behavioristic and humanistic approaches to treatment of speech, language, and hearing disorders.

Acknowledged applications of humanistic psychology in approaches to treatment of communication disorders belie the continuing absence of courses on counseling in college and university programs for speech pathology and audiology. However, since its beginning, literature of the communication disorders discipline has contained valuable information and references to psychological and emotional reactions to disorders of speech, language, and hearing.

Another valuable resource is R. E. Hartbauer's *Counseling in Communicative Disorders* (1978). Hartbauer's work offers the reader the views of several professionals on case management of psychological and emotional problems in treatment of a broad spectrum of communication disorders. The book is easy to read and provides insight into the experiences of practicing clinicians with examples of their patient relationships. The reader can understand and appreciate the narrative descriptions and explanations of counseling or helping patients and their families. Hartbauer's book clearly shows that counseling or helping as defined by Rogers is a critical, integral part of both traditional and modern prevention and intervention for communication disorders.

In their study of what makes therapy helpful, Rogerian psychologists identified the therapist's personal characteristics as singularly the most significant factors in helping the client (Carkuff & Berenson, 1967). To be effective in helping communication-disordered clients, then, speech-language pathologists and audiologists must first recognize themselves as their most significant and constant therapeutic tools. They need to identify their personal strengths in communication relationships, to understand and appreciate their own reactions and feelings, and to practice counseling or helping skills. Clinicians need to treat the whole person rather than the single disordered behavior. They need to understand and appreciate the power of empathy, warmth, concreteness, congruence, and genuineness while seeking to develop creative, adaptive, and autonomous individuality in their clients (Chabon, 1982; Clark, 1982; Moses, 1985).

❦ ❦ ❦

THE CLINICIAN AS THE MOST SIGNIFICANT THERAPEUTIC TOOL

The 1980s saw increased attention to the role of the clinician in terms of personal characteristics. Many authors have addressed issues of clinical supervision to establish the desired outcomes in graduate students participating in clinical practica. Many have discussed ways to enhance the desired traits of students and young clinicians during their Clinical Fellowship years. Although not an attempt to mold these aspiring professionals into uniformity, it is interesting to note the similarities among desirable traits of practitioners identified by a variety of authors.

Essentially, the most desirable personal traits of competent clinicians identified in the literature of the communication disorders discipline reflect the basic tenets of Judeo-Christian philosophy. Descriptive terms used to designate those traits (Table 1.4) correspond with those used to describe the counselor in psychological literature since the middle of the twentieth century (Table 1.5).

The list of desirable personal characteristics for the communication disorders clinician in Table 1.4 is lengthy. While it is possible the reader may

Table 1.4
Desired traits of clinicians in communication disorders

Adaptable	Encouraging	Introspective	Sense of humor
Articulate	Enthusiastic	Literate	Sensitive
Caring	Feeling	Modest	Supportive
Cheerful	Flexible	Non-judgmental	Tactful
Committed	Friendly	Nurturing	Tolerant
Compassionate	Genuine	Objective	Understanding
Concerned	Good listener	Open	Warm
Cooperative	Healthy	Patient	Well-groomed
Courteous	Honest	Professional	
Creative	Humble	Reassuring	
Dependable	Interested	Resourceful	

Note. Compiled from: Clark, 1982; Cornett & Chabon, 1988; Fortier & Wanlass, 1984; Ling-Phillips, 1981; Mendelsohn, 1981; Neidecker, 1987; Northern & Downs, 1984; Sarason, 1985; Schmaman & Straker, 1980; Stein & Jabaley, 1981; Stream & Stream, 1978; Van Hattum, 1980.

Table 1.5
Desired traits of clinicians in psychology

Admirable	Empathic	Respecting	Self-reinforcing
Comfortable	Genuine	Rewarding	Sensitive
Compassionate	Immediacy	Self-aware	Tolerant
Concrete	Integrated	Self-confident	Understanding
Confrontational	Loving	Self-directing	Unique
Congruent	Pleasant	Self-disclosing	Warm
Coping	Prizing	Self-expressing	

Note. Compiled from: Bailey, et al., 1986; Carkuff & Berenson, 1967; Dillard, 1983; Dillard & Reilly, 1988; Evans, Hearn, Uhlmann, & Ivey, 1975; Gazda, Balzer, Childers, & Walters, 1984; Kagan, 1961; Rogers, 1961; Tomm, 1987.

possess all those traits, the composite seems instead to suggest that the competent communication disorders clinician, counselor, or helper is a perfect human being, an ideal *Everyman* as is espoused in Morality Plays of the fifteenth and sixteenth centuries. However, much of this broad description of personal traits of clinicians may be related to the scarcity of definitive research particularly addressed to the core facilitative dimensions of the speech-language and hearing professional. On the other hand, review of the two lists cited in Tables 1.4 and 1.5 presents many similarities.

Carcuff and Berenson (1976) explained that communication cannot be neutral. When two or more people gather, they cannot avoid communication (Galvin & Book, 1975). In clinician-client communications, as in those of daily life, each interpersonal exchange is either facilitative or detracting. Research on effective counseling or helping during the 1960s and

1970s identified seven core facilitative dimensions of the counseling or helping process: empathy, respect, genuineness, concreteness, self-disclosure, immediacy, and confrontation. Spielberg (1980) summarized these seven and added three more dimensions: potency, warmth, and self-actualization. Because of the importance of these 10 core facilitative dimensions, borrowed from psychology literature, the definitions are provided here:

- *Empathy:* the ability to perceive and communicate accurately what another person is feeling
- *Genuineness:* outward evidence of inward feelings and attitudes
- *Respect:* regard for the client as an individual who can make choices, grow, and change
- *Concreteness:* the ability to specify feelings, experiences, and actions
- *Confrontation:* the ability to indicate lack of consistency or congruence between verbal expressions and nonverbal behaviors
- *Self-disclosure:* the sharing of information about the self to facilitate self-exploration by the client
- *Warmth:* concern and regard for the client expressed both verbally and nonverbally
- *Immediacy:* the sharing of feelings between client and clinician
- *Potency:* the ability to show confidence and have an impact on client and therapy
- *Self-actualization:* the state of being a fully functioning individual

The traits, knowledge, skills, and techniques that counselors use to empower their clients to act and to change vary from individual to individual. It became important to discover ways to teach these core facilitative dimensions of counseling or helping to interested students. Of particular interest is the work of Allen Ivey (1971, 1983), whose investigations led to development of *Microcounseling.* During 10 years of efforts to identify teachable components of the effective helping session, Ivey and his colleagues repeatedly demonstrated that effective interviewing, like effective helping, involves the components of effective interpersonal communication. From his work on communication in interviewing, Ivey developed a "training-as-treatment" model, which had been suggested by his mentor, Bernard G. Guerney, Jr. In this approach, analysis of effective counselor behaviors provided a basis for identifying individual helping skills and designing a method and materials to train others in those skills.

Here the discussion comes full circle to provide humanistic treatment for clients by accounting for and enhancing clinician behaviors. Ivey and Authier (1978) indicated that successful microcounseling depends on several essential propositions. First, learning skills one at a time reduces the complexity of counseling. Second, all trainees must have the opportunity to perform and analyze their use of the designated behaviors and their effectiveness. In addition, videotaped models of each skill are helpful in teaching the form and manner of using the skills in a wide variety of disciplines. Students also benefit from roleplaying, and engage in interviewing as the process gives way to relating actual concerns and events.

Clinician behaviors targeted in *Microcounseling* (Ivey & Authier, 1978) include individual attending skills and influencing skills. *Attending skills* are patterns of eye contact, body language, verbal following, vocal tone, rate and loudness of speech, client-clinician positioning (proxemics), closed questions, open questions, non-verbal encouragement (minimal encourage), paraphrasing, reflection of feelings, and summarization. Influencing skills are those that involve giving directions, expressing content (instruction or advice), expressing feelings, summarizing (of clinician's and client's interactions), and interpreting (renaming client's behaviors).

A comparison of these behaviors with those listed in Table 1.1 demonstrates that Ivey offers a more concrete resource for identifying aspects of effective and ineffective therapy. Microcounseling behaviors have undergone considerable study since their inception and that data substantiates the initial psychoeducational hypothesis of "training as treatment." Also, Microcounseling emphasizes counselor-client interpersonal communication, a subject that seems to have been subsumed in much of the speech, language, and hearing disorders literature.

Introducing recognizable and countable clinician communication behaviors as instruments of counseling or helping seems a logical means to step away from the pervasive list of abstract qualities in Table 1.4. This is not to deny that personal traits of clinicians are significant in speech, language, and hearing therapy, but rather that there is not an accurate, objective way to teach or measure most of the attributes on that list.

In his early work, Ivey indicated that a major contribution of Microcounseling's approach to helping was its move toward demystifying counseling or helping. Such demystification is essential to open discussion of counseling or Rogerian helping in the field of communication disorders. This implies that speech-language pathologists and audiologists who are called upon to assume a counseling role in their daily professional lives should be able to benefit from analyses and enhancement of their own behaviors which facilitate their work and preserve their energies, while engendering desired positive change in communicatively handicapped clients and their families.

Determining one's personal and clinical strengths is essential in considering career options and in preventing burnout. Clinicians who know their abilities, strengths, interests, and limits are better prepared to make informed career decisions, to conserve energies in the presence of circumstances that cannot be changed, and to act positively and effectively upon a true need for career change.

EXERCISES

1. Discuss the sequence of treatments for human communication disorders during the past 200 years. Which dysfunctions were first perceived as needing intervention?
2. List your strengths. Try to identify specific skills or activities you perform well or attributes you perceive as strengths. Some may be casual, others deliberately learned.
3. As you consider your own strengths, identify one or two actions, behaviors, or modes of thought you want to change. Write them down and tuck them away for later use.
4. Carefully observe someone you know well. List the personal strengths you have observed in that person.
5. Review the definition of therapy in terms of the following case. Your client is a 75-year-old male Caucasian with mild dysarthria and a unilateral moderate sensorineural hearing loss. His communication disorders have biomedical etiology. However, his memory and intelligence are unimpaired. Your client's career gave him and his wife opportunities for worldwide travel. They collected many treasures in their travels and books about places they have visited. His wife is healthy, alert, and very interested in helping rehabilitate your client. Create a series of topics that might be used to design therapy materials for the client.
6. Explain how you would use the therapy materials described in #5 to counsel the client and his wife. Describe how this focus might help the client as he comes to understand new limits and needs for coping with some degree of permanent disability.

REFERENCES

Arkof, A. (1974). Some workers in improvement. In D. L. Avila, A. W. Combs, & W. W. Purkey (Eds.), *The helping relationship sourcebook* (pp. 19–50). Boston: Allyn and Bacon.

Armitage, A. (1975). *Social welfare in Canada.* Toronto: McClelland and Stewart.

Backus, O., & Beasley, J. (1951). *Speech therapy with children.* Cambridge, MA: Houghton Mifflin.

Bailey, D. B., Simeonsson, R. J., Winton, P. J., Huntington, G. S., Comfort, M., Isbell, P., O'Donnell, K. J., & Helm, J. M. (1986). Family-focused intervention: A functional model for planning, implementing, and evaluating individualized family services in early intervention. *Journal of the Division of Early Childhood, 10,* 156–171.

Bernstein, A. (1965). The psychoanalytic technique. In B. B. Wolman (Ed.), *Handbook of clinical psychology* (pp. 1168–1199). New York: McGraw-Hill.

Beutler, L. E. (1979). Values, beliefs, religion, and the persuasive influence of psychotherapy. *Psychotherapy: Theory, Research and Practice, 16,* 432–440.

Boome, E. J., Baines, H. M. S., & Harris, D. G. (1950). *Abnormal speech* (2nd ed.). London: Methune and Company.

Boorstin, D. J. (1987). *Hidden history.* New York: Harper and Row.

Bronte, C. (1982). *Jane Eyre.* New York: Penguin Books. (Original work published 1847)

Bronte, E. (1956). *Wuthering Heights.* Boston: Houghton Mifflin. (Original work published 1848)

Carkuff, R., & Berenson, B. (1967). *Beyond counseling and therapy.* Toronto: Holt, Rinehart, and Winston.

Carkuff, R., & Berenson, B. (1976). *Teaching as treatment.* Amherst: Human Resource Development Press.

Chabon, S. S. (1982). Client preparation: A counseling imperative. *ASHA, 24,* 603–608.

Churchill, W. S. (1964). *The island race.* London: Cassell and Company.

Clark, D. (1982). Counseling in a pediatric audiology practice. *ASHA, 24,* 521–526.

Commanger, H. S. (1950). *The American mind.* New Haven: Yale University Press.

Cornett, B. S., & Chabon, S. S. (1988). *The clinical practice of speech-language pathology.* Columbus, OH: Merrill.

Darwin, C. (ND). *Origin of species by means of natural selection* and *The descent of man* (Modern Library ed.). New York: Random House. (Original works published 1859 and 1871, respectively)

Dickens, C. (1961). *Oliver Twist* (3rd ed.). New York: The New American Library of World Literature.

Dillard, J. M. (1983). *Multicultural counseling: Toward ethnic and cultural relevance in human encounters.* Chicago: Nelson Hall.

Dillard, J. M., & Reilly, R. R. (1988). *Systematic interviewing.* Columbus, OH: Merrill.

Durieux-Smith, A., Manion, I. G., & Finkelstein, M. (1988). Counseling parents of children with communication disorders. In S. E. Gerber & G. T. Mencher (Eds.), *International perspectives on communication disorders* (pp. 190–205). Washington, DC: Gallaudet University Press.

Eisenstadt, A. A. (1972). Weakness in clinical procedures: A parent's evaluation. *ASHA, 14,* 7–9.

Eldridge, M. (1968). *A history of the treatment of speech disorders.* London: E. and S. Livingston.

Ellis, A. (1973). My philosophy of psychotherapy. *Journal of Contemporary Psychotherapy, 6,* 13–18.

Evans, D. R., Hearn, M. T., Uhlmann, M. R., & Ivey, A. E. (1975). *Essential interviewing.* Monterey, CA: Brooks/Cole.

Fischer, J. (1978). *Effective casework practice: An eclectic approach.* New York: McGraw-Hill.

Flower, R. (1984). *Delivery of speech-language pathology and audiology services.* Baltimore, MD: Williams and Wilkins.

Ford, D. H., & Urban, H. B. (1964). *Systems of psychotherapy.* New York: Wiley.

Fortier, L. M., & Wanlass, R. L. (1984). Family crisis following the diagnosis of a handicapped child. *Family Relations, 33,* 13–24.

Frankl, V. (1965). *Man's search for meaning.* New York: Peter Bedrick Books.

Galvin, K., & Book, C. (1975). *Person to person.* Skokie, IL: National Textbook Company.

Gazda, G. M., Balzer, F. J., Childers, W. C., & Walters, R. P. (1984). *Human relations: A manual for educators* (3rd ed.). Boston: Allyn and Bacon.

Glasser, W. (1965). *Reality therapy.* New York: Harper and Row.

Goldberg, H. K. (1979). Hearing impairment: A family crisis. *Social Work in Health Care, 5,* 33–40.

Goldstein, K. (1959). Functional disturbances in brain damage. In S. Arieti (Ed.), *American Handbook of Psychiatry* (Vol. 1, pp. 770–794). New York: Basic Books.

Hartbauer, R. E. (Ed.). (1978). *Counseling in communicative disorders.* Springfield, IL: Charles C. Thomas.

Hughes, M. V. (1980). *A London home in the 1890s.* Oxford: Oxford University Press.

Ivey, A. E. (1971). *Microcounseling.* Springfield, IL: Charles C. Thomas.

Ivey, A. E. (1983). *Intentional interviewing and counseling.* Monterey, CA: Brooks/Cole.

Ivey, A. E., & Authier, J. (1978). *Microcounseling* (2nd ed.). Springfield, IL: Charles C. Thomas.

Kagan, N. (1961). *Influencing human interaction.* Washington, DC: American Personnel and Guidance.

Kierkegaard, S. (1962). *The point of view for my work as an author: A report to history.* New York: Harper Torchbooks.

Ling-Phillips, A. H. (1981). Early habilitation: A blend of counseling and guidance. In G. T. Mencher and S. E. Gerber (Eds.), *Early management of hearing loss* (pp. 136–149). New York: Grune and Stratton.

Luterman, D. (1984). *Counseling the communicatively disordered and their families.* Boston: Little, Brown.

Marx, K., & Engels, F. (1978). *The Communist manifesto* (Samuel Moore, Trans.). Chicago, IL: Charles H. Kerr. (Original work published 1848)

Maslow, A. (1968). *Toward a psychology of being.* Princeton, NJ: Van Nostrand Reinhold.

May, R., Angel, E., & Ellenberger, H. (Eds.). (1958). *Existence: A new dimension in psychiatry and psychology.* New York: Basic Books.

McWilliams, B. J., & Smith, M. (1973). Psychosocial considerations. *ASHA Reports, 9,* 43–52.

Mendelsohn, J. Z. (1981). The parent-professional: A personal view. In L. K. Stein, E. D. Mindel, & T. Jabaley (Eds.), *Deafness and Mental Health* (pp. 56–61). New York: Grune and Stratton.

Mill, J. S. (1975). *On liberty.* New York: Norton and Company. (Original work published 1859)

Moses, K. L. (1985). Dynamic intervention with families. In E. Cherow (Ed.), *Hearing-impaired children and youth with developmental disabilities* (pp. 82–100).

Neidecker, E. (1987). *School programs in speech-language pathology: Organization and management.* Englewood Cliffs, NJ: Prentice-Hall.

Northern, J. L., & Downs, M. (1984). *Hearing in children* (3rd ed.). Baltimore, MD: Williams and Wilkins.

Padden, E. P. (1970). *A history of the American Speech and Hearing Association: 1925 to 1958.* Washington, DC: American Speech and Hearing Association.

Pannbacker, M. (1977). Parental preoperative ideas of speech after surgical management of cleft palate. *Rehabilitation Literature, 38,* 352.

Perkins, W. H. (Ed.). (1982). *General principles of therapy: Current therapy of communication disorders.* New York: Thieme-Stratton.

Perls, F. S. (1969). *Gestalt therapy verbatim.* Lafayette, CA: Real People Press.

Rogers, C. R. (1958). The characteristics of a helping relationship. *Personnel and Guidance Journal, 37,* 6–16.

Rogers, C. R. (1961). *On becoming a person.* Boston: Houghton Mifflin.

Rousey, C. (1974). *Psychiatric assessment by speech and hearing behavior.* Springfield, IL: Charles C. Thomas.

Sarason, S. B. (1985). *Caring and compassion in clinical practice.* San Francisco, CA: Jossey-Bass.

Scheuerle, J. (1979). Communication behavior change. Unpublished paper presented to Florida Cleft Palate Association.

Schmaman, F. D., & Straker, G. (1980). Counseling parents of the hearing-impaired child during the post-diagnostic period. *Language, Speech, and Hearing in the School, 11,* 251–259.

Schwartz, B. D. (1978). The initial versus subsequent theoretical positions: Does the psychotherapist's personality make a difference? *Psychotherapy: Theory, Research and Practice, 16,* pp. 344–349.

Shadden, B. B. (1987). Precrisis intervention: A tool for meeting the needs of significant others involved with aphasic older adults. *Topics in Language Disorders, 7,* 64–76.

Shipley, R. H. (1979). Implosive therapy: The technique. *Psychotherapy: Theory, Research and Practice, 16,* 140–147.

Skinner, B. F. (1957). *Verbal behavior.* New York: Appleton Century-Crofts.

Spielberg, G. (1980). Graduate training in helpful relationships: Helpful or harmful? *Journal of Humanistic Psychology, 20,* 57–70.

Stein, L. K., & Jabaley, T. (1981). Early identification and parent counseling. In L. K. Stein, E. D. Mindel, & T. Jabaley (Eds.), *Deafness and mental health,* (pp. 10–31). New York: Grune and Stratton.

Stream, R. W., & Stream, K. S. (1978). Counseling parents of the hearing-impaired child. In F. N. Martin (Ed.), *Pediatric audiology* (pp. 126–140). Englewood Cliffs, NJ: Prentice-Hall.

Strupp, H. H. (1980). Humanism and psychotherapy: A personal statement of the therapist's essential values. *Psychotherapy: Theory, Research, and Practice, 17,* 396–400.

Tomm, K. (1987). Interventive interviewing: Part I. Strategizing as a fourth guideline for the therapist. *Family Process, 26,* 3–14.

Travis, L. E. (1957). The psychotherapeutic process. In L. E. Travis (Ed.), *Handbook of speech pathology* (pp. 229–242). New York: Appleton Century- Crofts.

Van Nathum, R. J. (1980). *An introduction to communication disorders.* New York: Macmillan.

Van Riper, C. (1939). *Speech correction.* Englewood Cliffs, NJ: Prentice-Hall.

Van Riper, C. (1972). *Speech correction* (5th ed.). Englewood Cliffs, NJ: Prentice-Hall.

Wolpe, J. (1958). *Psychotherapy by reciprocal inhibition.* Stanford, CA: Stanford University Press.

CHAPTER TWO

Hidden Talents: Ordinary Interactive Behaviors As Helping Skills

Issues

ༀ *Speech-language pathologists and audiologists use interactive behaviors in treatment of communicatively impaired clients and their families.*

ༀ *Helping skills are identified and described as interpersonal communicative behaviors to enhance the treatment of communication disorders.*

ༀ *Proficient use of helping skills requires clinicians to recognize and understand their own communicative behaviors.*

ༀ ༀ ༀ

INTERACTIVE BEHAVIOR IN TREATMENT OF COMMUNICATION DISORDERS

Chapter 1 traced social change to discover why the discipline of communication disorders emerged in the 20th century as a dynamic, growing field among the helping professions. A similar rationale applies to the emergence of characteristics that are now prized and revered in individuals who establish careers in communication disorders, whether they deal with treatment, research, teaching, administration of training, or service programs.

Professionals in the discipline of communication disorders share interest in a common body of knowledge. In addition to that knowledge, each speech-language pathologist or audiologist embodies a unique combination of variables that affect career goals, daily endeavors, extent of professional and community influence, and ultimately professional and personal satisfaction. Those variables are neither accidentally acquired nor incidentally grouped. Instead they consist of personal traits, skills, attitudes, goals, ambitions, and values that the professional has acquired, nurtured, adapted, and prioritized throughout life. We cannot expect that all individuals who display characteristics identified in Table 1.3 in chapter 1 or those who declare interests in communication disorders are equally able to perform all types of activities required within the discipline. Daily experience in the field of communication disorders, as in other such disciplines, indicates that the best results occur when individuals apply specific strengths to activities that correspond with those strengths.

The focus of this book is the role of the speech-language pathologist or audiologist as counselor/helper in clinical treatment. However, that professional role has similarities to other fields. For example, research in social work and business administration shows that the use of helping skills creates a climate of mutual respect among members of an institution or office staff. This climate enables members to achieve institutional goals, minimizes worker stress, and encourages the creative participation of students or employees. Additionally, the broad application of interpersonal communication reported in research literature has led to identifying a significant aspect of the role of clinician/helper as that of listener and interviewer. Thus, helping skills are useful to clinicians, supervisors, teachers, researchers, and administrators alike in the field of communication disorders. In addition, as often indicated in the fields of psychology and social work, the keys to effective counseling/helping are good communication skills on the part of the helper and improvement of the client's communication skills in the counselor/client relationship.

Graduate students and professionals are expected to be knowledgeable and proficient in many ways. The communication disorders discipline draws on almost every modern field of knowledge. Besides being knowledgeable, the clinician who treats clients with communication disorders must develop the ability to interact with strangers to achieve desired behavioral changes. Such skills—the "what do I do?" part of treatment— have not been systematically taught within the discipline of communication sciences and disorders. Like the educators and psychologists of the mid-1900s who sought to train helpers/therapists, in communication disorders we continue to seek better ways to prepare clinicians to meet and cope with the varying needs of clients. Training must address the diverse ages, cultures, and ethnic groups of clients, as well as the wide assortment of treatment settings.

Some authors have compared the goal of clinical preparation to the role of a detective seeking ways and means to solve mysteries. However, besides solving the mystery of the communication disorder, the clinician must also treat the person with the disorder. The clinician must identify, diagnose, and assess the observable communication disorder itself. These steps are significant both at the outset and in ongoing remediation. However, even more significant at the beginning of the rehabilitation process, the clinician must establish an adaptive environment that invites the client's trust and encourages the client to participate in activities that demonstrate successful communication practices as a starting point for treatment. Ideally, therapeutic change evolves from the two-way interaction of the clinician and the client. The changes that occur during treatment often become permanent parts of the personal makeup of both individuals.

On the other hand, if therapy addresses only the behavior that is labeled *the disorder,* the client and the family may not develop the behavioral and attitudinal context needed to sustain the acquired communication skills. This lack of adjustment can lead to the client's failure to carry over learned skills into daily life. If this happens, the client has a realistic chance, after being dismissed from therapy, not only of reverting to pretreatment communication behaviors, but also of experiencing a sense of failure.

Rollin (1989) reminds us that speech-language pathologists and audiologists are not entirely altruistic. Each professional has a variety of motives for entering and remaining in the field. Those motives typically comprise a driving force for long hours and arduous work. Other factors influence what each clinician learns and remembers, the types of disorders studied, the setting selected as a work site, and the preferred methodologies, materials, and style.

Who Becomes an SLP or AUD

Students admitted to academic programs in communication disorders must demonstrate above-average intelligence and good speech, language, and hearing skills that include freedom from or expert control of communication disorders. They must have the desire to help people rather than to work with objects, plants, or animals. Candidates for this profession must have a basic knowledge of biology and psychology, and should have a compelling interest in those disciplines. They enter the profession with the understanding that treatment of communication disorders has a growing market with continually developing opportunities for employment and even the potential for independent practice.

The experienced clinician demonstrates similar interests. Practicing speech-language pathologists (SLP) and audiologists (AUD) believe that they help people with communication disorders. They recognize a market demand that provides a reasonable livelihood and allows for changes in job placement and career interests. In a variety of settings, they enjoy increasing recognition from other professionals as well as the public. Above all, they can often see the demonstrated effectiveness of their work and enjoy the appreciation of their clients.

The most striking characteristic of students and seasoned clinicians alike is their commitment to helping others attain the clear, meaningful communication they regard as a life-long need of all people. They believe that communication is intertwined with self-identity, socialization, independence, self-esteem, and self-maintenance throughout life. They understand that, from infancy through old age, nonverbal and verbal communication are essential for interaction with environmental elements and influences. Through experience they know that people can change and that change will occur more efficiently with a helper than alone. They believe that improved interpersonal communication diminishes the handicap of a communication disorder.

Needless to say, the effectiveness of therapy can vary widely among clinicians, beginning as well as experienced. Professors in training programs have long debated exactly what those differences are (Blakeley, 1989). Some say that the clinical helping skill is an art, while the knowledge of principles and theory of the discipline is a science. Some claim this skill involves establishing rapport. Others indicate that an individual's accumulated treatment techniques learned through trial and error explain that seasoning results from experience. Still others have identified the helping skill as a natural talent, something that cannot be taught. These many viewpoints underscore the confusion over what the successful SLP and AUD does, that is, the actions performed during client treatment sessions, and the issue continues to generate interest among all members of the discipline. Regardless of the many views of this undefined aspect of treatment for the communicatively handicapped, clinicians have an early and lasting desire to help individuals and their families. This desire reinforces the need to understand what *helping* is, and what it is not; how one person succeeds in helping another; and how to enhance one's helping skills.

What Is Helping?

Rogers (1961) described *helping* as open, honest communication evolving from and based on the trust and respect shared by two people. The helper/counselor is characterized as: (a) genuine and transparent; (b) warm, accepting, and prizing of the other person; and (c) sensitive to the client's world as the client sees it. Rogers characterizes clients in terms of how they will change or what they will become, do, understand, and feel as they respond and relate to the helper.

To assure open and honest communication is no easy matter. The process of transplanting an idea from one mind to another is complicated at both foci of the transmission because communication is a two-way system. Complications may lie in the idea itself, the generation of language to express it, the expression and the media through which it will travel, or the condition, availability, comprehension, or associations of the receiving mind. Figure 2.1 presents a scheme of this activity and some of the impediments that can confuse the process.

Figure 2.1
Scheme of potential impediments to communication

INTERNAL ENVIRONMENT
experience / culture
cognition / emotional state / attitude
hearing / vision / homeostasis

INTERNAL ENVIRONMENT
experience / culture
cognition / emotional state / attitude
hearing / vision / homeostasis

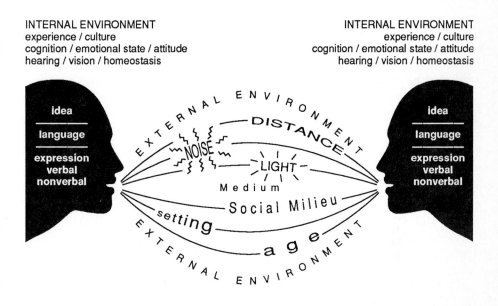

Proponents of parallelism among the many roles of the clinician as counselor, helper, therapist, listener, and interviewer realized early that teaching students in human services disciplines to be genuine, warm, and sensitive was a very difficult and time-consuming task. Students who enter academic programs of helping professions already proficient in ways that demonstrate genuineness, warmth, and sensitivity are welcome but rare cases. More commonly, even academically strong candidates need training and experience in those three abstract clinical traits to become effective counselors. This need led to the design of teaching technologies that are now widespread in training human service personnel. The terms *counselor, helper, therapist, listener,* and *interviewer* came to be used interchangeably.

The earliest methodologies for teaching genuineness, warmth, and sensitivity were developed in university psychology departments. The predominant method consisted of the student and teacher conducting brief trial interviews, discussing and reviewing the session, and then repeating the interview. Depending on the philosophical approach to psychological treatment, the use of this interview-review-interview technique was modified somewhat from university to university. However, the actual role of the therapist-in-training was fairly consistent across training programs in the mid-20th century. This cycle of counseling-critique-counseling provided students the opportunity to learn to modify their interactive communication behaviors in ways that would bring about desired changes in clients.

The added use of audio- and videotaping improved this learning process and provided an aid for more accurate recall during the critique of the content and the sequence of interaction in the trial interview. This system of teaching continues in use today in many settings where human service professionals are trained. On the other hand, this technology did not reduce the time professors must spend conducting performance reviews and critiques with individual students. In fact, the added need to protect confidentiality of the recordings created an air of secrecy and mysteriousness as well as a need for long-term specialization in counseling.

During this same mid-century period, the number of school-age children in the United States increased greatly as children resulting from the post-World War II "baby boom" entered the education environment. One result of the increased enrollment at that time was the research that led to a classroom teaching methodology called *microteaching* (Allen, 1967; Aubertine, 1967). Microteaching is a system of teaching small increments of information in a structured sequence within a determined amount of time. Allen, Ryan, Bush, and Cooper (1969) compiled a list of microteaching skills and categorized them into the five clusters shown in Table 2.1: giving responses, asking questions, creating student involvement, increasing student participation, and using presentation skills. A review of those five clusters of behaviors shows many similarities to clinical behaviors used in remediation of communication disorders.

These microteaching skills were combined with other interpersonal communication skills and built into a two-way exchange system for use in counseling (Ivey & Rollin, 1972). Analysis and observation of the successful use of interpersonal communication behaviors demonstrated the essential nature of human relations through skills that people use in daily living. Like the recognized goal of speech-language pathology and audiology, those researchers in the early 1970s saw the basic need for a helper to be a proficient communicator who teaches and engenders communication

Table 2.1
Skills applicable to microteaching

Giving responses: Verbal, nonverbal, verbal and nonverbal
Asking questions: Fluency in asking questions, probing, higher order questions, divergent questions
Creating student involvement: Set induction, stimulus variation, closure
Increasing student participation: Reinforcement, recognizing attending behavior, silence and nonverbal cues, cuing
Using presentation skills: Completeness of communication, lecturing, use of examples, planned repetition

Note. From Allen, Ryan, Bush, & Cooper, 1969.

abilities in the client. Anything that gets in the way of such a relationship is categorized as *what is not helpful.*

Elements in communication that are not helpful can occur at any time and from any source. As Figure 2.1 suggests, the interpersonal cycle is fraught with possible bipolar interference, which adversely affects the clarity of "idea transplant." As mentioned, interference may arise from the generation, delivery, reception, or comprehension of the message.

Helping Behaviors or Skills

Ivey (1971) initiated *microcounseling* as a method for teaching single helping skills. He searched for attending and influencing behaviors that could be demonstrated, observed, identified, taught, practiced, videotaped, and counted. His work has been built upon and expanded by many researchers, resulting in the identification of facilitative behaviors or skills of helpers. These behaviors are presented in alphabetical order in Table 2.2.

Table 2.2
Helping skills

Accept without judgment	Give directions	Refrain from interrupting client
Active listening	Give instructions	Restatements
Adjust tense/time of language to here and now	Identify incongruities	Self-disclosure
	Interpretation	Sharing oneself
	Minimal encourages	Silence
Attend selectively to positive aspects of client	Minimal verbalization	Target client reference to "first person"
	Movement	
	Paraphrasing	Touches client
Body language	Passive listening	Unstructured/open questions
Challenge incongruities	Position	
Constructed/closed questions	Posture	Verbal and nonverbal matching of client messages
	Promptness – timely action	
Eye contact	Recall previous content	Verbal clarifying
Facial expression	Recall previous interaction	Verbal elaboration
Facial scanning		Verbal following
Find and verbalize assets of client	Reflection of client's feelings	

Note. Compiled from: Bandler & Grinder, 1985; Blakeley, 1989; Bryant, 1984; Cecchin, 1987; Egan, 1975; Evans, Hearn, Uhlemann, & Ivey, 1984; Haase & Tepper, 1972; Hepworth & Larsen, 1982; Ivey, 1987; Kagan, 1975; Maccoby & Maccoby, 1954; Matarazzo, Phillips, Wiens, & Saslow, 1965; Mehrabian, 1972; Morganstern & Tevlin, 1981; Priestly & McGuire, 1983; Sathre, Olson, & Whitney, 1977; Skinner, 1953; Tanner, 1980; Tomm, 1987a, 1987b; Weber, McKeever, & McDaniel, 1985; Webster & Newhoff, 1981; Winton, 1988; Zimmer & Anderson, 1968; Zimmer & Park, 1967; Zimmer & Pepyne, 1971.

Professionals in other human service disciplines became interested in the applications of microtraining as they sought to develop more efficient ways to prepare graduate students in education and psychology (Gustafson, 1978). Microtraining has been used in the preparation of teachers, counselors, paraprofessional counselors, social workers, and health care providers such as medical students and residents, speech therapists, and physicians' assistants. Other uses involve municipal and corporate agency personnel, middle- and high-school students, psychiatric patients, and cross-cultural groups. By themselves, the helping skills do not make a helper. However, recognizing and practicing these behaviors in supervised settings has proven beneficial to facilitating communication and modifying interactive behaviors.

The helping behaviors listed in Table 2.2 should be familiar to the average person in most cultural groups. These behaviors occur in daily social communication among friends and acquaintances, although the typical user may be minimally aware of selecting a behavior for use in that context. Individuals adopt these behaviors during childhood and adolescence in accordance with societal customs. However, in a natural conversational setting, people give little consideration to the frequency, intensity, duration, or context of a behavior or its communicative significance or power in particular environments.

Facilitating interpersonal communication serves a common purpose in any human relationship (Heider, 1958). Regardless of the helper's academic background or technical strengths, the relationship, mutual regard, trust, and communication between the client and clinician are the most effective elements in achieving a positive therapeutic change. Thus, we need to consider these identified helping skills as part of the treatment of communicatively handicapped clients and their families. Further, the clinician must recognize the need for selective application of helping skills as being quite different from their casual use in social intercourse.

❦ ❦ ❦

IDENTIFICATION AND DESCRIPTION OF HELPING SKILLS

Among the helping skills listed in Table 2.2, the reader will recognize many behaviors that are easily observed in treatment sessions for communication disorders, while others may seem less obvious. In less restrictive terms, the listed behaviors are all familiar, ordinary interactive behaviors that are also useful skills of counseling or helping. Until they are recognized as treatment tools, these behaviors lie hidden.

In diagnosis and treatment, clinicians place communicative and therapeutic value on each helping skill according to whether it can positively influence the client at a particular moment. That is, each helping behavior in and of itself is neither good nor bad, right nor wrong. Instead, the clinician in the selection and use of each skill determines its appropriateness, influence, and communicative significance. In practice, the helper will use the skills in various combinations. However, in this discussion, it is not feasible to suggest all the possible combinations of behaviors that can be used in counseling. Instead, following the single skill concept of Ivey (1971), individual helping behaviors are presented.

To facilitate discussion, the skills can be separated into categories: nonverbal and verbal. *Nonverbal helping skills* are those that are complete without use of words. *Verbal helping skills* are those that require the appropriate use of linguistic expression, including sign language. Composites of these skills require simultaneous nonverbal and verbal expression or complex communication behavior and strategies, such as writing, reading, or augmentative communication instrumentation. However, including such complexities is not useful in this discussion.

The brief discussion of helping skills that follows does not intend to be either a definitive analysis or a "cookbook" of behaviors. Instead, the discussion represents an introduction to the helping aspects of behaviors that are found in ordinary interpersonal communications and an indication of the therapeutic value of those behaviors. It would not be possible to devise a standard set or sequence of behaviors that is appropriate for all therapy. Instead, this discussion provides the reader with a general understanding of the helping/counseling tools available for clinicians to use in the treatment of clients with communication disorders.

The following organizational steps will simplify the discussion of individual helping skills. The term *client* designates either the client alone or both the client and the family. The order of behaviors listed in Table 2.2 is changed to allow a clear description of the actions involved in each skill. To avoid gender bias, the male gender is used in discussions of nonverbal skills, and the female gender is used in discussions of verbal skills. Also, the terms *helper, counselor, clinician, therapist, listener,* and *interviewer* are used interchangeably.

Nonverbal Helping Skills

Nonverbal communication predominantly expresses emotion or affect. Table 2.3 lists nonverbal helping skills, which as a group are considered attending behaviors. Communication research has reported that 93% of social meaning comes from nonverbal messages (Gavin & Book, 1975; Mehrabian, 1972). The influence of nonverbal behaviors is widely recognized as both communication and meta-communication. Published since the late 1970s, *The Journal of Nonverbal Behavior,* like other scholarly journals of psychology, social behavior, and personality, reflects the interest of researchers in the role of nonverbal actions in human behavior. For example, Butterworth and Hadar (1989) and McNeill (1989) critiqued and replied to criticism of analysis of the interrelationship of certain gestures

Table 2.3
Nonverbal helping skills

---

1. Minimal responses
   1.1 Body language: movement, position, posture
   1.2 Vocalization
   1.3 Eye contact
   1.4 Facial monitoring
   1.5 Facial expression
2. Passive listening or acceptance
3. Proxemics
4. Refrain from interrupting
5. Silence
6. Timing: Action/waiting, promptness, rate/speed

---

with specific speech. Sebeok (1986) discussed communication primarily through nonverbal means based on semiotic theory. The components of semiotic communication are the message producer, message or sign, message receiver, and underlying processes. The verbal message cannot occur alone in human dialogue. Analyzing verbalization as a singular phenomenon strips it of essential meaning that is ordinarily imbedded within the delivery matrix.

In daily living, individuals communicate personal information by appearance, grooming, position, posture, respiration patterns, gait, and other nonverbal behaviors. In the treatment setting, the clinician learns to observe, interpret, and make inferences from many of those behaviors in the client. Those observations provide clues to diagnosis and treatment planning. However, this discussion focuses on the clinician's nonverbal behaviors as skills that enrich the client-clinician relationship and facilitate client progress in therapy. Clinicians must be aware of their own nonverbal behavior because clients as communicators perceive and react to nonverbal behaviors in clinicians (DePaulo, Kenny, Hoover, Webb, & Oliver, 1986; Gnepp & Hess, 1986; Saarni, 1982). Becoming familiar with personal habits of gesture, facial expression, and acquired mannerisms that depict socio-cultural influences allows the helper to strengthen the most useful behaviors and learn to use them selectively. In this way, the clinician's nonverbal behaviors become aids rather than impediments to client-clinician communication. Further, the clinician will more easily learn to recognize these experience-driven behaviors in clients.

The client usually receives the clinician's nonverbal messages through visual and auditory channels and sometimes through the tactile sense (Brown, 1984; Butler & Lewis, 1986). While clarity of articulation, extensive vocabulary, and standard syntax are essential to good oral-aural communication of ideas, nonverbally expressed messages carry meaning about the sender, the world as he sees it, and the way he perceives himself in that world. Although this chapter considers the verbal and nonverbal components of communication separately, the reader should remember that the match or congruence between the two is essential for the accurate transmission of the intended message of the sender. This congruence has been identified in client-centered therapy as elementary to genuineness.

1. Minimal Responses. This somewhat awkward collective term refers to actions of short duration that require minuscule amounts of physical energy. Minimal responses may be used alone or in combination with other nonverbal skills, or they may accompany verbal behaviors. In general, the message of a minimal response is, "I'm listening to what you are telling me. I understand what you are saying. Tell me more." Minimal responses include the clinician's body language, nonverbal vocalization, eye contact, facial monitoring of the client, and facial expression.

1.1. Body Language refers to the messages sent by the way a person cares for, presents, and manages his body. Work of such well-recognized anthropologists as Malinowski (1929), Sapir (1949), Mead (1956), and Hall (1959, 1976) laid the foundations for modern cross-cultural interpretation of body tension or relaxation, alignment or posture, and gesture or movement. Research and observation indicates that the accepted and preferred body language of the helper expresses relaxed attentiveness.

As a rule, the ideal position and posture for the helper reflect a relaxed body. When standing, he balances his weight evenly on both feet. While sitting, he places his body well back in the chair, supporting his weight in an upright manner and allowing him to bend his knees and cross his ankles. He may rest his hands and arms on the chair arms or in his lap. While working at a table or desk, he may place his body forward in the chair, feet slightly apart and set squarely upon the floor, with forearms and hands resting on the table. Each of these positions provides appropriate support for the body, aligns the skeleton and joints, and gives freedom to muscles to relax or initiate movement as needed. This state of relaxation is perceived as an attentive stillness that expresses awareness, preparedness, and readiness to act in any direction, with no evidence of somnolence.

Position also implies the direction in which the clinician faces. The clinician usually needs to be able to observe the face of the client. Sitting at the two joining sides of a table corner (Figure 2.2) generally provides more satisfactory clinician-client placement than sitting across a table (Figure 2.3). If mirror work is to be done, they may sit side-by-side (Figure 2.4). However, decisions about the seating arrangement for each client will vary according to the individual circumstances, such as the disorder involved, handedness of the participants, materials used, furniture available, and setting.

Figure 2.2
Position at table corner

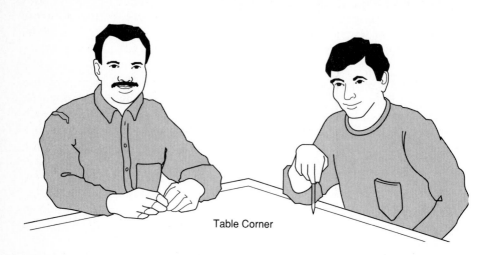

Table Corner

As in casual communication, movements during a helping session most often involve the head and upper limbs. Gestures such as nodding, rotating the head from side to side, pointing, measuring the air, and clapping the hands are quite common in casual communication. In counseling, the clinician uses these gestures conservatively, without hurry or force and within a limited space. Helpful gestures or movements embellish the message of clinician attentiveness and encourage the client to continue his performance. During oral-aural communication, hands that are held still or almost still are perceived as comfortable and comforting. The use of sign language, of course, requires more extensive movement of the arms and hands. Signs should be as rapid, abrupt, energetic, and sharp as needed for clarity of meaning, but they must remain controlled and the clinician should be relaxed.

A great deal has been written about closed and open body language. Crossed arms and legs suggest closed posture. Hands in the lap or on the arms of the chair and feet set on the floor or arranged with ankles crossed indicate open posture. Stance with feet in tandem and the weight on the balls of the feet with arms resting at the sides is considered open posture, while feet apart and hands on the hips is seen as aggressive posture. For further consideration of body language, the reader may refer to Hall (1976) and Fast (1971).

Changing posture and moving limbs are sometimes necessary to prevent numbness or muscle cramps, even in a relaxed clinician. Acquiring and arranging appropriate furniture prior to the therapy session can help alleviate the need for excessive postural adjustment. Body movements are often reflexive. Affective discomfort, like physiological discomfort, triggers changes in musculoskeletal alignment. The client will perceive an excessive amount of movement by the clinician as an indication of discomfort, a desire for the session to be over, or some other escape message. The clinician should study and understand what body language he displays and how others read it.

1.2. Vocalization without the production of words is often heard as a grunt, a hum, or an inflected vocalic tone. Generally, the utterances are not morphemic, although with vocal inflection some have been assigned meaning, for example, um-hum, ummmm, oh, ahhhh. In fact, the vocal melody carries the meaning, not the morpheme approximation. The clinician may use such minimal phonatory expression during client verbalization without interrupting the speaker or causing a distraction from the topic. Like other minimal responses, these vocalizations are perceived by the client as indications of the clinician's interest, recognition, and comprehension of the message content and its importance.

The clinician must remember that vocal characteristics must be modulated to accommodate the auditory needs of the client. Also, during verbal communication, the messages carried in vocal characteristics, whether deliberate or incidental, are often comprehended better and remembered longer than the words spoken.

Figure 2.3
Position across table

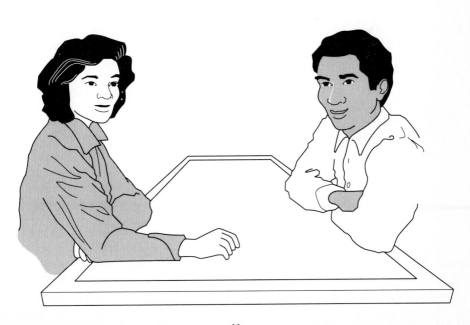

Figure 2.4
Using a mirror

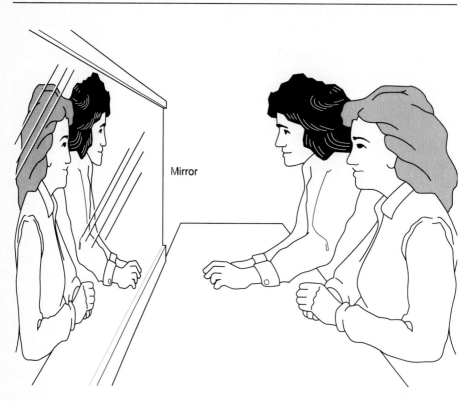

Mirror

1.3. Eye Contact. Although the communication disorders discipline concentrates on the oral-aural aspects of human interaction, the visual perception of a speaker also enhances the listener's understanding of oral language. In a therapeutic setting, the clinician needs to glean every bit of client information available at every moment. Since it helps the clinician accomplish this and provides direct visual attention to the client, eye contact has been identified as a critical helping behavior (Hamlet, Axelrod, & Kuerschner, 1984). An immediate problem, however, is that it is impossible to establish and maintain eye contact with both eyes of the client simultaneously, since human eyes focus on a single point. Knowing this, the clinician can switch his gaze back and forth between the speaker's eyes to monitor the focus of visual attention.

Eye contact also implies relaxed visual monitoring of the client's eyes. Eye contact breaks will occur. For example, the relaxed clinician will typically blink his eyes 4 to 16 times per minute and may look away from the client's face momentarily at various times. Direction of the client's gaze and breaks in eye contact depend largely on the style of communication that is most comfortable for the clinician. Sometimes the clinician wants the client to look at written or graphic materials, such as a picture, a paper, or some other object. To guide the client's gaze, the clinician may shift his own gaze from the client's eyes to the material (Hamlet, Axelrod, & Kuerschner, 1984). This type of direction through gaze control also occurs in pre-verbal communication of infants who want something that is out of reach. When the helper uses gaze in this manner, he breaks eye contact with the client for the therapeutic purpose of instruction or returning to the topic.

A fixed gaze or stare is not a helping behavior, nor is a continually wandering gaze. Either of these two extreme behaviors may signal the client that the clinician lacks interest, is ill at ease, or is bored. Breaks in eye contact occur more frequently and consistently in speaking than in listening. Wearing contact lenses causes some people to blink their eyes more often, resulting in frequent breaks in eye contact. A clinician with contact lenses may require consultation with an ophthalmologist to be sure there is no organic reason for this undesirable behavior. A clinician can best accomplish self-monitoring and modification of habitual gaze patterns using the microtraining technique of single skill videotaping (Ivey, 1971). No other tool allows the clinician to observe and count his own habitual eye contact breaks as effectively as videotape recording.

Some cultures consider direct eye contact impolite or even taboo. The wise clinician will act cautiously in the early stages of acquaintance to ascertain the client's degree of acceptance of eye contact. In some therapies, the client must visually monitor the clinician's speech mechanism. In doing so, the client focuses on the clinician's lower face while the clinician watches the client's direction of gaze, thus alleviating the potential problem of shyness or cultural bias in maintaining eye contact.

1.4. Facial Monitoring. This skill is just as important as eye contact in maintaining interpersonal communication. The helper monitors the client's face and facial expressions to ascertain nonverbally communicated reactions within the context of the setting and the client-clinician relationship (Kenny and Mallory, 1988). The client's face reveals so much about his inner reactions that the helper cannot afford to be distracted from that vital source of information. Facial monitoring also gives the clinician direct information about the client's ability to monitor selectively the visible environment. The areas of the face around the eyes and the mouth especially reveal reflexive and/or learned expression of affective status.

To succeed in both eye contact and facial monitoring, the helper must become aware of and develop a technique for facial scanning. Figure 2.5 shows one method of facial scanning that proves useful. The clinician gazes at (a) one eye, (b) the other eye, (c) the lower third of the face, and then traces the triangular area again. This technique of triangular scanning of the face allows the viewer to observe changes in tone, color, and stretch of the facial skin due to contraction of underlying musculature.

Figure 2.5
Face scanning pattern

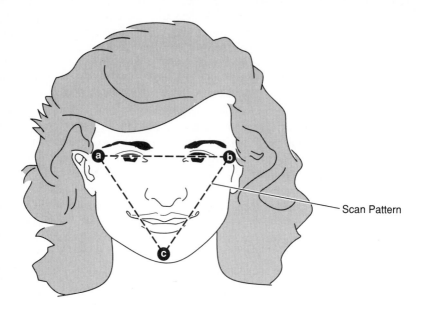

Scan Pattern

In children, changes in the face are usually instantaneous and fleeting. The clinician must be conscientious in observing those changes while he is talking, while the client is speaking, and when both are silent. In mature clients, the development of facial lines can provide clues for reading facial expression. Since wrinkles result from repeated patterns of muscle contraction, wrinkle patterns often display reflexive and habitual facial configurations. The clinician's use of gaze for facial monitoring and eye contact are critical to proficiency in comprehending the messages expressed in the client's face.

1.5. Facial Expression. The human face is highly mobile; it changes by reflex or by conditioned neuromuscular actions. The actions may result from the stimulation of any or all of the senses or from enculturation and social learning. The variety, intensity, and meaning of facial expressions are almost limitless. Table 2.4 contains an alphabetical list of terms that identify actions commonly witnessed in the face. These terms were gathered from many casual and formal sources and checked for definitions in the *American Heritage Dictionary*. The range of facial motion represented here emphasizes that speakers and listeners interpret the facial expressions of their communication partners whether or not the partner is aware of having made or changed the expression. This is seen as important information in that only 4 of the 63 facial expressions listed are considered unequivocally positive messages: *calm, grin, still,* and *twinkle. Calm* and *still* are facial expressions of the ideally relaxed listener. The other two terms refer to neuromuscular reflexes of the mid-face (*grin*) and orbital (*twinkle*) regions of the face. The other listed terms are not to be considered as expressions that convey negative messages. Instead, they are equivocal in meaning, and the environmental and communicative contexts in which they are used will determine their values.

In treatment, the clinician's facial expression may comprise a visual antecedent to stimulate client communication behavior or convey an informative, inquiring, or confirming message. While reflexive changes of facial configuration reveal inner feelings, young children in some social groups are taught to control or mask negative expressions and even to pose positive facial expressions. This practice results in such rules as, "big boys don't cry" and "nice girls don't show anger in public." Regard for the use and meaning of facial expression varies in different cultures (Ekman, Sorensen, & Friesen, 1969). Reflexive and posed facial expressions are more accurately read by older children and adults than by young children (Soppe, 1988). This is in agreement with Piaget's (1955) description of the development of moral judgment or intentionality.

Because the use of facial expression is so complex and yet so vital in communication, the clinician should learn about his own facial expressions. Like direction of gaze, facial expressions are often fleeting and thus can be identified and studied most successfully by use of videotape recording and review. In using this technique, the clinician should remember that the appropriateness of any passing or sustained facial configuration

Table 2.4
Facial expressions

Beam	Flutter	Look hang-dog	Snicker
Bite lip	Frown	Lower eyebrows	Sparkle
Blanch	Gape	Open mouth	Squint
Blank face	Gawk	Pale	Stare
Blink	Glare	Peek	Stick out tongue
Blush	Glimpse	Peer	Still face*
Bug eyes	Glower	Pout	Sulk
Calm face*	Goggle	Pucker	Twinkle*
Chew lip	Grimace	Purse lips	Weep
Chew tongue	Grit teeth	Put nose in air	Widen eyes
Clench jaw	Grin*	Raise eyebrows	Wince
Close eyes	Grind teeth	Scowl	Wink
Cry	Laugh	Simper	Wrinkle brow
Eyes mist	Lick lips	Smile	Wrinkle face
Eyes tear	Lick teeth	Smirk	Yawn
Flush	Look daggers	Sneer	

* unequivocally positive facial expressions

depends on its context and the client's ability to comprehend the intended meaning. For example, consider the message you convey by winking at a friend who is 6 feet away from you in a department store. Now consider the message you send by winking at a stranger who is 6 feet away from you in a cocktail bar. The environmental context modifies the message of the wink.

In a professional setting, individual clients also may interpret the same facial expression in different ways. While the clinician concentrates on applying his knowledge and expertise to therapy, the client observes concomitant nonverbal behaviors. The client perceives those behaviors as affirmation of the clinician's self-image, indications of his expectation for treatment outcomes, and his respect for and trust in the client.

2. *Passive Listening or Acceptance.* Fully listening to the communication of another person requires attention to verbal and nonverbal expression. Passive listening occurs when the helper is alert and relaxed, still, and "tuned in" to the client, yet is not participating actively in the transmission of messages. This in no way implies lack of interest or understanding. Passive listening offers non-judgmental quiet acceptance of whatever the client has to offer or wishes to communicate. The listener recognizes the other's rights and responsibilities to be truthful while revealing personal and often confidential information. The client's revelations or comments may not agree with or be compatible with the knowledge, beliefs, or philosophy of the clinician.

Information divulged by the client may reveal self-perceptions, knowledge of the world, or fears of the unknown. Simple acceptance of this information means that the clinician does not impose values on what is being told; is not influenced by the client to value the content either positively or negatively; and is not led by the disclosure to judge the conversational content, the client's attitude toward it, or the client himself. As a result, the clinician is able to interact with the client on a continuing professional basis, unbiased by the influence of self-imposed value judgments. Thus, the revelations of the client do not create barriers between the communicating partners. At the same time, listening to the spontaneous discourse of a client can guide consultation and referral decisions of the clinician.

Passive listening often occurs naturally in the clinical treatment room after a client returns from an absence such as a vacation, an illness, a new baby at home, a new car, or the loss of a loved one. The client may need to relate an adventure or an experience or renew acquaintance with the clinician. Since communication disorders therapy encourages verbalization, passive listening is an excellent tool to assess a client's level of re-entry into treatment or determine the need to undertake formal re-evaluation. Certainly, when a client is motivated to talk about daily life, the clinician will not wish to stifle that effort. In fact, the client may well provide excellent materials for the clinician to design subsequent treatment sessions.

In passive listening, the helper's facial expression is typically a minimal smile, with a steady gaze directed toward the client's face and gestures. Once the helper adds animation or verbalization, passive listening ceases and active listening begins.

3. Proxemics.   A widely recognized study by Festinger, Schachter, and Back (1950) demonstrated the effects of proximity on formation of friendships. Proximity tends to increase the probability of liking people or objects (Heider, 1958). This principle of proximity and liking may partially explain why many clients prefer to return to the same clinician, and many patients, to the same physician. On the other hand, Ebbeson, Kjos, and Konecni (1976) showed that proximity can increase disliking as well as liking. Thus, a clinician may sometimes find it necessary to refer a client to a colleague to complete a therapy program.

Proxemics is the science of personal spaces and distances that are acceptable to assume and move through in different settings. Personal space is the amount of space around an individual's body that others may not invade. Personal space varies among cultures (Hall, 1976). In western culture, comfortable distances for human interaction in different settings are:

Public speaking distance: 12 to 25 feet
Social distance: 4 to 12 feet
Personal distance: 1.5 to 4 feet
Intimate distance: Contact to 1.5 feet

Children develop personal-space zones by the age of 12 years. Anxiety, stress, social stigmas, and some personality disorders tend to cause individuals to require larger personal-space zones. Friendship tends to reduce reserved personal space (Evans & Howard, 1973; Hayduk, 1978). Personal space provides protection against stress, reduces stimulation overload, and regulates privacy and intimacy. The clinician's manner of greeting clients and his position in the treatment setting are behaviors that involve proxemics of both client and clinician.

In the clinical setting, some variability will occur in individual distancing behavior. Typically, seating for participants in therapy falls within the personal distance range (DeBeer-Kelston, Mellon, & Solomon, 1986). However, for the very young, very old, physically handicapped, or ill client, closer distances are often preferable. The watchful clinician will note these distances and monitor changes in them as the client-clinician relationship matures and as he determines the client's needs.

The handshake is an important culturally imposed behavior for the helper to learn, assess his performance of, and perfect. In most cultures, the handshake is now an accepted form of greeting by adults of both genders. A gracious handshake is an indication of good will and friendship.

Handshakes tell a great deal about the participants. Hands that are warm and dry are a sign of self-assurance, comfort and relaxation. Hands that are sweaty, whether hot or cold, send a message of internal stress, distress, anxiety, or pleasurable excitement. Hands that are cold and dry may be physiological signs of low blood pressure.

Handshakes that do not include finger and thumb pressure around the hand being shaken are considered limp or "dead fish," and the opposite is a "knuckle-buster." Ideally, the professional, friendly handshake presents an energetic grasp of a right hand by a right hand. The grasp of each hand encircles the other with a discernible squeeze expressed by bending the fingers and pressing the back of the hand with the thumb.

Like excesses in many other behaviors, too much or too little pressure in a handshake or too long or too short a clasp of the hand sends a message about the individual involved in the behavior and his relationship with the environment. In addition, a strong grasp can be very painful for a client who has arthritis, has sustained an injury, or is recovering from an illness, although the grasper may have the best of intentions. Also, a careless handshake with long fingernails or heavy jewelry may even result in injury to a client.

In some treatment settings, the clinician will encounter a client with paralyzed upper limbs. Some clients offer the left hand; the clinician should simply take the client's left hand in his right hand in a modified grasp. Other clients may not offer a hand to shake or not accept the clinician's offered hand; the clinician may accept that behavior and go on to the next procedural step. Sometimes it is appropriate for the clinician to place his hand in a gentle manner or easy grasp on the unmoving hand of the client.

Some cultures consider a slight bow preferable to a handshake. These are primarily Oriental cultures. If the clinician does not know the client's custom, he may follow the lead of the client or simply ask the client the appropriate or preferred form of greeting.

To avoid all too frequent errors in this introductory interactive social behavior, professionals of all human service disciplines should develop the "art" of handshaking. Practicing handshakes with peers and supervisors is an excellent way to gain experience and understand the differences in grip pressures.

4. *Refraining from Interrupting.* Just as its title indicates, this helping behavior allows the client to continue, to complete, or to digress according to his needs and preferences. The clinician must conscientiously refrain from any of the nonverbal or verbal behaviors that would disrupt the flow of thought and communication from the client. Instead, the helper devotes full attention to listening. There is no greater reinforcement to communication than attention. The helper also gains insight into language content, spontaneous language formulation, client thoughts, feelings, and attitudes as well as speech production, that is, the overall communication ability and style of the client.

Interruption by the listener disrupts the orientation of the speaker and breaks his train of thought. Interruption also reveals to the client that the interviewer is inserting his world into that of the client and therefore is not fully attending the client.

5. Silence.   Although silence refers particularly to the absence of sound, it also infers alert stillness of the relaxed clinician. Silence may generate feelings of discomfort in the beginning clinician, but it is a very useful tool. During silence, the client can gather his thoughts, reconsider a previous event, or add information to his prior remarks. The clinician can observe or read significant informative nonverbal behavior to recall and review for later discussion.

While developing the use of silence, the clinician should keep the duration short and carefully monitor the client's reactions. Because all helping behaviors are selected to move therapy forward, the wise clinician manages silence in the same manner as with other helping skills, using silence when it will help the client in achieving the desired change.

Recording reactions to silence on videotape is very instructive. During initial sessions, the time lapsed during silence often seems long, but a recording will show it lasted only seconds. Close and enduring relationships utilize extensive periods of silence shared between the communication partners.

6. Timing.   The alert, relaxed listener neither rushes nor retards interpersonal communication. The proper pacing of each behavior in the interaction is important in preparation for moving on to the next behavior. A pause in the information exchange is sometimes more valuable than an immediate verbal answer, even though a prompt response may give assurance as well as information. The rate of interpersonal communication is regulated by the attributes of both partners. Each clinical session establishes a unique communicative environment that dictates the rate of the helper's speech and nonverbal expressions, activity and pause, and the initiation and ultimately the termination of the session.

A characteristic of great actors is their sense of timing. They use this expertise to transmit a message simultaneously to large numbers of listeners. Indeed, only truly great communicators can achieve that astounding feat. Clinicians, of course, do not have to become great actors; however, like actors, they must pace all aspects of each communication to accommodate the needs and abilities of the client. Otherwise, the attempt at communication is a wasted effort.

Verbal Helping Skills

Verbal helping skills, those that are language-based, can be organized into six clusters by function. Table 2.5 presents the clusters in order of their discussion. Each helping behavior builds on preceding behaviors as we progress through the sequence. As indicated prior to the discussion of nonverbal helping behaviors, *client* is used to mean both the client and the client's family, and the female gender is used in the discussions of verbal behaviors. In therapy with some hearing-impaired clients, these same verbal helping skills are utilized through gesture-language, for example, American Sign Language, Signed English, or Cued Speech, in the visual-motor mode.

Verbal messages cannot occur without nonverbal messages. Verbal messages may differ in form and manner of presentation depending on the background of the sender. These can occur in the verbal behavior of the clinician or the client. In any case, the clinician's role largely involves the use of helping skills to minimize the impediments to idea transplantation that are shown in Figure 2.1 (p. 33).

1. Semantic Focus. As a category, semantic focusing or refocusing provides the clinician a technique to use to move or maintain the client's center of attention on the reality of the moment, the therapy session, or the

Table 2.5
Verbal helping skills

Function	Skill
1. Semantic Focus	1.1 Adjust tense or time of client's language to here and now
	1.2 Target client use of first person
2. Inquiry	2.1 Ask constructed or closed questions
	2.2 Ask unstructured or open questions
3. Reinforcement	3.1 Verbalize assets of client
	3.2 Attend positive aspects of client
	3.3 Minimal verbalization
	3.4 Recall of content and interaction
4. Semantic Clarification	4.1 Reflect client feelings
	4.2 Match client's message
	4.3 Restatements
	4.4 Verbal clarification
5. Add Information	5.1 Instruction and directions
	5.2 Self-expression
6. Semantic Exploration	6.1 Challenge incongruities
	6.2 Verbal exploration
	6.3 Interpretation
	6.4 Verbal following

planned activity and on herself and her behaviors. To do this, the helper utilizes linguistic cues. Selection of verb tenses and pronoun forms focuses the interpersonal communication on the client and her present status.

1.1. Adjust Tense or Time of Client's Language to Here and Now. Speech-language pathologists and audiologists provide treatment that deals with behavior as it is exhibited. Some refer to this as keeping the client on task. The helper monitors and maintains the focus of the client's attention by providing interesting and challenging materials in appropriate increments of difficulty. If distractions occur or if the client digresses into verbalization of memories or asides, the clinician refocuses their common efforts on the task or topic at hand.

In some clients, distractions may indicate (a) a perception of the task's importance or difficulty, (b) a characteristic of the diagnosed disorder, or (c) a stress reaction to an experience that preceded the therapy session. In other clients, revelation of memories from the past, dreams of the future, or verbalization of unrelated comments may indicate a need to (a) address a personal or family situation, (b) share unrelated personal concerns, or (c) escape from the demands of the treatment exercise or the clinical room. Information provided by the client at such times offers the clinician unsolicited opportunity to gain a greater understanding of the client as a person; an estimate of the disorder and therapy progress as reflected in spontaneous communication; content for client-specific treatment materials; and awareness of experiences, humor or pathos, that can be shared to further the interpersonal relationship in the therapy setting.

On the other hand, the best of therapy cannot change the client's past or promise specific outcomes for the future. Instead, memories and dreams must be recognized for what they are and used, if possible, to build upon. However, the clinician also has the responsibility to refocus the client's attention on the task at hand, the here and now. The helper may accomplish this with the use of present, present progressive, and future tense verb forms. For example:

PRESENT TENSE: Please place your hands on the table and look at me.
PRESENT PROGRESSIVE TENSE: You are continuing to speak with no breath support.
FUTURE TENSE: We'll try this next.

Attention to present reality helps the client to observe her own performance, demonstrate her ability, practice new skills, acknowledge achievement, and discover potential for change.

When the client initiates a distraction related to another time, the clinician can say in a positive tone, "Thank you for sharing that story with me. Now, we are ready to . . ." or "Very good. Today we are working on . . ." In this way, the clinician acknowledges the right and need of the client to digress, to express her thoughts and feelings. The clinician shows respect for the client by attending her message and modifies the treatment plan or setting as indicated, allowing therapy to continue.

If the client repeatedly initiates distractions, the clinician should consider whether there is cause for the client to repeat the distractions. For example:

Child: My mommy does it another way.

Clinician: This is how we make the sound.

Child: I want to do it mommy's way.

Clinician: There are many ways to make sounds.

Child: I want to do it like mommy showed me.

or

Adult client: Oh, Yes. I don't want to do that. We tried that last week. I couldn't do it and didn't like it.

Clinician: That's right. We decided last week to set it aside. Today we'll try it again in a slightly different way even if it's difficult.

Adult Client: Well, I never could do it. I don't even need to try.

Any of a number of inner processes, for example, feelings, memories, or needs, may cause unanticipated client behavior. The treatment program on a particular day may be difficult or boring. The client may be demanding freedom to demonstrate that she has needs or wants that have not been addressed. At a particular time, the client may require attention to some condition previously unknown in the therapy relationship. Whatever the cause, the client's behavior signals the observant clinician that something is amiss. Responsibility for responding to the situation and helping to resolve it is a part of the clinician's professional commitment. Successful clinicians bring to bear the client's knowledge, disorder, and developmental considerations. To do this, the clinician uses other helping skills, either nonverbal or verbal, to discern the client's whole message prior to adopting an arbitrary resolution.

As a helper, the clinician recognizes that a client's needs vary. The client's behavior is influenced by a deep-seated need to participate in the control of her own activity—as well as what she may or may not have eaten for breakfast or lunch. The client generally expresses a desire for control of her own life simply as agreement or willingness to participate in treatment activities suggested by the clinician. However, the helper must respect the client's right to withhold or suspend the agreement to participate. When the client consistently refuses to participate in the treatment process, the clinician must meet the challenge of regaining the client's compliance. In some cases, the clinician may find it necessary to make alterations in content, materials, and methods of treatment, or restructure the treatment session to meet the client's needs. In rarer cases, the helper may discover that the client's distractible behavior signals the presence of a problem besides the communication disorder that must be given priority or concomitant treatment. Proper treatment may necessitate referral to an interdisciplinary team, a mental health professional, an educator, or some other individual or agency.

1.2. Target Client Use of First Person. Since rehabilitation of speech, language, and hearing impairments requires the client to change, the primary focus of treatment must be the client. Although therapeutic endeavors often influence home and work environments, the focus and direction of change remains centered on the client. In that way, what the client does, believes, thinks, feels, says, aspires to, and hopes for are essential to the progress of therapy. These concerns will necessarily mention and at times concentrate on relationships with third parties, such as a client's peers, family, or co-workers. However, even during discussions of third parties, the primary target of the discussion is the client, her perspective, and her responses to her environment. For example:

Client: Th-th-those g-g-g-uys at wo-wo-wo-wo-work ma-mak-k-ke fun of m-m-m-me. Th-th-they're m-m-mean. I-I-I-I haaaate 'em.

Clinician: You're really upset about being teased by people where you work.

In this example, the client is focusing on her co-workers' behavior. The clinician rephrases or paraphrases the client's message and presents the content in the second person, referring to the client. In this way, fluency therapy can incorporate the feelings of the client by directly addressing her attitude, feelings, and behavior in the despised situation. This also brings the communication content into the present, the here-and-now. In that way, the client and clinician can explore the thoughts and feelings of the moment and construct ways to meet similar situations in the future.

Consider an adult female client with a voice problem due to vocal abuse. This client's physician referred her for therapy to reduce her vocal nodules. The client's chart contains an intake interview with a history of long-term use of a loud, strained voice both at home and at work. She is a single mother of two children in elementary school. She works as the head of inventory control for the largest department store in the city. Her vocal condition suggests the presence of family strife and work conflicts, both stressful and unpleasant. However, the clinician cannot know the cause of the ongoing strife or conflict, but only the client's version of her experience in the settings. It may be that the stress management problem is internal to this client and would be constant for her in any environment.

Neither the client nor the clinician can set out immediately to judge or change the home or work environments to any great extent. Instead, they must look together for realistic behavioral options that are available to the client and determine how to apply those options in- and outside the clinical setting. Such clients need to learn their own response behaviors, the environmental influences that trigger those responses, and the ways those responses elicit reactions from others. By maintaining on-target assessment and treatment protocols, the clinician helps the client deal realistically in both the here-and-now and the first person, the only contexts with which both participants can work knowledgeably. Through such efforts, the client learns to modify her control over her role in environments outside the therapy setting.

2. Inquiry. The clinician uses inquiry behaviors to elicit information or behavior from the client. Some are clinician-directed or closed and involve the helper selecting or targeting the information she wants from the client. Others are client-centered or open and indicate expectations that the client will provide some response without specific directions from the helper.

2.1 Ask Constructed or Closed Questions. The clinician formulates these interrogative statements to elicit specific information on designated topics. Intake interview protocols consist largely of closed questions that elicit concise responses to content-oriented questions, such as name, address, weight, height, eye color, occupation, hobbies, and work experience. In therapy, the clinician often uses closed questions to help the client identify a targeted behavior: "Jean, what sound are you working on? Is that an easier one than your last sound?"

Because closed questions are usually simple grammatical structures, they are short in length and in the time needed to utter them. Such questions can address a wide range of topics in a relatively small amount of time. Typically, the response is a word, a brief phrase, or a short list of terms, and is easy to record, check later, and tabulate. Closed questions are very useful in gathering necessary information when the goal is to create categories, files, or data banks. They provide references to *what* and *who* and generate information that is essential to formalize reports.

The use of closed questions poses two major problems for the beginning interviewer. On the one hand, the responsibility of formulating the question falls on the shoulders of the clinician. To ask a competent closed question, the clinician must select the topic, add the condition being questioned, and formulate an interrogative statement that carries the interviewer's exact intent to the listener. Additionally, she must ask the right question in the correct intonation and inflection patterns to achieve her purpose for asking it in the first place. To help with clarity of communication, interviewers may use standardized interviewing protocols, which can be purchased from reputable suppliers. Not all protocols will satisfy the needs of every interview situation, so clinicians should select and use published protocols with care.

On the other hand, a complete and truthful response to a properly formulated closed question may reveal only a partial truth about a topic in the client's life. The client may need to qualify an answer or elaborate on the application of a question to her particular circumstances. For example, the clinician may ask the simple question, "Where do you live?" The client may respond truthfully, but the client may also know without revealing that, by the end of the week, her address will change. A client responding to the question, "Do you drive a car?" by saying "No" may not elaborate to explain that, since her automobile wreck last week, she won't drive a car until she gets a new one. Some clients will not give information unless it is specifically elicited.

The closed-question form of communication offers strong advantages when used properly. However, the experienced helper recognizes the limitations of using closed questions alone.

2.2. Ask Unstructured or Open Questions. Unlike closed questions, open questions are essentially an invitation to the client to talk. Open questions commonly use introductory phrases such as, "Tell me about . . ." or "How do you feel about . . ." to elicit verbalization from the client. The formulation of open questions focuses on a topic introduced by the client. Responses to open questions depend upon the traits and the current state of the client. Thus, these devices invite the client rather than the clinician to select the content. Skill in the use of open questions depends upon the interest and ability of the clinician to gain insight into the world of the client.

Properly formulated open questions address the client's interests and invite her to verbalize them. The topic or its referent becomes a fulcrum about which the client reveals a great deal about herself, her cognitive and affective perspectives of the topic, and her knowledge, understanding, experience, and language related to the topic. In response to a successful open question, the client expresses much about her inner self. The client provides information about how she thinks, how she relates to the topic, the clinician, and others related or unrelated to the topic, and how she perceives herself in those relationships.

As indicated, a successfully designed open question may not be a question at all. Rather, it may be a statement, such as, "Tell me more about that." or "I'd like to hear what you think about . . ." Some counselors avoid controversial topics such as religion or politics, but each helper must be the judge of the topic content of eliciting questions. In general, the most successful questions or invitations to talk focus on a known interest or concern of the client. One can easily ask a parent about her child, a dog lover about her pet, or a student about school. When asking those questions, the clinician must be prepared to hear both positive and negative responses or discourse on subjects that are more pressing for the client at the moment. Although an open question may determine a topic or subject, the invitation to talk does not restrict the respondent. The clinician may use a variety of nonverbal and verbal helping skills to keep the communication on topic or within certain bounds.

3. *Reinforcement.* In every human relationship, the presence and behaviors of one person influence the behaviors of the other. Attention is a powerful reinforcement for children and adults alike. The clinician uses verbal reinforcement to influence the behaviors of the client, to provide the client insight into unrecognized or unprized attributes, and to increase behaviors that are desired as outcomes of the treatment program.

3.1 Verbalize Assets of Client. In many social groups, talking about one's own assets is considered taboo. From earliest childhood, teachings of politeness and decorum may insist that it is better for a child to let others compliment or praise her than for her to tell others about her good points. This often results in a child growing up with a deficit of language and a lack of experience for recognizing, acknowledging, or accepting positive aspects of herself and her abilities. To identify these aspects of the client, the clinician provides verbal and nonverbal language that describes and approves of the client, her characteristics, abilities, and attributes. A statement that verbalizes the client's assets may be as simple as, "You have excellent posture" or "You're always right on time." The clinician may include her own reaction to an asset in a statement, for example, "I like your . . ." or "I like the way you . . ."

Assets that can be verbalized vary from client to client and from time to time in one client. The clinician must be realistic and honest in making observations and statements. Genuine acceptance and regard for the client's assets provide egocentric language for the client, indicate the clinician's approval and acceptance, and comprise a critical link in the desired interpersonal relationship that is basic to therapy. Maintaining awareness of the client in this way helps the clinician keep the whole person in focus. The practice also gives the client a better chance to learn about and accept her strengths in realistic ways as she tries to modify her communication ability and reduce its disorder.

3.2 Attend Positive Aspects of Client. In addition to verbalizing the client's assets, the helper attends to positive aspects of the client, including many previously recognized by the client. This skill is a reinforcement of desired behaviors, which increases their incidence and thereby reduces the occurrence of less desirable behaviors. As the helper gives attention to different aspects of the client, she is demonstrating awareness and responsiveness to the client in a holistic way. These acknowledgements of client attributes add to the client's realistic self-appraisal and make it easier for the client to accept herself and the changes in attitude and behavior brought about through treatment.

Some writers describe this skill merely as the use of direct comments on the client's efforts in completing assignments, such as, "Good work!" or "Well done!" An observant clinician will also manage to look for and reinforce other characteristics especially those prized by the client, such as a pleasant smile or bright eyes. Additionally, the clinician may decide to use other forms of reinforcement to acknowledge positive aspects of the client. Many of the other helping skills discussed in this chapter are recognized as strong reinforcers.

3.3. Minimal Verbalization. This skill refers to the use of single words or brief phrases. In the use of this skill, the helper acknowledges the client and signals that she is listening to the client's message. The listener's full attention encourages the client to continue relating information. This helper response is part of *active listening,* and the clinician's vocal inflection and the duration of the minimal verbalization enhance its effect. For example:

Client: Our daughter is coming to visit us.

Clinician: Oh?

Client: Yes, and she is bringing our new grandson.

Clinician: A new grandson.

Client: My husband and I can hardly wait to see him.

Minimal verbalization does not imply refusal to talk, nor does it impose judgment on the statements or messages of the client. Instead, this skill signals the client that whatever she is doing or saying is accepted, appropriate, and important and that the proper behavior is to continue what she is doing.

3.4. Recall of Content and Interaction. At the beginning of a therapy session, the clinician may find it beneficial to review material, techniques, or achievements from previous sessions, assignments, or homework. This practice is especially helpful during the early stages of getting acquainted or when the clinician introduces new materials, techniques, or other information. Recall and review enables the client to understand the objectives of specific treatment stages and remember content and methods of approach. For example:

Clinician: I brought the Visi-Pitch again today so we are going to watch it record the sound of your voice.

or

Clinician: This is the . . . We started to talk about it during the last session. At that time we discovered that it will help with . . .

or

Clinician: Three weeks ago, although we worked very hard, we didn't finish a paragraph. But today you read a whole paragraph and explained what it means without any help.

or

Clinician: Remember how much fun we had when we prepared for Thanksgiving? It's time to get ready to celebrate Valentine's Day.

In ongoing treatment, recall of information and activities helps keep learned information and behaviors fresh in the minds of both client and clinician and enriches their relationship. Reminders of their mutually shared history reflect a growing regard and respect for each other, their accomplishments, and their relative roles in the relationship.

4. Semantic Clarification. In conversational exchange, each participant strives to gain full understanding of the message intended by the partner. (Note: Although this helping skill category is verbal, to clarify semantic content the clinician must address both verbal and nonverbal communication of the client.) This category involves redundancy. By repeatedly reviewing the information received, the clinician helps compare the received message to the client's intended one. Identifying or exposing differences invites the sender to revise the message. This is an application of the helping skills to the natural communication process shown in Figure 2.1. In counseling, the helper must clearly understand the meaning of the client; the client must match verbal messages with intended messages so as to present her meaning clearly; and both participants must learn to recognize the changes that have been made in the message and/or its transmission.

4.1. Reflect Client Feelings. This helping behavior can be pictured as wrapping language around an expressed, but unnamed, feeling. Although at times the client expresses feelings both verbally and nonverbally, this verbal helping behavior is used to:

1. Clarify vaguely expressed feelings of the client.

Client: Mrs. Johnson gave me a C and I deserved a B.
Clinician: You're angry about your grade.

2. Question the accuracy of the client's verbalization about her feelings.

Client: My tawk's awrite, I guess.
Clinician: You're feeling unsure about the way you talk.

3. Confirm or agree with the client's statement of feelings.

Client: I'm so tired, I can't think about my voice.
Clinician: You sound tired all over.

4. Modify or vary the client's statement of her feelings.

Client: I'm Joan-the-Giant-Killer!
Clinician: You're wound up and ready for tough jobs.

or

Client: I can't do that.
Clinician: This seems difficult.

In reflecting feelings, the clinician must be alert to the affective state of the client regardless of the words being spoken. Nonverbal communication carries the predominant emotional message. Linguistic supra-segmentals (i.e., pitch, stress, and juncture), vocal variation, rate and rhythm of speech patterns, gesture, and facial expression are all meaningful signals of emotional state. When the speaker's nonverbal emotional expression does not match her spoken language, the helper must identify the incongruity and confront the client with the observed difference. (See paragraph 6.1, Challenge Incongruities, for related information.)

4.2 Match Client's Message. This helping skill involves paraphrasing, and its use in verbal communication is similar to its use in writing. The helper extracts meaning, content, feeling, attitude, or insight from the client's message and verbally presents her interpretation of that meaning. In doing this, the clinician deliberately and cautiously represents her understanding of the client's message. If the client then perceives an accurate match between her intended message and the listener's representation, she can and usually does continue her discourse. If the helper's interpretation does not match the intended message, then the client has the opportunity to reiterate or revise her original message.

Paraphrasing brings about an interchange of communication that contributes to a mutual sharing of ideas and information. It not only helps to establish, clarify, and maintain the client's world, but also expands that world by including the understanding of the helper. Paraphrasing also provides the helper an opportunity to verify her understanding of the client. Paraphrasing also allows the client to affirm, rephrase, restate, reconsider, or even discard language or ideas that have been expressed.

In professional literature, some explanations of paraphrasing clients' expressions have limited the role of the interviewer to verbalization of content alone. However, because so much meaning is transmitted nonverbally, the accurate paraphrase of a message will necessarily include information from its nonverbal aspects. This demands that the helper be aware of and use both nonverbal and verbal communication in an accurate paraphrase.

Examples of content paraphrase in print cannot provide the same value as observation and practice of nonverbal elements to demonstrate the full impact of this skill. The reader may want to ask a partner to role-play the following exchange between a client and clinician to get a better idea of the impact of paraphrasing. In this exchange, the clinician paraphrases the message and also reflects the feelings of the client. For example:

Client: I don't know where to turn. When I was little, I could just be quiet and watch what was going on. But now I'm growing up. Being hearing-impaired and 16 are the worst possible combination.

Clinician: Your hearing impairment is interfering with things you care a great deal about.

Client: Yeah. My friends talk a lot and fast whether I'm looking at them or not. I just can't keep up with a group discussion.

Clinician: You feel like you miss a lot even if you're part of the group.

Client: I guess I do miss a lot. Last night, Kera laughed at me when I said the same thing someone else had just said.

Clinician: You feel bad that you missed what was said and even worse that Kera laughed at you.

4.3. Restatements. Sometimes the helper finds that the client has not correctly or clearly stated an idea. At such times, one way to check the client's meaning is to quote back to her what she has just said. This is one form of reflecting content. To do this, the clinician makes only minimal changes to the client's statement in lexicon, syntax, and nonverbal expression. For example:

Client: I saw what I know.
Clinician: You saw what you know.

or

Client: The machine we used had red and green dials.

Clinician: The machine you used had red and green dials.

This skill requires the helper to engage in role-playing, using linguistic supra-segmentals, rate, and inflection pattern to reflect the meaning expressed by the client. The clinician must take on the character and attitude of the client and imitate the client's production. The client may gain a clue about how to clarify her own statements by hearing her words echoed by another speaker. This skill may not be useful with certain language disorders, or when the client's native language is not the same as that of the clinician.

4.4 Verbal Clarification. Sometimes the clinician will find it helpful to add words to a client's statement to exchange a term for one that more closely reflects an event, phenomenon, attitude, or feeling. The clinician may add words or phrases to complete the meaning of the client's statement or to explain clearly a situation with which the helper has no direct experience. Verbal clarification is the practice of introducing language that focuses particularly on a topic or an element of a topic to expose its attributes. Such a practice tends to promote the correct use of words, decrease exaggerated over- or understatements, eliminate equivocation, and increase shared understanding. For example:

Client: I'll see you tomorrow.

Clinician: Your next session is on Thursday.

Client: Yeah! Right!

Clinician: So, since today is Tuesday, I'll see you day after tomorrow.

Client: Oh, okay. We'll skip a day.

or

Client: You want me to take a deep breath?

Clinician: Yes, and then say "ah" and hold it as long as you can.

Client: How can I hold my breath and say anything?

Clinician: You're right. You can't do that. Just take in a deep breath and then slowly breathe out while you're saying "ah." Hold that sound as long as you can.

Client: Like this? aaaaaaaaaaaaaaaahhhhhh.

Clinician: Exactly. Now do it again so I can time your "ah."

5. Add Information. Instructing the client is required as part of the treatment of any communication disorder. Clinicians find it necessary in almost every therapy session to give instruction or to review, revise, modify, or adapt information for the client.

5.1. Instruction and Directions. These helping behaviors relate to one another because they both deal with providing new information to the client. Directions generally explain how to achieve a task or to reach a location. Instructions may involve management of a process or procedure or new cognitive information about an item already familiar or new to the client.

In the treatment of communication disorders, directions or instructions often involve an instrument or device, making demonstration possible. Demonstration, modeling, and trial use by the client are all recommended procedures found in many therapy programs. Accurate and adequate communication of new information to the client is critical to the success of the next steps in therapy. The clinician must use vocabulary and syntax appropriate to the client's comprehension level. The client's understanding can best be verified with two skills that will be discussed later, interactive clarification and verbal exploration. Verbal or gestural exchange is used most frequently in directing and instructing.

For clients who use a gesture language or augmentative communication devices, the helper must provide directions and instructions in their specific language modes. Some clients may have difficulty replicating new procedures or remembering new material. The wise clinician will distribute information in smaller segments over a number of treatment sessions, with repetition as indicated. This practice will avoid placing stress on the comprehension or retention capacities of the client. Also, the clinician should test for comprehension and retention before introducing new information.

5.2. Self-expression. Sometimes the clinician may want to reveal something about herself. This behavior is different from statements about her reactions to the client. Self-expression involves statements about the clinician herself, revealing information that the client would not know otherwise. The information may relate to the clinician's opinions, judgment, preferences, feelings, concerns, knowledge, or experiences.

The content of self-expression depends on the context of the treatment session. Use of this behavior opens the world of the helper to the client. Because the openness reveals something about herself, the clinician needs to be sure that the shared information is appropriate, accurate, and timely. As with other skills, the clinician must be sure that self-expression is the helping skill that will be most effective at a given time in positively influencing the behavior of the client. For example:

Client: I have such a hard time understanding what is being said when there is any noise in the room.

Clinician: In some noisy places, I do, too.

or

Client: I get home so late at night; and then with supper to get and the kids to get to bed, I don't have time to relax, do my exercises, and take care of myself.

Clinician: I remember when my children were little. There was never enough time to get everything done. Some things just got set aside.

With self-expression, the helper can let the client know that she is not alone in an experience or feeling and that, whatever the problem, others have found ways to deal with a similar problem. The clinician shows the client another point of view and may suggest an alternate mechanism for addressing the circumstances.

Clinicians should take care in the use of self-expression. It may appear easier to give the client advice about a problem than to help the client reach her own solutions and conclusions. In the long run, such advice is usually less effective than the client's own solutions. Also, a manipulative client can quickly turn a treatment session into a period of social exchange or emotional venting if the clinician is not alert to the timing and extent of self-expression.

6. *Semantic Exploration.* This category helps the client to clarify impressions, feelings, ideas, and thought processes and the language used to express those inner reactions.

6.1. Challenge Incongruities. The clinician may witness two or more conflicting messages transmitted simultaneously by the client. For example, a smiling client may be gritting her teeth, a client whose vocal quality sounds belligerent may have tears in her eyes, or a client who says she has done her homework may be unable to describe or perform those same tasks in the clinical setting. The helper identifies the observed conflicting messages and verbally describes them to the client. These dual messages are called mixed messages. Because both are presented by the client, the clinician should not choose or judge which to attend first or in one preference to the other. The fact of the conflict must be recognized and the incongruity clarified, and the client is the only one who can make that clarification. The role of the helper is to verbalize the observed mixed messages and ask for clarification on the part of the client, for example, "I hear you saying that you're happy to be here, but you seem very tense today."

When mixed messages are pointed out, the client may recognize and explain that a temporary conflict is interfering with the usual or expected ease of participation in the therapy session. On the other hand, the client may have difficulty accepting the clinician's description of the contradicting messages. When this happens, the client may deny the presence or intent of one of the messages and try to explain it away as related to some recent insignificant but worrisome event or a longstanding habit. There is a risk that the client will elect to address only the aspect of the message that is most comfortable or skirt the issue altogether if given the opportunity. Any such reaction may provide an opportunity for the counselor to further interpersonal interaction through the use of other helping skills. In this case, the mixed message may result in bringing the client and clinician into a closer helping relationship. In other cases, the client's reaction may indicate that the communication disorder under treatment is but one component of a more complex problem. The clinician may want to re-evaluate the communication problem or consult with a colleague in another profession.

6.2. Verbal Exploration. Often a client will make statements that seem to hint at something, but do not clearly specify a meaningful message. At such a time, the helper needs to elicit more information from the client. Some clients will have a great deal of knowledge and be able to generate lengthy discussions and descriptions when stimulated to do so. Other clients may have little knowledge or language, but may have strong feelings about an idea or impression that needs to be clarified. In some cases, a client may contradict earlier statements.

When clear or limited information about treatment appears to interfere with the client's progress, the clinician should explore the extent of the client's understanding of the matter. Verbal exploration involves the use of open questions, restatements, or paraphrases. For example, the clinician may say, "Earlier, you mentioned . . . Tell me more about that." Or the helper may simply indicate confusion: "I thought you had said that . . . Now you are telling me that . . ."

Verbal exploration provides the clinician and client a chance to test subtleties of word meaning, preferences for word choice, and emphasis on nonverbal language. It also allows an opportunity for the confirmation of ideas, attitudes, feelings, and interests as well as for the retraction of false statements and impressions. From the perspective of the speech-language pathologist, and audiologist, verbal exploration is also one way to identify and assess receptive and expressive language.

6.3. Interpretation. When a helper makes an interpretation, she speaks in a new and different way about a client-originated idea, behavior, or observation. The clinician modifies the manner and focus in which the idea was framed by the client. To do this, the helper generates language that adds something of herself—thoughts, perspective, creativity, imagination, or experience—to the client's original message.

Interpretation provides a new frame of reference or linguistic format for the client, allowing her an opportunity to consider the central ideas with a fresh perspective. Interpretation includes a reflection of expressed feelings, the content of the client's statement, and pertinent information added by the clinician.

Client: I'm sorry I didn't do my assignment.

Clinician: You feel bad (reflection of feelings) about not keeping your part of our bargain (paraphrase) and you think you won't do well today (interpretation).

Through this added point of view, the client may gain insight into her thoughts and feelings and their impact on her current behavior. If the failure to carry out assignments has occurred before, the clinician may respond as in the following exchange.

Client: I'm sorry I didn't do my assignment.

Clinician: You feel bad (reflection of feelings) that you didn't do another assignment (paraphrase) and you're wondering how I may react.

Some writers have described interpretation as "getting a new angle" on things. A risk involved in interpretation is that the clinician necessarily inserts her understanding or self-expression of the client's message within the context of the time and setting. The client may then accept or reject the interpretation in whole or in part. Because of the conflict of ideas that may accompany interpretation, the clinician should check the accuracy of any interpretation used. Paraphrases, reflections of feelings, and restatements are helpful in approaching subtle and covert meanings in statements made during therapy.

6.4. Verbal Following. The clinician may use this skill to recall earlier exchanges or specific expressions of the client. This may involve using active listening skills or recalling an item from an earlier portion of the discussion. The helper may repeat an idea, a statement, or a particular word. In that way, the helper causes the topic to resurface and refocuses the client on that topic so she can discuss it further. This behavior asks the client for more information, alerts her that the clinician wants to stay on the topic that the client introduced, and encourages her client to explore that topic more thoroughly.

Verbal following facilitates the therapeutic process in a way that may be *immediate,* using minimal responses or minimal verbalizations, or *distant,* using inquiry or statements to recall communication from a current or previous treatment session. Regardless of the subject, this behavior serves the function of telling the client that the helper is "tuned in" to the message, accepts it, and wants more information about it. Such interest and attention reinforces the client's behavior by demonstrating that the client is the focus of interest.

❦ ❦ ❦

PROFICIENT USE OF HELPING SKILLS

Attending behaviors are those that acknowledge the client's worth and importance, ideas, efforts, feelings, interests, and responses. *Influencing skills* are those that bring about change in the client. In practice, some helping behaviors will exert a more powerful influence than others. Each clinician establishes a hierarchy of influencing behaviors through practice and determines a comfort level with each skill. This hierarchy becomes the practitioner's clinical style. It would be quite difficult to separate the listed behaviors according to their utilization of attending or influencing.

Behaviors considered in this chapter are rarely, if ever, performed alone. For example, passive listening, the least active skill, incorporates facial monitoring and eye contact. If both are not incorporated, passive listening immediately changes to a negative communication skill, an aversive stimulus, and may cause the client to think, "I don't like to talk to . . . He just sits there." At the other extreme, the active skill of challenging incongruities or confrontation informs the client that the clinician is attending multi-modal expression. However, if confrontation occurs without other skills, it becomes a negative stimulus, likely to elicit an antagonistic response.

Of course, in quite the opposite frame of reference, in some planned therapy programs, the clinician will elect to apply communicative stress to test the endurance and resistance of the client's acquired behaviors. Many of the identified helping skills can be adapted for use in this way. Each behavior in and of itself has little value, but its application can either provide untold benefit or do immeasurable harm.

Observing highly skilled, experienced clinicians in treatment is an easy and effective method to discern use of helping behaviors in the typical clinical operations (Table 1.1). An analysis of five videotaped treatment sessions for each of two experienced clinicians showed their skill in distributing the use of counseling behaviors across the clinical operations. Table 2.6 provides a checklist of the nonverbal helping skills observed in each clinician, and Table 2.7 indicates their use of verbal skills. The distribution of behaviors shows that some helping skills, such as body language, were used in more clinical operations than were others, such as vocalization. Also, observing two clinicians made it possible to discern variations in their use of skills in different clinical operations. For example, both clinicians used several of the nonverbal helping skills in all operations, but neither used a single verbal helping skill in all the operations. Differences in the selection and use of helping behaviors depend on the client, disorder, and setting, but more particularly on the clinical style and personal traits of the clinician. What works best for one clinician may cause disaster for another. The secret of success in the use of helping skills is for clinicians to understand the impact of communicative skills that incorporate their clinical strengths.

Each clinician establishes a clinical repertoire or style in which three aspects of skill management come into play: (a) selection of the skill to use, (b) timing of its use, (c) manner of application, all of which yield therapeutic power. The concept of therapeutic power is not new or unique in the field of communication disorders. Such power is discussed in all areas of human services, and abuse of this power is well documented in professional and legal literature. The reader is encouraged to refer to Hubbell (1981, chap. 5) and Rollin (1989, chap. 9).

Clinicians must remember that the goal of treatment is improving the communication abilities of the client. In therapy, the client will use or learn to use a battery of behaviors similar to those of the clinician. Interpersonal communication in treatment sessions as elsewhere is managed to a large extent by meta-communication. The following points should be useful in learning to apply helping behaviors to the treatment process.

Table 2.6
Nonverbal helping skills observed in two experienced clinicians (X, Y) during videotaped treatment sessions

	Clinical Operation												
Helping Skill	Observation	Assessment	Demonstration	Elicitation	Instruction	Reinforcement	Diagnosis	Planning	Referral	Discussion	Recommendation	Summarization	Dismissal
1. Minimal responses													
1.1 Body language	XY	XY	XY	XY	XY	XY	XY	XY	XY	XY	XY	XY	XY
1.2 Vocalization	X		XY		XY					Y			
1.3 Eye contact	XY	XY	XY	XY	XY	XY	XY	XY	XY	XY	XY	XY	XY
1.4 Facial monitoring	XY	XY	XY	XY	XY	XY	XY	XY	XY	XY	XY	XY	XY
1.5 Facial expression	XY	XY	XY	XY	XY	XY	XY	XY	XY	XY	XY	XY	XY
2. Passive listening	XY	XY		Y			XY						
3. Proxemics	XY	XY	XY	XY	XY	XY	XY	XY	Y	Y	Y	XY	XY
4. Refraining from interrupting	XY	XY		XY		XY	XY	X		XY	Y		
5. Silence	XY	X	XY	XY			XY	X				X	
6. Timing	XY	XY	XY	XY	XY	XY	XY	XY	XY	XY	XY	XY	XY

Note. From Scheuerle, 1985.

Table 2.7
Verbal helping skills observed in two experienced clinicians (X, Y) during videotaped treatment sessions

Helping Skill	Observation	Assessment	Demonstration	Elicitation	Instruction	Reinforcement	Diagnosis	Planning	Referral	Discussion	Recommendation	Summarization	Dismissal
1.1 Adjust time to here and now	XY	Y	XY	XY	XY	XY	Y	Y			Y	XY	Y
1.2 Target use of first person	XY	Y	XY	XY	XY	XY	XY	XY			XY	XY	XY
2.1 Ask closed questions	XY	XY	XY				XY	XY		Y			
2.2 Ask open questions	XY	Y	XY	X			XY	XY					Y
3.1 Verbalize client assets	XY	Y	XY	X	XY	Y	XY	X			XY	XY	XY
3.2 Attend positive aspects	XY	Y	XY		XY	XY	Y	Y			Y	XY	XY
3.3 Minimal verbalization	XY		XY		Y		Y						
3.4 Recall of content/action	Y	Y	XY	XY	X		XY	XY	XY	XY	XY	XY	XY
4.1 Reflect client feelings	XY	Y	XY	X	XY	XY	XY	XY			X	XY	XY
4.2 Match client's message	Y		XY		Y	XY	Y	XY			X	XY	XY
4.3 Restatements	Y		XY	X	X		XY						
4.4 Verbal clarification	X	Y	XY	Y	X	X	XY	XY	XY	Y			Y
5.1 Instruction and directions	XY	XY			XY		XY	XY	XY		X	X	X
5.2 Self-expression				X	Y		XY	XY	XY	X	X		XY
6.1 Challenge incongruities	XY		XY	Y		XY	Y	X			X	X	
6.2 Verbal exploration	XY		XY			X	Y			Y			
6.3 Interpretation	XY	XY		XY		X	XY	Y	Y	Y		XY	XY
6.4 Verbal following	XY		XY		X	X	XY	Y					

Note. From Scheuerle, 1985.

1. Focus attention of both the clinician and the client (nonverbally and verbally) on the client.
2. Generally, the participant in the therapy session who talks most, that is, works most, benefits most.
3. With so many behavioral options in the helping battery, each clinician tends to settle into a unique clinical style that includes the most comfortable combinations and varieties of these behaviors.
4. So many helping skills are used in each clinical operation that it would be difficult, if not impossible, to do everything wrong, that is, to perform only incorrect or unsuccessful skills.

5. The successful use of helping behaviors varies with each client, disorder, setting, and clinician.
6. Clinicians are their own best and always-present clinical tools. Clinicians need to know themselves as well as expert workers know their tools.
7. Clinicians must know their strengths and weaknesses so they can draw on them selectively in professional practice.

Becoming a Counselor or Helper

The change from student to clinician, from novice to self-directed, experienced clinician, is often slow and difficult. Through many years of schooling, students absorb information and impressions from teachers and mentors. Students gather, consider, integrate, discuss, and conclude. They observe, compare, infer, hypothesize, question, decide, and imply. Professional researchers and teachers largely continue to use these same skills. Helpers must act, react, do, and perform, but not from a script. They must initiate, elicit, respond, reflect, infer, intuit, and act. They carry out what is needed at the moment, not only for themselves but also for their charges, the clients and their families. They must give information, demonstrate knowledge and confidence, develop alternatives and solutions, take responsibility for the well-being of themselves and others, give counsel when it is needed, recognize and acknowledge when to make referrals. Unlike researchers or academic scholars, clinicians must adapt their acquired academic abilities as ingredients to use in therapy, integrate those abilities with the power of interpersonal communication, and achieve demonstrable change in the client.

A common question for beginning clinicians to ask is: How do I learn what my strengths in helping skills are? The answer is not easy or simple to achieve. However, it is possible. The following steps provide some clues.

Begin by learning to recognize these skills in the actions of family members, friends, and social acquaintances. Observe the communication style of several acquaintances. You may be surprised if you observe how often helping skills occur in the communicative behaviors of popular individuals compared with people who are unpopular. To make observations, select one subject at a time and count one behavior at a time as it occurs. Of course, you can count only one at a time, but a 5-minute count during active participation in communication will suffice. Then select and count a different behavior in the same person.

Next, select one of the skills you counted in a person's behavior as described in the previous paragraph. A nonverbal skill is usually easiest at the beginning. If you decide to try a nonverbal behavior, practice that skill in front of a mirror to establish an associated kinesthetic sense of the expression and its varying intensities. By visually monitoring your expression as you practice it, your body will be better able to recognize that action later when you are involved in conversation. Use your selected behavior as often as you can during a particular communicative effort with someone you know well and with whom you feel comfortable. Awareness of the behavior and your use of it will be invaluable in monitoring the responses of your conversational partner.

The use of videotapes provides a more thorough but complex way to learn to identify skills that are helpful, maintain awareness of them, and use them selectively. Study videotapes of experienced counselors during treatment sessions or videotapes of your own interaction with a client. Many of the helping skills are minute increments of behavior. They are fleeting, momentary, and quickly gone. With a videotape, you can use the capabilities for *pause, slow-forward,* and *rewind* to identify and replay pertinent segments. For detailed methodologies using video-training for single skills and for combining skills, the reader can refer to microteaching (Allen, 1967), microcounseling (Ivey, 1971), and microtraining (Gustafson, 1978).

❧ ❧ ❧

RISKS INHERENT IN USE OF INTERACTIVE SKILLS

The indiscriminate use of any behavior can have negative effects on both the clinician and the client. In the therapy setting, the helper is expected to influence positive change in the client. However, the extreme of any aspect of interpersonal interaction can subvert the outcome. Modern society tends to hold the opinions of professionals in high regard. As recognized professionals, speech-language pathologists and audiologists must use caution and practice within the bounds of ethical standards to protect their clients.

Consider the power wielded by the practitioner who can change others. Personal and professional power depend on a society's cultural values. Personal power may lie in charisma, charm, influence, position, title, credentials, reputation, or family or social connections. In fact, professional power is founded on those same characteristics as perceived by a specific body of people, the clients. In each power base, the line between expert and extreme is narrow and often dim. Society generally admires cognitive ability, persistence, endurance, creativity, integrity, promise, generation of trust, constancy, assuredness, and confidence, but most of all recognizes success. How success is measured introduces an entirely different element into the perception of professional practice.

Like the original list of helping behaviors described by Rogers (1961), these bases of power are not magical. Instead, the power of the practitioner lies in the perceptions of the beholder. Focusing the power on the good of the client produces ideal results. Abusing the power serves only to deceive the client, the profession, the community, and even the practitioner.

EXERCISES

In the alternative exercises suggested here, the reader is asked to follow instructions step by step. All the suggested exercises utilize the following client/family member statements.

Client/Family Member Statements

1. A telephone voice: Hello, this is Mrs. Heinz. I'm the wife of Otto Heinz. Otto won't be in for therapy today. He had another stroke on Monday. (Mrs. Heinz is 67 years old.)
2. Father of an 8-month-old boy: Yentl can't be deaf. He's just like his older brother used to be. I don't believe you.
3. Mother of 2-1/2-year-old twins, Mina and Margie: They jabber a lot to each other and sometimes to me, but I usually don't know what they're saying. I just have to guess. What's wrong with them?
4. An 18-year-old female, a cheerleader: Hello. My name is Gretchen. My voice sounds awful. Dr. Ortiz said I should bring you this medical report and you'd tell me what to do.
5. Mr. and Mrs. Kapowski are holding their 3-year-old son whose condition has been diagnosed as cerebral palsy. They have just moved to your community. Mr. Kapowski says, "Thank you for seeing us on such short notice. We're very eager to continue Noah's interdisciplinary treatment."
6. Mr. Rasheem has brought his 8-year-old son, Josiah, to see you for professional services. "Josiah is having trouble in school with reading and spelling. Otherwise, Josiah's been a fine healthy boy since he outgrew those awful earaches."
7. Lin Ku is a 10-year-old girl whose face bears scars from a cleft lip repair. She has run into your treatment room. She has been crying. She sniffles, "He's a bully! He called me a dummy and said I was ugly, too."
8. Mrs. Esposito is 57 years old. She reports ringing in her ears and sometimes feeling dizzy. Her audiological evaluations confirm a high-frequency hearing loss and tinnitus. She says, "I'd like one of those little bitty hearing aids that no one else can see. You notice I don't have to wear glasses."
9. Reggie Brown Johnson is a 35-year-old rising junior executive from a major international corporation. He speaks with a heavy dialect. You have been working with him for 2 months. Your work has concentrated on reduction of the dialectal characteristics. He laughs and says, "My mamma wouldn't know me, or maybe she wouldn't want to."

10. Vera Robinson, a 26-year-old woman, has completed her treatment for spastic dysphonia. She knows how to care for herself and how to maintain vocal quality. She reports to you that she has been offered a job in walking distance from her apartment. She finishes recounting her adventure by stating, "I met Mr. Latham, who would be my boss. I'm not sure I'm ready to take on so much responsibility. Maybe I shouldn't try to work away from home any more."

The exercises are constructed to (a) assist the reader in identification of hidden talents, that is, helping skills that are already in use, (b) develop the ability to vary habitual use of interpersonal communication behaviors, and (c) adapt new behavioral concepts for use in clinical practice as well as in daily life.

The first set of exercises is a two-step sequence. The first step focuses on spontaneous communicative responses. The second step focuses on the selection and use of helping skills. You will need a pencil, paper, and a tape recorder to complete these exercises.

Spontaneous Communicative Responses

1. Read each statement carefully as though the originator were speaking directly to you.
2. Respond to each statement as you normally would and record your response.
3. Review your responses and categorize them according to the verbal helping skills categories.
4. Count the incidence of the different behaviors that you used. Keep a record of this count.

Selection and Use of Helping Skills

1. Read each statement carefully again as though the originator were speaking directly to you.
2. This time, deliberately identify a helping behavior that seems appropriate. Try to select a response that differs from the one you used in the first step of this exercise; be sure to record your responses.
3. Review your responses and categorize them according to the verbal helping skills categories.
4. Make and keep a record of the incidence of skill distribution.

The second set of exercises should be completed in class.

With videotaping capability

1. Select a partner. Determine who will be the client and who will be the counselor. Participants may select odd- or even-numbered statements or draw lots for assignment of characterizations. Each communicator will role-play five characters. If possible, use two video cameras and split-screen capability so that each partner gets a full-face view of the other coordinated with the timing of interactions, both verbal and nonverbal.
2. Record the interpersonal communication interactions for all 10 of the client/family member statements.
3. Review the videotape. Identify the helping behaviors used. Count and record them.
4. Discuss with your partner the effectiveness of the helping behavior you used.

Without videotaping capability

1. Form groups of three. In the triad, the individuals will assume roles as (a) client/family member, (b) counselor/helper, and (c) observer—the living camera who records listener behaviors. The three participants in the group can rotate role-playing these functions so that each has at least three opportunities to perform each.
2. The observer records listener responses and attempts to describe both verbal and nonverbal behaviors.
3. When interactions are completed, the observer reviews the recorded descriptions of each helper/client interaction.
4. Identify the behaviors used and keep a count of them by category of skill.
5. The observer may also be able to relay information about the client/family member's perception of the listener's behaviors. Some groups find it most helpful to carry out the review, behavior count, and categorization after each helper/client interpersonal communication.

The third set of exercises should be completed in class.

1. Select or assign one of the client/family member characters suggested in the statements or other individuals whom you have observed. Extend the scenario suggested by that character. Sustain and videotape the characterization and the helper actions for a 3- to 5-minute period.
2. Review the full tape to identify and count the helping behaviors used. Discuss the effect of the behaviors used in terms of client/family member continuation of the communicative exchange. This method is particularly useful in that during review the client can provide input to effec-

tiveness of the clinician's selection of helping behaviors during the role playing attempt.

REFERENCES

Allen, D. (Ed.). (1967). *Microteaching: A description*. Stanford: Stanford Teacher Education Program.

Allen, D., Ryan, K., Bush, R., & Cooper, J. (1969). *Teaching skills for elementary and secondary school teachers*. New York: General Learning.

Aubertine, H. (1967). The use of microteaching in training supervising teachers. *High School Journal, 51*(1), pp. 99–106.

Bandler, J., & Grinder, R. (1985). *The structure of magic I*. Palo Alto: Science and Behavior.

Blakeley, R. W. (Ed.). (1989). Great clinicians. *Seminars in Speech and Language, 10*, p. 2.

Brown, C. C. (Ed.). (1984). *The many facets of touch*. New Brunswick, NJ: Johnson and Johnson Baby Products.

Bryant, C. (1984). Working with families with dysfunctional children: An approach and structure for the first family therapy interview. *Child and Adolescent Social Work, 1*(2), pp. 102–117.

Butler, R. N., & Lewis, M. I. (1986). *Aging and mental health*. St Louis, MO: C. V. Mosby Co.

Butterworth, B., & Hadar, U. (1989). Gesture, speech and computational stages: A reply to McNeill. *Psychological Review, 96*(2), pp. 168–74.

Cecchin, G. (1987). Hypothesizing, circularity, and neutrality revisited: An invitation to curiosity. *Family Process, 26*(3), pp. 405–414.

DeBeer-Kelston, K., Mellon, L., & Solomon, L. Z. (1986). Helping behavior as a function of personal space invasion. *Journal of Social Behavior, 126*, pp. 407–409.

DePaulo, B. M., Kenny, D. A., Hoover, C., Webb, W., & Oliver, P. V. (1986). Accuracy in person perception: Do people know what kind of impressions they convey? *Journal of Personality and Social Psychology, 52*(4), pp. 303–315.

Ebbeson, E., Kjos, G., & Konecni, V. (1976). Spatial ecology: Its effects on the choice of friends and enemies. *Journal of Experimental Social Psychology, 12*(4), pp. 505–518.

Egan, G. (1975). *The skilled helper: A systematic approach to effective helping*. Monterey, CA: Brooks/Cole.

Ekman, P., Sorensen, E. R., & Friesen, W. V. (1969). Pan-cultural elements in facial displays of emotion. *Science, 164*(1), pp. 86–88.

Evans, D. R., Hearn, M. T., Uhlemann, M. R., & Ivey, A. E. (1984). *Essential interviewing: A programmed approach to effective communication* (2nd ed.). Monterey, CA: Brooks/Cole.

Evans, G. W., & Howard, R. (1973). A methodological investigation of personal space. In W. J. Mitchell (Ed.), *Environmental design: Research and practice (EDRA)*. Los Angeles: University of California Press.

Fast, J. (1971). *Body Language*. New York: Pocket Books.

Festinger, L., Schachter, S., & Back, K. (1950). *Social pressures in informal groups: A study of human factors in housing*. New York: Harper.

Gavin, K., & Book, C. (1975). *Person to person*. Skokie, IL: National Textbook Company.

Gnepp, J., & Hess, D. L. R. (1986). Children's understanding of verbal and facial display rules. *Developmental Psychology, 22*(1), pp. 103–108.

Gustafson, K. (1978). Microtraining as used in other settings. In A. E. Ivey & J. Authier (Eds.), *Microcounseling* (2nd ed.). Springfield, IL: Charles C. Thomas.

Haase, R., & Tepper, D. (1972). Nonverbal components of empathic communication. *Journal of Counseling Psychology, 19*(3), pp. 417–424.

Hall, E. (1959). *The silent language*. Greenwich, CT: Fawcett Publications.

Hall, E. (1976). *Beyond Culture*. Garden City, NY: Doubleday.

Hamlet, C. C., Axelrod, S., & Kuerschner, S. (1984). Eye contact as an antecedent to compliant behavior. *Journal of Applied Behavioral Analysis, 17*(4), pp. 553–557.

Hayduk, L. (1978). Personal space: An evaluation and orienting overview. *Psychology Bulletin, 85,* pp. 117–134.

Heider, F. (1958). *The psychology of interpersonal relations*. New York: Wiley.

Hepworth, D., & Larsen, J. (1982). *Direct social work practice: Theory and skills*. Homewood, IL: Dorsey Press.

Hubbell, R. D. (1981). *Children's language disorders: An integrated approach*. Englewood Cliffs, NJ: Prentice-Hall.

Ivey, A. (1971). *Microcounseling: Innovations in interviewing training*. Springfield, IL: Charles C. Thomas.

Ivey, A. (1987). *Intentional interviewing and counseling*. Monterey, CA: Brooks/Cole.

Ivey, A., & Rollin, S. (1972). A behavioral objective curriculum in human relations: A commitment in intentionality. *Journal of Teacher Education, 23*(2), pp. 161–165.

Kagan, N. (1975). *Influencing human interaction*. Washington, DC: American Personnel and Guidance.

Kenny, D. A., and Malloy, T. E. (1988). Partner effects in social interaction. *Journal of Nonverbal Behavior, 12*(1), pp. 34–57.

Maccoby, E., & Maccoby, N. (1954). The interview: A tool for social science. In G. Lindzey (Ed.), *Handbook of Social Psychology* (Vol. 1). Cambridge, MA: Addison Wesley.

Malinowski, B. (1929). *The sexual life of the savages.* New York: Halcyon House.

McNeill, D. (1989). A straight path—To where? Reply to Butterworth and Hadar. *Psychological Review, 96,* pp. 175–179.

Matarazzo, R., Phillips, J., Wiens, A., & Saslow, G. (1965). Learning the art of interviewing: A study of what beginning students do and their patterns of change. *Psychotherapy: Theory, Research, and Practice, 2*(1), pp. 49–60.

Mead, M. (1956). *New lives for old, cultural transformation.* New York: William Morrow.

Mehrabian, A. (1972). *Nonverbal communication.* New York: Aldine Atherton.

Morganstern, K., & Tevlin, H. (1981). Behavioral interviewing. In M. Hersen & A. Bellack (Eds.), *Behavioral assessment: A practical handbook* (2nd ed.). New York: Pergamon Press.

Piaget, J. (1955). *The moral judgment of the child.* New York: Macmillan.

Priestly, P., & McGuire, J. (1983). *Learning to Help: Basic skills exercises.* London: Tavistock.

Rogers, C. (1961). *On becoming a person.* New York: Houghton Mifflin.

Rollin, W. J. (1989). *The psychology of communication disorders in individuals and their families.* Englewood Cliffs, NJ: Prentice-Hall.

Saarni, C. (1982). Social and affective functions of nonverbal behavior: Developmental concerns. In R. S. Feldman (Ed.), *Development of nonverbal behavior in children.* Berlin: Springer-Verlag.

Sapir, E. (1949). *Selected writings of Edward Sapir in language, culture, and personality.* Berkeley: University of California Press.

Sathre, F. S., Olson, R. W., and Whitney, S. I. (1977). *Let's talk: An introduction to interpersonal communication* (2nd ed.). Glenview, IL: Scott, Foresman.

Scheuerle, J. (1985). *Helping skills mesh with clinical techniques.* Paper presented to Hillsborough County Public Schools.

Sebeok, T. A. (1986). The doctrine of signs. *Journal of Social and Behavioral Structures, 9*(3), pp. 345–352.

Skinner, B. F. (1953). *Science and Human Behavior.* New York: Macmillan.

Soppe, H. J. G. (1988). Age differences in the decoding of affect authenticity and intensity. *Journal of Nonverbal Behavior, 12*(2), pp. 107–119.

Tanner, D. C. (1980). Loss and grief: Implications for the speech-language pathologist and audiologist. *ASHA, 22*(11), p. 916.

Tomm, K. (1987). Interventive interviewing: Part I. Strategizing as a fourth guideline for the therapist. *Family Process, 26*(1), pp. 3–14.

Tomm, K. (1987). Interventive interviewing: Part II. Reflexive questioning as a means to enable self-healing. *Family Process, 26*(2), pp. 167–184.

Weber, T., McKeever, J. E., & McDaniel, S. H. (1985). A beginner's guide to the problem-oriented first family interview. *Family Process, 24*(4), pp. 357–364.

Webster, E. J., & Newhoff, M. (1981). Intervention with families of communicatively impaired adults. In D. S. Beasley & G. A. Davis (Eds.), *Aging: Communication processes and disorders*. New York: Grune and Stratton.

Winton, P. J. (1988). Effective communication between parents and professionals. In D. B. Bailey, Jr., and R. J. Simeonsson (Eds.), *Family assessment in early intervention*. Columbus, OH: Merrill.

Zimmer, J., & Anderson, S. (1968). Dimensions of positive regard and empathy. *Journal of Counseling Psychology, 15*(5), pp. 417–426.

Zimmer, J., & Park, P. (1967). Factor analysis of counselor communications. *Journal of Counseling Psychology, 14*(3), pp. 198–203.

Zimmer, J., & Pepyne, E. (1971). A descriptive and comparative study of dimensions of counselor response. *Journal of Counseling Psychology, 18*(5), pp. 441–447.

CHAPTER THREE

❦ ❦ ❦

Serving Clients Across Ages

Issues

❦ *Normal human development progresses in a chronological sequence across the life span and can be discussed in relation to determiners of behavior.*

❦ *The life span can be arbitrarily subdivided into stages and substages, which reflect the development of traits that greatly influence the interactive behavior of the counselor and the counseling needs of the client and family.*

❦ ❦ ❦

HUMAN DEVELOPMENT ACROSS THE LIFE SPAN

Communication impairments have been found in every human society. The incidence of speech-language and hearing disorders tends to be highest at the extremes of the life span, the young and the old. Smaller numbers of adult and middle-aged clients may be related to the availability of records and the status of neurobiology, among other factors. Observations and records are more readily available for (a) young children treated in pediatric medical facilities or schools and (b) elderly men and women treated in nursing homes and retirement centers. In the very young, their acquisition of the communicative function can be observed and catalogued; in the aged, especially those who are ill, their decreased communication function likewise reduces the task of charting expression and reception of language.

No two people, even identical twins, are exactly alike. On the other hand, the fields of psychology, education, and medicine have identified and accepted clusters of attributes as predominantly associated with certain age groups across the life span. Those basic markers of development can provide the clinician with a point of departure for objective observations and inferential reasoning during diagnosis, treatment, and counseling of the client and family. Developmental sequences and milestones are well documented in many disciplines. This chapter presents an overview of the

79

patterns of maturation. The presence or absence of normal progressive changes in a client's life at or near specific ages will help the clinician formulate a holistic perspective of care. (Appendix B suggests age-related interactive stimulus materials. Appendix C includes a short list of supplementary readings that invite students to explore attitudes, feelings, and ideas in different cultures. The list is only introductory; many other sources are equally useful in understanding the worlds of other people.)

Norms of speech, language, and hearing development from birth onward provide the clinician with a tool to gauge initial expectations of client communicative proficiency, interactive behaviors, therapy goals, and materials for client treatment. The clinician then makes adjustments to diagnostic and treatment strategies that may be simpler or more complex as the client displays different aspects of the communication impairment over time. The clinician learns standards for normal communication and treatment of communication disorders initially in academic and clinical courses in college and university programs and later through a lifetime career in the discipline. In addition to the client's speech, language, and hearing, the clinician who is a counselor or helper recognizes the client's other personal interests and incorporates them into the treatment paradigm. The clinician gathers this information in the client's case history and in ongoing conversations. Topics that may indicate the client's personal interests include home, family, personal history, beliefs, opinions, attitudes, experiences, and abilities. Thus, (a) the student of communication sciences and disorders learns about normal development of speech, language, and hearing as a basis for understanding disorders; and (b) the helper or counselor needs to be knowledgeable about the sequence of personal attributes normally expected to emerge and fade across the life span.

In chapter 1, Tables 1.2 and 1.3 list personal characteristics that the clinician, client, and client's family bring to the treatment setting. Those attributes suggest that the humanness of each person molds and shapes interpersonal relationships. Those complex lists encompass far more than can be discussed in a single chapter. Instead, this chapter presents a simplified scheme to place developmental markers at specific points in the life span.

A workable scheme for tracing human development can be formed by creating a matrix composed of progression through time or chronology and variables of development or determiners of behavior (Atchley, 1980; Erikson, 1963; Levinson, 1978; Piaget, 1952; Shaie & Willis, 1986; Sheehy, 1976). Chronological stages of development arbitrarily arrange the life span into six categories, five of which are further divided into substages. Table 3.1 lists these developmental stages of the life span and a range of ages assigned to each. The overlap of ages from one developmental stage to the next suggests that the stages are not clear-cut, but blend across the years.

Table 3.1
Chronological stages of development

Stage	Substage	Age Range
1. Young child	1.1 Infant-toddler	0-3
	1.2 Preschool age	3-6
2. Pre-adolescent	2.1 Elementary school age	6-10
	2.2 Pre-pubescence	10-13
3. Adolescence	3.1 Early teenage years	13-16
	3.2 Late teenage years	16-20
4. Adulthood	4.1 Young adulthood	20-35
	4.2 Mature adulthood	35-50
5. Middle age		50-65
6. Old age (Aging)	6.1 Young old	65-75
	6.2 Old	75-90
	6.3 Very old	90-105+

While chronological stages are a useful device for organizing ideas about development, the reader must remember that the divisions are arbitrary and nominal only. These stages do not include the critical prenatal period, nor do they describe discrete steps in sensation or action, emotion, attitude, or ability. Instead, chronological stages represent a set of time markers or guideposts onto which to drape information that is of consequence to clinical proficiency in helping communicatively impaired clients and their families.

In the developmental matrix, the second set of markers that comprise reference points for the clinician are determiners of human behavior. Like chronological stages, these are applicable to clinicians themselves as well as to clients and their families. As we progress through this matrix, the reader should find developmental markers that are applicable to personal experience. Also, the reader may want to add to the characteristics of staged determiners as presented here. By modifying the matrix in a personal way, the reader will see the need to modify this scheme, like others, for each individual client.

Determiners of human behavior can be clustered into four broad composite and overlapping categories: biology, cognition, psycho-social adaptation, and environment. These terms are complex and may be used in a variety of ways. The following definitions will clarify the use of each term in the matrix.

1. *Biology* refers to the chemical and cellular mass that comprises the human body and its systems, maintains its integrity and ability to function, grows and develops according to a genetic program or code, is influenced by and responds to external and internal stimuli.

2. *Cognition* refers to what you do with what you know. This determiner includes learning, that is, the establishment of new relationships or the strengthening of relationships between two events, actions, or objects.
3. *Psycho-social adaptation* considers the ability of the biological and cognitive being to interact with elements of the environment to assure survival and guarantee satisfaction, if not pleasure.
4. *Environment* includes internal and external influences that impinge upon the complex neurobiological mechanism to challenge and support its function and maximum development.

Interference with the normal development driven by each determiner can initiate or aggravate a disorder in communication. Table 3.2 presents a distribution of communication disorders, the behavioral determiners to which they are most closely related, and modes of potential interference with normal development. As a general rule, the earlier the onset of the disorder, the more far-reaching and dramatic its effect; the more severe the disorder, the greater the handicap; and the more complex the disorder, the longer and more complicated the remediation or habilitative process. The delineation of disorders as presented in Table 3.2 is not exact. For example, the characteristics of disorders overlap, such as a hearing disorder affecting language, and the influence of one determiner on the others is very powerful, such as brain damage affecting cognitive abilities. However, this chart provides a structure to which the clinician can add refinements as needed.

❧ ❧ ❧

PERSONAL ATTRIBUTES RELATED TO CHRONOLOGICAL AGE: STAGES OF DEVELOPMENT

1.1 Infant-Toddler—Birth to 3 Years

At this stage, diagnosis and intervention for communication disorders are directly applied to the child. Indirect intervention is carried out through interacting with, counseling, and training the caregivers and consulting with other professionals involved in the client's care.

Biology. This is the period of most rapid postnatal growth. Neurobiological development progresses normally from the head to the feet. This is easily observable in gross motor movement and body and limb control during the first 3 years of life. Sensation apparently matures in somewhat the same fashion, except that the special senses of sight and hearing are acutely active from birth. Within an hour after birth, neonates demonstrate response to environmental sound and their eyes selectively focus on the human face. Developmental milestones, biological and other, are recorded in pediatric literature and reflected in assessment scales such as the Bayley Scales (Bayley, 1969), the Brazelton Behavioral

Table 3.2
Behavioral determiners and related communication disorders

Behavioral Determiner	Potential Interference	Communication Disorder
1. Biology	Genetic	Sensory deficit
	Environmental	Receptive disorder
	Congenital	Hearing impairment
	Disease	Deafness
	Trauma	Vision impairment
	Radiation	Blindness
	Chemical	Structural deformity
		Cleft lip/palate
		Craniofacial anomaly
		Hearing loss
		Neurological
		Cerebral palsy
		Aphasia
		Language-learning disability
		Agnosias
		Deafness
		Attention deficit disorder
		Dementia
		Mental retardation
		Neuro-motor
		Dysarthria
		Dyspraxia
		Dysphonia
		Oral-pharyngeal incoordination

Assessment Scale (Brazelton, 1973), and the Cattell Infant Intelligence Scale (Cattell, 1947). Recognized advances in development occur so rapidly that they are chronicled by weekly and then monthly increments in descriptive literature and assessment scales.

Newborn crying and accompanying vocalization, facial contortion, Moro reflex, turning to sound, and tearing of eyes demonstrate intact neurological substrata of respiration, phonation, muscles of facial expression, and hearing. All of these are important to acquiring oral-aural language. Each newborn is rated on a 10-point scale called the APGAR, an acronym for the components of the test:

A = Appearance (color of skin)
P = Pulse (rate and rhythm)
G = Grimace (facial expression following aversive stimulus)
A = Activity (muscle tone)
R = Respiration (regularity of breathing)

Table 3.2 (continued)
Behavioral determiners and related communication disorders

Behavioral Determiner	Potential Interference	Communication Disorder
2. Cognition	Physical Emotional Psychological	Mental retardation Language disorder Perceptive Auditory, visual Memory Recall Formulation Encoding
3. Psychosocial adaptation	Temperament Personality Genetics Stress Culture Family	Autism Depression Schizophrenia Elective mutism Nonverbal disorders Pragmatic disorders Selective attention Elective deafness
4. Environment	Deprivation Overprotection Rejection Carelessness Stress	Language Speech articulation Pragmatic disorders Vocal disorders Rate and rhythm disorders Noise-induced hearing loss

Of the newborns who are tested on the APGAR scale in the United States, 90% score 7 or better. APGAR scores correlate with prenatal and later development (Serunian and Broman, 1975). More recently, pediatricians are being encouraged to examine the oral cavity for the presence of structural anomalies that may interfere with suckling and may need immediate referral for treatment. This reduces incidence of both "failure-to-thrive" babies and parental distress.

Limited movement of the neonate's arms and legs may be observed, but generally a warm, dry, well-fed newborn sleeps most of the time—17 to 20 hours in 24 hours. In fact, the cutaneous sensory receptors for warmth and dryness as well as proprioceptors for gastro-intestinal comfort act as the initial regulators of homeostasis. Through these neurological components, the child utilizes external stimuli of swaddling, rocking, crooning, patting, and warmth to regulate body functions such as breathing, heartbeat, movement, and wakefulness. The locus of control is truly external.

Within the first 3 months, the baby shows dramatic change in appearance and activity. Cervical strength steadies the head on top of the vertebral column. Now the head can be rotated to survey and scan the visible environment. Sitting up by the age of 6 or 7 months requires greater body control and allows more freedom from support and access to new environmental stimuli. Grasping, reaching, and babbling are common by then. The urge to acquire something out of reach seems to drive the infant on to scoot or crawl. Laryngeal, pharyngeal, and oral motor function are maturing noticeably, as seen in babbling and the imitation of adult inflection patterns. Turn-taking, nonverbal communication, and the use of generic terms for common objects and persons develop rapidly.

Locomotion on all fours opens the baby's world more than previous motor skills, but not as wondrously as walking, which will soon follow locomotion. Most babies begin to walk at the age of 12 to 14 months. The toddler is now free from need for the constant support and consequent restriction of a vehicle or caregiver. The newly mobile creature reacts eagerly to adventure, curiosity, and mischief. The child spends vast amounts of energy exploring, testing, trying, and repeating pleasurable and interesting activities. Such use of energy requires frequent infusions of a variety of nourishing foods. The body grows at a fairly steady pace. Pediatric charts indicating growth in height, head circumference, and weight are standardized for these aspects of development among Caucasian infants and toddlers (Behrman & Vaughn, 1986).

Sensory reception and cortical perception of the ever-expanding environment involve children in learning more about their world and behaving so as to influence it in exciting and satisfying ways. Caregivers of young children know all too well that, toward the end of this stage, naps get shorter and busy activities fill the day.

Infants and toddlers whose congenital and developmental biology varies from the expected pattern are often identified by medical experts through well-baby pediatric monitoring. However, subtle differences and subclinical disorders of communication may not be noticed by the busy medical professional with a primary focus on wellness, health, immunizations, and normal growth and development. Also, there remains an alarming number of young children who are not seen by any medical specialist. In the latter case, a communication disorders professional may be the first to discover a hearing disorder or a structural or a neurobiological condition that requires early interdisciplinary preventive intervention (Scheuerle, 1989).

Cognition. These early years are described as the sensory-motor period. Piaget (1952) limited this cognitive age to 0 to 2 years. He described the child's behavior as initially reflexive, but becoming organized in relation to the environment.

A psychoanalytic approach to child development traces the young child through the oral (satisfaction from sucking) and anal (gratification in defecation, toilet training) stages. Infants are egocentric and do not differentiate themselves from the outside world. They view environment in much the same way that ancient civilizations believed that the sun and stars moved around the earth. That is, the environment exists for the gratification of the child.

Observation of the normal infant-toddler reveals that some babies are quiet and content, while others are restless and irritable. Thomas, Chess, Birch, Hertzig, and Korn (1963), Carey (1981), and Chess (1967) discussed temperament or behavioral style as inborn. This style normally includes regularity of body function; acceptance of change in environment and routine; sensitivity to intense noise, light, and temperature; cheerfulness; reaction intensity; distractibility; and degree of persistence. Individual babies vary greatly across these traits, but barring dramatic or traumatic experience, the maturing individual continues to exhibit a behavior style present in infancy.

Infants and toddlers tend to pay more attention when something unexpected or unusual happens. Within hours of birth, auditory and visual functions are observed. Neonates tend to habituate to physical and social surroundings. As early as 2 months of age, infants display differentiation of the mother's face from that of others; discrimination of sounds, odors, and tastes; and variations in body temperature and increasing perception of pain. Even at this young age, children begin to organize information, adapt responses to find new ways to solve puzzles, incorporate new ideas, and change actions to manage new objects in daily situations. Toddlers increasingly utilize verbal communication, reducing the need for continual proximity of a parent or other caregiver.

Besides learning to manipulate toys and other objects, toddlers coordinate and integrate information from sight, hearing, touch, taste, and smell. They understand that all these sensory messages can come from one object and do not represent separate entities. They typically exhibit goal-directed behavior, take turns in communicative activities, and organize as well as imitate the phonemes of the native language. By age 3, toddlers have command of some 900 intelligibly spoken words.

In the modern world, intellectual prowess is greatly honored. Infants and toddlers who demonstrate slowness in cognitive development or communicative activities may be incidentally or incorrectly labeled and carry that label through life. Rather than a generic title assigned to a composite of behaviors, a definitive diagnosis of disabilities is much preferred. Careful sharing of information with other professionals in the child's world is very important. In this way, all care-management personnel focus their interests and attention appropriately and minimize duplication or waste of time.

Psycho-social Adaptation. Erikson (1963) based his stages of maturation on cultural and societal influences. Each stage represents encounter-
ing and resolving specific crises. According to Erikson, how these crises
are resolved is determined by and, in turn, affects psycho-social development. Two of these stages apply to children between birth and 36 months
of age.

Crisis I, according to Erikson, describes the creation of trust versus
mistrust in infants up to 18 months. Trusting babies sleep deeply, eat well
and regularly, and evacuate the relaxed bowel with little variation in
schedule from day to day. This regulation of biological functions, or homeostasis, demonstrates the secure feelings of the infants by the absence of
inhibitions in the neurological management of the sensory-motor mechanism.

During the 12 months following birth, caregiving adults give babies a
sense of comfort by alleviating hunger and wet-cold distress and by listening to, talking to, touching, and holding them. The baby's pleasure is min-
gled with dependency on the caregiver. The shared experience is known as
bonding between infant and caregiver (usually the mother). The quality of
that bond is critical to the ongoing development of the child. Speech-language pathologists and audiologists are the experts who can readily identify poor or absent interaction between infant and caregiver. Intake interviews, observation, and counseling interaction with the caregiver can help
determine what the child's communication environment is like. The quality of the child-caregiver relationship is affected by the personality
attributes of each. However, mutual trust that evolves in the relationship
is basic to the further development of the child. For example, mutual trust
enables the child to separate from the mother because the child accepts
and understands the certainty that the mother will return.

The second of Erikson's stages addresses autonomy versus shame or
doubt. This occurs between 18 and 36 months. During this time, children
explore their physical space and test the limits of behavior. They need
realistic limits that are monitored by the trusted parent. This continued
interaction establishes boundaries for self-control in the young child and
gives assurance that the trusted monitor can be counted on for guidance
and safety by maintaining limits. Herein is easily recognized the *terrible
twos* of both genders. Assured that the watchful parent, through continued external control, will "keep them good," children dare to discover the
world. Their behavior is influenced by body chemistry, gender, temperament, family size, birth order, and the personalities of role-models, monitors or caregivers, and others who comprise the psycho-social environment.

Babies born to alcoholic or diseased mothers, or those born addicted to
drugs, present an initial condition that will need to be addressed individually. Any neurobiological damage acquired in utero cannot be reversed,

but the plasticity of the young central nervous system may provide a period of compensatory adaptation.

Environment. The ideal neonate-infant-toddler environment and its parameters have been described in health and health-related disciplines. That environment should provide for the continually changing physical, psychological, and social needs of the immature human being. In the traditional family structure of mother-father-children, the mother dominates the young child's environment. The mother is the acknowledged partner in the child's adventure with all aspects of maturation. Interestingly, the ability to succeed in the complex role of parenting is taken for granted in most western cultures. Except for memories of personal experience and observations from their own childhoods, most young first-time parents have no instruction or training in normal-child care, child development, or the establishment of interpersonal relationships with their infant-toddlers or older children. This means that the interaction between parent and child ultimately depends on the mixture of their dual personalities, temperaments, biological, cognitive, creative, and psycho-social adaptive abilities.

Physical care of the baby consumes a great deal of time and energy during day and night. Other family duties and household chores also require the parents' attention and energy. These distractions from the baby vary from family to family and from day to day in each family. In some social groups, physical care is the only aspect of infant-toddler care that is understood. In such cases, much-loved offspring are well-nourished but unstimulated. They become quiet and passive watchers and abide by imposed external controls without overt protest.

The parent's ability to cope with hundreds of demands, familiar and new, greatly influences the course of the normal baby's development. Like food and sleep, stimulation is essential in appropriate amounts during waking hours. All family members may participate in the many phases of care for the young child. Those who do so will contribute additional elements to the environment and influence the maturation of the infant.

It would be unacceptable to leave discussion of this critical period of the child's life without brief comment on the changing aspects of home environments. Many families have a single parent of either gender, and some have two parents of the same gender. In 1988, among all births registered in the United States Bureau of Census, 56% of African American babies and 15% of white babies were born to single women, many of whom were teenagers.

Both parents in a two-parent family or the single parent may work outside the home. This situation leaves the infant with a non-parent caregiver or in a nursery with many other small children for a large portion of the day. Child care for young children of working parents did not become a critical national concern until the last two decades, although it had been a problem for many years prior to that.

At the opposite extreme, many infants are born into poverty to unemployed single mothers who immediately go on public welfare and receive Aid for Dependent Children from public funds. Another consideration for the helper/counselor is that improved obstetrical care has encouraged many women to postpone pregnancy until their mid- to late 30s. Many first-time mothers are now much older than first-time mothers in the past. During the late 1980s, one third of the women having a first child were older than 30 years of age. These older women tend to be highly educated and have careers to which they return soon after the baby is born. This situation often requires a surrogate parent or nanny to monitor the formative years of the infant-toddler.

Another consideration that may affect child development is the recent evolution of national, international, and interracial practices in adoption, fertility clinics, genetic selection, and surrogate pregnancies. These legal developments in progeneration may contribute unexplored intellectual, emotional, and physical factors to the infant's world. The counselor's awareness of potential differences in the home environment of the infant-toddler may be helpful in deciding which behavioral factors to reinforce, treat, or refer to colleagues in other disciplines.

❦ ❦ ❦

COUNSELING CONSIDERATIONS

At 8 months of age, Raiesa is a quiet baby, does not respond to voices or other sounds, and has ceased babbling. Her only sounds are reflexive laughter or crying. Medical and audiological assessment find that she is severely hearing-impaired, with bilateral hearing loss between 84 and 89 dB across frequencies of the speech range. After the battery of diagnostic tests is completed, the audiologist, speech-language pathologist, and the parents become the primary treating team. Amplification, auditory training of residual hearing, receptive and expressive language, and socialization through pragmatic skills become the immediate focus of concentration for treatment of the complex communication disorder.

The mother is a 38-year-old corporate lawyer in a local firm, and the father is a certified public accountant or CPA in private practice. Raiesa is their second child; Boris is her 4-1/2-year-old brother. Her grandparents live more than 3,000 miles away and manage to visit only a couple of times each year.

Training and counseling of the parents and other caregivers are essential to help the family accept and understand the child's disorder and to cope with the many ramifications of infant deafness. The following suggestions indicate a method of approaching the client and family to interact in a reasonable and professional manner. Before reading the suggestions, make note of how you feel about interacting with this family.

1. Consider how Raiesa differs now from others her age.
2. How will these differences modify her development according to all the determiners?
3. What interactive counseling skills must be incorporated in the initial client-clinician relationship?
4. What concerns, considerations, and problems will the mother and father bring to this first meeting?
5. Identify the emotions that may comprise the affective state of the parents during this initial interview.
6. What do the parents need or want to know at this time?
7. What information, and how much, is appropriate to share with the parent during this initial interview?
8. Will Raiesa's deafness affect Boris? How? When?
9. What can the family do to maximize interaction of the siblings?
10. What community services do the parents need to know about now?
11. Who else in the community may be of help to the family?
12. Write a dialogue that reflects this initial interview. In the margin, identify and code the message of the parent, the counselor, and the client.

1.2 Preschool Age—3 to 6 Years

Diagnosis and treatment focus on the child. Both the child and primary caregivers need counseling and guidance. Parents and surrogate parents, like the physical environment, must be adaptive and accommodate the child's needs (Greenspan, 1983).

Biology. Growth and physical development continue at a rapid rate, but begins to slow down from that of the previous stage. Many boys and girls begin to show differences in developmental strengths. Skeletal, muscular, and nervous systems show marked maturation and integration of action. Boys tend to have greater muscle strength and body control for accuracy of such things as throwing balls. Whole body coordination of large muscle function leads to running, skipping, hopping, jumping, and climbing. Throwing and catching a ball are great fun and often involve a companion in play. Girls are often introduced to dance movements during this age. Boys and girls alike begin to participate in circle/dodgeball, kick-ball, and other recreational group activities. Families who enjoy individual activities such as skating and swimming may begin to encourage their children to participate in sports.

A typical 3-year-old Caucasian child weighs between 35 and 38 pounds and is about 38 inches tall. Standards for children of other races are not readily available and those which are sometimes used are poor. However, on average, African American children tend to be larger than white, and oriental children smaller. Growth and development are closely related to nourishment. During this period of continued rapid growth, the deciduous teeth should complete eruption. This enables the child to chew better and aids intake of a larger variety of nourishing foods. International recognition of the problem of feeding entire populations of children has long been a focus of UNESCO, The Peace Corps, and various religious groups.

Children at this stage begin to refine fine motor abilities. Using crayons to color drawings or make original drawings is quite popular. Arrangement of puzzle pieces, lock-together toys such as Tinkertoys or Lego blocks utilize manual dexterity. Use of scissors and small lightweight tools is creative and enjoyable. Realistic use of kitchen implements in first or repeated successful efforts to prepare food are very rewarding. Likewise, when available, large empty cardboard cartons, paper, scraps of cloth, transparent tape, and string become fascinating. In fact, children of this age are constantly active. Unfortunately, this constant activity may be a partial contributor to reduced parental tolerance and widespread child abuse which prevails in society in the late twentieth century, as it did in previous eras.

Children between 3 and 6 years of age sleep less during the day than younger children and 8 to 10 hours per night. Children select and regulate their activities within the limits set by caregivers. In nursery schools, a favorite activity corner is the household or playhouse, where miniature furniture and utensils invite children to manipulate familiar objects.

Cognition. This stage of learning matches the Piagetian preoperational phase of cognitive development. Advancing language abilities provide children with a symbol system by which to represent objects and experiences in their absence. Preoperational symbolic function is demonstrated through deferred imitation, symbolic play, and language. After watching a parent put gasoline in the car, a child pretends to put fuel into his tricycle, illustrating deferred imitation. Symbolic play is exemplified in a child knowingly using one thing to represent another. On average, vocabulary or language increases from 900 to 2,500 words during these years, and adult syntax is acquired. These achievements add to children's freedom. Besides becoming locomotively independent, their minds develop the ability to dart back and forth among ideas and assimilate and coordinate new combinations of ideas. Further, they can share their mental experience through exchange of language with others.

Thought processes of children in the preoperational stage of development have unique characteristics. Children at this stage are egocentric; that is, they can comprehend the world from only their own point of view. They focus on one aspect of a situation (centration) to the neglect of others. They demonstrate irreversibility, such as a child denying that his sister has a brother. They see a series of actions as separate, not as a sequence. Fantasy is locked into experience in that children will mentally review and mingle a series of real phenomena to create unreal imaginings. Children do not always generalize from discrete repeated points of information, that is, every object is "the" object (Piaget, 1951).

Preschool-age children serialize some things by size; they classify and label by color, shape, and size. Guilford (1959) created a matrix of 120 different intellectual abilities in categories of operations, products, and contents. Many intelligence tests have been designed to assess those abilities, either singly or in clusters. Measures of language competency and assessment of language-learning disabilities are derived from such tests. Tests commonly recognized in work with preschool populations include the Stanford-Binet (3–8 years of age) and the Wechsler Preschool and Primary Scale of Intelligence (WPPSI) (4–6-1/2).

Cognitive function permeates the psycho-social adaptive behaviors of this age group. The interdependence of these two determiners of behavior is readily noted when children are observed in group interaction.

Psycho-social Adaptation. Interaction between the child and the parent or caregiver remains central to the child's acquisition of appropriate psycho-social adaptive behavior. Selective physical and verbal reinforcement by the parent of the child's desired traits strengthens those that are socially and culturally approved and reduces less desired ones. Verbal humor is readily accepted in this age group and children appreciate the unexpected as in riddles, such as "knock-knock" jokes, and the obviously inappropriate as in puns. Boys and girls of this age imitate role models and enjoy pretending. They create imaginary friends with whom they share real and imagined experiences, even involving them in family affairs.

Preschoolers may exhibit a wide range of play behaviors in a group of their peers, such as neighborhood play groups, nursery school, or kindergarten. Recognizing a child's many approaches to play is useful for the clinician who works with individuals and groups of preschool clients. Parten (1932) identified the following six distinct classifications of such behaviors that continue to be observed in preschool children.

1. *Unoccupied Behavior* describes children who are not apparently playing. They are watchful, following the teacher or clinician around, playing with their own body, getting on and off chairs, or sitting and gazing around the room.
2. As *onlookers,* children watch other children play. They may talk to others about what they are doing, but do not undertake to enter into play activities.
3. In *solitary independent play,* children play alone with toys different from those used by others. Although they may be near other children, they make no effort to interact.

4. *Parallel activity* defines children playing independently, but with toys and in ways like the other children who are present. They do not try to influence others nor are they influenced by them. They play *beside* rather than *with* other children.
5. In *cooperative play,* children play with others, talk about common activities, share materials, and carry out similar behaviors, such as rolling cars. Children do the activity because they choose to do so, rather than because it is a role to be carried out within a group. In general, their interest tends to lie in the association with others instead of the activity itself.
6. *Cooperative* or *organized supplementary play* describes children participating in a role within an organized goal-oriented group activity. There is a sense of belonging, and one or two children are the acknowledged leaders. There is a division of labor so that cooperative efforts are required to complete the whole task.

Play at this stage serves a function like that of work at later stages. Many theories have been formulated to explain how play functions in child development, for it involves use of the body, interactive behavior, emotions, intellect, and socio-cultural influences. Ideally, according to some of those theorists, the preschool child moves through the six play behaviors described by Parten and emerges a socially compatible creature ready to participate in the imposed structure of formal schooling.

During this preschool age, Erikson's (1963) third crisis of initiative versus guilt is noted. Curious, adventurous 4- to 6-year-old children identify behaviorally with a parent or caregiver of the same sex. They gain greater body strength and size, and they realize they are no longer babies. They undertake to express self-reliance and become involved in risk-taking. Fears emerge, some deliberately taught by parents for safety, such as fear of fire, deep water, fast cars, or gifts from strangers, other fears growing out of experience, imagination, and incomplete understanding of phenomena that children observe.

Environment. In addition to home environment, formal preschool or academic programs and eventually kindergarten, a large portion of the preschool population experiences some form of day care. Preschool children 3 years of age and older may participate in half-day organized school activities two or more times a week. These experiences, especially kindergarten for 5-year-olds, have proven to be valuable assets in readiness for entry into academic activities in primary grades.

Many 3-, 4-, and 5-year-olds spend from 4 to 18 hours a day in some form of child-care facility. Proficiency of the management, staff, and program of the preschool setting correlates with the location, clientele, and cost to the parents. Because increasing numbers of working parents are locked into traditional business hours of 8:00 a.m. to 5:00 p.m., and many single parents maintain two unskilled jobs, child-care needs demand more facilities and longer hours of service.

Since 1926 the National Association for the Education of Young Children (NAEYC) has drawn together and represented professionals who have long-standing concerns for the early formative years of the next generation. In the late 1940s and early 1950s the post-World War II baby boom escalated the need for unprecedented out-of-home child care. As is found in the history of centuries before, no organized effort was made to meet the needs of children. Each family pursued workable solutions regardless of the quality of care. Each year since that time has found growing child-care needs with minimal efforts toward resolution of the problem by employers, elected public officials, or from unification of the thousands of families caught in the conflict created by this unserved need for competent and knowledgeable child care.

Federal legislation has addressed the civil rights of minorities, women, handicapped citizens, and equal opportunity for employment. Still, the daily care needs of young children from most strata of industrialized society were not considered for assistance. In 1983, a group of interested men and women initiated a national citizens' effort, *The Child-Care Action Campaign* (99 Hudson Street, Room 1233, New York, NY 10013) to focus on child-care needs. This campaign, headed by Elinor Guggenheimer, was organized to alert the country to changes in family life, publicize the tragedy of inadequate child care, create a network of child-care advocates, and provide a resource for information to be funneled to those who shape national policy. Through such efforts, changes have begun in perspectives on the needs of children before school days begin.

The environmental problems of preschoolers have been exacerbated by the high rate of teenage pregnancies, which has increased since the 1960s and 1970s. Since then increasing numbers of single teenage mothers who live in poverty keep their babies to grow up in deprived home environments. The thousands of individuals who will enter the 21st century from this start in life can be expected to continue to exhibit developmental problems that must be addressed in schools and clinics for habilitative services. If these problems are not treated successfully, we will have a work force glutted with unskilled labor that is less and less in demand.

❦ ❦ ❦

COUNSELING CONSIDERATIONS

Bobby is in kindergarten. He is a very active and independent child with a great deal of energy. Because of his persistent hoarseness, Ms. McCord, his mother, took Bobby to an otorhinolaryngologist (ENT), who referred them to you. Dr. Marita Jardin, the ENT, sent a note explaining that Bobby has vocal nodules that she prefers not to remove surgically because of his age. Voice therapy is indicated. Dr. Jardin also indicated that Bobby is a healthy boy. She finds him spoiled and reports that he screams a lot at home and at after-school day care where he stays 3 hours, three times a week. According to Bobby's mother, teachers say that he does not scream at school.

Treatment of this functional voice disorder demands behavior change in the child, among other considerations. Is it significant that different behaviors are demonstrated in different settings? What can you infer from this? Besides testing and assessment of the child's hearing, speech, and language:

1. What information do you, the clinician, need to formulate a comprehensive treatment or management plan?
2. What helping behaviors are effective in eliciting important information from the client and the parent?
3. In addition to Bobby and his mother, who will need to become a part of the care-management team?

2.1 Elementary School Age— 6 to 10 Years

The adventure of leaving home to go to school is required and regulated by law in many countries. Families often find this experience a happy indicator that their child-rearing practices have been successful and the survival of their child is assured. Entering elementary school opens new horizons for child and family; it is an adventure that renews hope, but also adds stress. School and classroom discourse may introduce new realms for communication problems (Ripich & Spinelli, 1985). In treatment of communication disorders, the clinician extends services beyond the child and the family to school personnel who work with the child.

Biology. In general, health among children of elementary school age is much better than earlier in the 20th century. Inoculations and antibiotics have prevented crippling conditions and enabled children to attend school more regularly. In fact, by the 1980s death rates for all causes among 5- to 14-year-olds were reduced to one fifth of what they had been 50 years earlier.

Poverty continues to be the most serious health problem among American children. Prenatal malnutrition and related low birth weight are responsible for much of the continuing child mortality problem. Additionally, medical expertise in neonatal intensive care units maintains life in babies who would have died in past decades. While the skill and technology found in medical care of neonates and very young children attest to the devotion of society to preserving life, the numbers of children with disabilities are increasing faster than ever before. When these children reach the age of 6 to 10 years, they carry with them the biological problems retained or acquired since birth. School systems that receive federal funds are legally obliged to accommodate student needs regardless of disabilities. But even the best of schools generally segregate students with physical handicaps or mental or emotional disabilities from the general able-bodied school population. This is often done with the knowledge and agreement of parents.

One additional public policy consideration should be mentioned. When the school systems of many states stepped forward to accept responsibility for educating handicapped or disabled children in the 1970s, they did so with minimal preparation of programs, teachers, or facilities. A great deal of federal money was at stake, and the schools with proposals for programs that were ready to go, received funds to activate their programs. Needless to say, as time tested some of the curricula and teaching methodologies, revisions had to be made. Such add-on changes by generalists in any discipline may risk quality of overall programs and outcomes for expediency in developing data to demonstrate numbers served.

Normally developing elementary school children polish their skills in running, jumping, bicycling, reaching, throwing, kicking, and gymnastic activities. There are noticeable differences in teacher expectations by pupil gender and in the actual performance those differences are rewarded (Brophy & Good, 1974). Partially based on the verbal environment of elementary school, that setting is often thought of as a girl's world. Girls of this age are typically more compliant and verbal than are their male peers.

Six- to 10-year-olds lose their teeth, which curtails their cute appeal and distorts their speech articulation. They develop binocular coordination, and their faces reshape through forward growth of the mandible and elongation of the midface to more adult proportions. Whereas previously the face was on the lower third of the anterior surface of the head, now it occupies more than half of the front of the head. Growth rates of the different portions of the face regulate, and are normally regulated by, the match of the middle and lower thirds of the facial skeleton. Mismatches tend to result in disproportion of facial parts which may need physical manipulation by surgery or orthodontic appliances.

To maximize health, physical development, and coordination in school-age children, standards of performance have been developed. These were given impetus by rising interest in televised International Olympic Games. Popularity of the Games, particularly gymnastics, influenced large numbers of children and their families to become involved in physical activities, gymnastics, and organized sports whether at school or through private instruction. Increased private financial support for such activities was organized into national associations for raising funds and for training talented athletes. At the same time, national promotion of health and wellness focused the attention of many parents on diet, exercise, and long life for themselves and their families. During this same period, legislation was passed to outlaw discrimination by age for employment and by gender for participation in sports. In general, the 1980s ushered in a popularized commitment to eat right, stay well, get strong, and reduce the incidence of cardiovascular disease and other preventable causes of early death.

Outside of school, organized activities for children of elementary school age are common in many middle- and upper-class communities. Day camps and summer camps are popular. T-ball and soccer seem the most popular team sports. Parents act as coaches, and entire families attend games to cheer on the players. Involvement of the whole family adds to the exercise, outdoor activity, and physical development of all members of the household. Unfortunately, even at this early age of their children, some parents become aggressive in their emphasis on winning teams and thereby spoil the experience for others.

Unlike the middle and upper classes, children of low-income families endure substandard housing, poor diet, and inadequate medical and dental care. In general, their parents are busy, poorly educated, and have little skill in coping with their children's needs. A disproportionately large number of minorities live at or below the poverty level. The poor may turn to cheap alcohol or drugs to ease an acknowledged hopelessness that prevails in overcrowded urban ghettos or isolated and remote areas. The effects on biological and especially neurobiological development of children in such circumstances are devastating. Dialect, slang, and idiomatic language have been some of the notable differences among children in integrated school settings. In addition, previous and current hearing disorders, difficulties with central processing of language, and cultural pragmatics all confound the enculturation of minority children into the standard-English school community. Within some school districts as many as 40 or 50 non-English native languages and multiple non-standard-English dialects are spoken in homes. For those children, success in school requires acquiring a new language and adjusting to social interactions from a different culture.

Cognition.   Elementary school children are busily increasing their ability to use symbols, primarily in acquiring language, to carry out mental operations. According to currently popular learning theory, this tends to reduce their need for involvement in physical activities. These children are able to sit still and attend for increasing periods of time. Productivity becomes important, and play is replaced by work. Their manner of thinking becomes more logical, and they become better able to deal with abstractions. Different areas of understanding evolve during this period of concrete operations (Piaget, 1952). At about 10 years of age, the child who is developing normally is expected to have established realism, animism, artificialism, and conservation.

Realism refers to the ability to recognize symbols as separate from the objects they represent, and distinguish dreams or fantasies from actual experiences. The younger children's inability to make these distinctions represents a lack of separation of psychological events from objective reality.

Animism is the practice of assigning life characteristics to inanimate objects, especially moving things such as a stream of water or leaves being blown along the ground. By about 10 years of age, children recognize only plants and animals as living things. However, enjoyment of the fantasy of animation often continues into adulthood, as evidenced in the world-wide popularity among adults of Walt Disney's cartoon characters and Jim Henson's Muppets.

Artificialism embraces the notion that humans are not responsible for the universe, its contents, and activities. Children slowly begin to comprehend that people did not and do not control natural phenomena. This includes such constants as the change of day to night, the alternation of sun and moon in the sky, the seasons of the year, rain, snow, and other naturally recurrent happenings.

Piaget described *conservation* as the ability to recognize that equal quantities of matter remain equal in substance, weight, and volume even if the matter is rearranged in shape. To master this complex concept, children must be able to identify, quantify, compare, reverse, compensate, and infer. Exactly how children learn conservation is undetermined, but testing and measurement show that the process is apparently related to formal school experience (Greenfield, 1966).

Psycho-social Adaptation. Along with cognitive development, elementary school children begin to understand and appreciate the distinction of right and wrong. According to Piaget (1952, 1955) and Kohlberg (1964, 1969, 1984), the development of moral values is a rational process that coincides with cognitive development. Through the 6- to 10-year-old stage, interaction with family, teachers, classmates, and other peers provides children an opportunity to observe and participate in numerous decision-making opportunities. These serve as educational experiences upon which to base social learning and habituation of social behavior. Erikson (1963) suggested that industry and a desire for achievement during this period are accompanied by the risk of discovering one's own inferiority.

Six moral concepts that begin to formulate during this time deal with (a) recognition that others may have different perspectives or points of view; (b) separation of intentionality from outcomes; (c) recognition that rules exist to establish order and organizational coordination and that they can be changed; (d) respect for authority, peers, and self; (e) appropriateness of punishment that leads to restitution and reform of the culprit; and (f) distinction of natural misfortune from punishment (Kohlberg, 1964).

Traditionally, moral reasoning has been based largely on the tenets of various religions. Through education and psychosocial research it has become more broadly accepted that children from 6 to 10 years of age have not yet worked out a sense of moral values, nor can they exercise mature moral judgment for themselves or others. In the interest of competent counseling and guidance, it is important that clinicians have an understanding of their own value judgments so that they do not unwittingly influence these young clients with their biases, whether they are conscious or unconscious.

During this developmental stage, many children have difficulty adopting the role of others. Unlike pretending, the ability to adopt, describe, or explain someone else's role, perspective, or intent requires that the actor utilize a new and different point of view. Young children are not able to do this successfully. Clinically, this may have a significant impact on treatment of communication disorders such as severe hearing loss, disfluency, or dysphonia. Psychotherapists indicate that this is the time that children develop defense mechanisms, such as regression, repression, sublimation, projection, and reaction formation. These habits may carry over to adolescence and last throughout life.

In many households, parents or other caregivers do not understand the child's natural and normal limitations in making choices. In such households, blame and guilt become risks to normal development of the child's psycho-social adaptive self. Involved in this critical determiner of behaviors are the children's personality traits, such as impulsiveness or reflectiveness, as well as temperament. The combination of personality traits with the inability to justify decisions or behaviors can produce unhappy and even traumatic outcomes for children, outcomes that are unimagined by caregivers. Yet those effects can modify children's perceptions of themselves, their environment, and people around them for years to come. The more we learn about child development, the more critical it becomes to train and counsel current and potential parents as to abilities and limits of maturing children. In that way, it may be possible to prevent or modify negative family interactions before they scar the child deeply.

Environment. These children spend many waking hours in formal school settings. The physical space, its furnishings, the people, and the activities carried out there have a profound impact on the child's development in all areas. Schools vary according to factors such as geographic regions, tax structures, and whether the management or administration is public or private, or secular or religious. However, children's individual school experiences vary most with the ability of the particular teachers they happen to get.

Other factors that contribute to the learning environment of children from 6 to 10 years of age are class sizes, availability of specialists for teaching or tutoring in certain disciplines, equipment such as science laboratories and computers, libraries, and maintaining control and quiet in the classroom. Public schools provide more specialized services than most private schools, but the latter usually claim the benefits of lower pupil-to-teacher ratios. The choice of the type of school is usually left up to the parents. Within the school, the placement of students is typically determined by test results and class performance. Bilingual and disadvantaged or impoverished language are two educational categories for children whose home and school environments differ to at least a noticeable degree.

Most children singled out for special placement long remember the perceived differences between themselves and their classmates. Interviews with adults who have sustained childhood communication disorders into their post-adolescent years often describe the experience of having to leave their classrooms for special services as negative. Those assigned to "handicapped" classrooms also remember that "different" was not a good thing to be. Schools that view special services programs as an interference with the traditional or standard curriculum may have misplaced loyalties. Students who do not fit the traditional system comprise too large a segment of the population to allow their needs to be perceived as disruptive to the well-run organization. Of course, regardless of the school setting, each student fares according to the individual professionals and peers encountered in the educational setting.

Clinicians who treat elementary school children for communicative disorders are responsible for addressing their self-perception and self-concept needs. This requires interaction between the clinician and other school personnel to guarantee mutual support for each child. The clinician is a dramatic part of each client's school environment and can exert a tremendous influence on the positive shaping of the person with the communication disorder. Clinicians in schools, more than in any other setting, must practice counseling and helping skills with astute insight into the individual needs of clients and their families, classmates, and teachers.

Lastly, there is no guarantee that primary grades in elementary schools are ideal environments or that children there are free from physical and psychological abuse. Currently no means are available to assure that school or neighborhood environments remain free of illegal drugs or the people who entice young children to become involved with them. Likewise, there is no way to guarantee that the interactive manner and style of teachers and clinicians are sufficiently disciplined and sophisticated to meet the needs of every child who comes under their influence. Furthermore, there is no way to understand fully what kind of family situation the child experiences at home.

The children of today become the adults of tomorrow, and they take with them the attitudes, feelings, defense mechanisms, beliefs, hopes, and desires they acquire during these formative years. It is only reasonable that adults who deal with young children address the whole child in ways which are meaningful to that child.

❦ ❦ ❦

COUNSELING CONSIDERATIONS

Pierre is 8 years old. He has cerebral palsy, which affects his arms, legs, trunk, neck, and oro-pharyngeal complex. The school psychologist has reported finding an IQ of 132 when he tested Pierre last month. Currently, the child is learning to use a talking computer for expressive communication. He activates the computer by pressing keys with his left index finger or moving the mouse with his left hand. Pierre has had 5 weeks of therapy at your clinic for his communication disorders. During that time, your observation of his behavior has led to the recommendation for current complete vision and audiological evaluations. Those assessments are now completed. Results of those tests reveal normal vision and a moderate bilateral mixed hearing loss. Your job is to share the diagnostic information with Pierre and his parents and make appropriate recommendations.

1. Research the recommendations likely to be made for this child in all areas of communication disorders.
2. Research the application of any equipment that you may want to introduce to the family.
3. What counseling considerations should you include in the parent interview?
4. What counseling considerations should you use when you inform Pierre of the diagnostic findings?

2.2 Pre-pubescence—10 to 13 Years

This age group demonstrates broad variability in all aspects of development. Adaptability to genetically determined changes in their own bodies often establishes a pattern of social interaction that continues into teenage years. Often new and unexpected experiences in pre-pubescent years introduce conflict with which the child is unprepared to cope.

Biology. During this pre-pubescent period, growth and increase of body mass are noted in boys and girls. Black children of both genders tend to grow faster and be larger than white children. Girls tend to outgrow boys. However, there is no regularity in growth among children, each proceeds at an individual rate. During these years, tonsils shrink and faces elongate through skeletal growth. By age 13, some will be a whole head taller than their peers due to long-bone growth. Some boys and many girls will have fully developed secondary sex organs and wear adult styles of clothing. Differences in body size and contour can create feelings of self-consciousness and embarrassment. Reactions of pre-pubescent children to their own changing bodies depend largely on their interaction with family at home and peers at school.

As with body shape, facial configuration and complexion and hair texture and style become important. Changes in body chemistry in the endocrine glands cause differences in skin texture, body hair growth, and glandular secretions. Proper hygiene and knowledgeable care of these changes are needed to prevent unpleasant body odor and skin eruptions, and to treat acne, the scourge at this age and for years to come.

Fine motor coordination tends to improve throughout these years. Penmanship is one evidence of the student's dexterity. While schools place less emphasis on penmanship than in previous generations, students still tend to admire mannerisms such as writing style, especially in signatures and other identifying marks. Creative hobbies such as model building, sewing or knitting, and playing musical instruments or video games also involve well-coordinated fine motor control.

Tests of strength and endurance among groups of peers stimulate interest in team sports and group games. In any group, some will excel in athletic skills beyond the ability of others. This climate of competition and mutual support often creates best friends and greatly treasured life-long memories.

Permanent dentition continues to erupt. The cuspids or canines, first and second premolars or bicuspids, and second molars appear about this time. While only the cuspids are visible during speech and laughter, the 10- to 12-year-olds often think they have *funny-looking* teeth or may be teased about "growing fangs." Orthodontia is fairly routine in middle- and upper-class America, although this practice is not prevalent in many other countries nor in other socio-economic classes.

The 10-year-old frequently needs reminders to bathe and is usually not at all careful about hygiene. By 12 years of age, there may be an improvement in maintaining cleanliness, and showers are generally preferred, sometimes even several times a day.

Cognition. The percentages of students at this age found to be average and above average in cognitive skills are similar to those at the elementary school level. However, primarily due to lack of satisfaction with school, the drop-out rate is very high, even in middle school or junior high school. This societal problem has been recognized, but remains unresolved. The introduction or increase of peer and social pressures on children at this age can distract from future rewards of high academic achievement. Capable students often produce poor work or incomplete assignments, thereby deriving pleasure and peer recognition from getting away with less than what adults expect from them. Because of peer relationships, children whose cognitive abilities exceed those of their classmates often hesitate to show their mental prowess. Instead, they try to gain approval from the group, have fun, and perhaps expect to learn later.

The requirements for independent and abstract thinking that begin at about the third grade level are difficult for many students to meet. Many previously unsuspected language-learning disabilities are noted at this grade level. Quite often, girls are not encouraged to excel in the study of mathematics or science. Young boys may not be expected to excel in spelling or reading, but they are often expected to do well in science and math. Reality may have little to do with the match of gender to academic abilities; however, such social and cultural pressures are present and exert influences. Such attitudes may be found at home as well as at school. Expectations of student performance at this young age are often reflected later in the selection of studies in college and in career or job employment.

In spite of the lack of rewards and incentives for cognitive achievements among this age group, pre-adolescents are below the legal age of 16 to withdraw from formal schooling, except for some who are taught at home by their parents. Performance in athletics often becomes a major attraction for students remaining in school.

Psycho-social Adaptation. As pre-pubescent boys and girls increasingly see themselves growing into adulthood, identity with a parent or parent-figure of the same sex leads them to assert their independence. They want to make important decisions about their own affairs, friends, curfew, recreation, socialization, and even education. They develop idols among entertainers or other public and glamorous figures, and often adopt mannerisms of those individuals as presented through various media, especially television. Daydreams about media stars and heroes may occupy a considerable amount of time, especially for children who are somewhat inactive.

In this age range, boys and girls begin to explore what their real abilities are. Children with a musical talent or an ability with written or spoken language may begin to see that ability as a strength, different from that of peers. The same is true with an absence of ability or a disability, whether real or merely labeled as such. As with younger children, these sensitive 10- to 13-year-olds tend to live up or down to the expectations of those around them. If parents and teachers become excessively concerned with discipline, the mental and creative abilities of this energetic group may go untapped throughout the middle school years.

The sexual revolution that began in the 1970s has reached into the 10- to 12-year age group. Exploration of and experimentation with sex, for many a cultural taboo, has long been recognized as an area of informational awareness, even in younger children. However, impregnation of 12- and 13-year-old girls by boys their age or slightly older is not uncommon.

National television newscast titles such as "Children Having Children" or "Children Raising Children" are typical.

Perhaps the most trying puzzle for the pre-adolescent child is the experience of being on the threshold of growing up. Anticipation of becoming a "big" person with recognized power to be independent is in the realm of fantasy, and is hard to await patiently. This anticipation is free of the understanding of constraints imposed by accompanying responsibilities. Impatience may lead to outbursts of anger and frustration at apparent unfairness and injustice by authorities. Wisdom and understanding are essential for the clinician to help guide girls and boys through this difficult and scary age.

Environment. While retaining many of their previous possessions, habits, and practices, pre-adolescent children enter the world of talking, talking, talking. Conversations with best friends or new acquaintances tend to dominate their time. For many, conversation replaces most of the physical activity they had formerly exhibited. Telephones are very useful and quite busy. Computers with connecting telephone modules enhance the intrigue of communication, as do walkie-talkies and ham radios. Conversation with parents may decrease, but not necessarily. The amount of communication at home seems reduced only in comparison with that which goes on with non-family friends.

Quiet, contemplative children may need to be monitored during this period to assure that their quietness is not a defensive device for shielding a sense of insecurity and inadequacy from others. Children who are quiet but happy have positive self-esteem. Children who are quiet but alone and sad need help to get through the period of massive chemical upheaval in their bodies and torturous times of peer pressures.

Much of verbal communication may be saturated with slang that is popular with a particular group or adopted from a motion picture or television program. Slang terms and their use, like other fads, change often. Less time is spent with family members, and more time and loyalty are given to peers. Friends and best friends share play, ideas, overnight stays, and secrets. Pre-adolescents create a large segment of their environment, which extends to reality, fantasy, and imagination.

❦ ❦ ❦

COUNSELING CONSIDERATIONS

Lori Jo Cooper is a 12-1/2-year-old girl, the oldest of three siblings. Her father and stepmother are in your office and are very concerned about her poor performance in school. Lori Jo is not present. The father is a medical doctor, a radiologist; Lori Jo's natural mother is executive director of a regional television network; Mrs. Cooper, the stepmother of two years, is a housewife and homemaker. The natural parents share legal custody of Lori Jo. School records show good quality work in the first and second grades. Since then, Lori Jo's grades have continued to fall in spelling, reading, and social studies. Math grades have been average, but they are lower now than at this time last year. Three teachers have indicated to the parents that they suspect that Lori Jo may have a learning disability. Because of their interest in the child, the teachers have referred the parents to you for testing, observation, and recommendations concerning Lori Jo's school performance. Dr. Cooper vigorously disagrees with the teachers. Mrs. Cooper sits quietly, not expressing her thoughts on Lori Jo's ability.

1. What influences can be inferred to be active in Lori Jo's development?
2. What feelings do you detect in the father?
3. What feelings do you detect in the stepmother?
4. Discuss the precautions you must take to prevent complicating Lori Jo's problem with the parents' problems.
5. What counseling skills can you use with the father?
6. What attitudes and behaviors are desirable in the father and stepmother? What are some of the impediments to achieving these quickly?
7. How do you feel toward the current parents?
8. How do you react to the expressed concerns and disbeliefs?

3.1 Early Teenage Years—13 to 16 Years

Middle school and entry into secondary school move the teenager into the near-adult world. While external controls are still powerful influences in everyday life, the normally developing young teen exercises increasing internal responsibilities for regulating events and reactions to events in daily life. Counseling activities are directed primarily toward the teenager, with appropriate information and recommendations provided to parents or guardians and involved professionals.

Biology. Rapid physical change in height and body contour are observed in this age of transition. Endocrine physiology, which began maturing between 10 and 12 years of age, now reaches its full function. Unexpected and startling modifications of physiological response patterns may require medical or counseling supervision for some adolescents and for those with whom they live.

Height and weight changes are particularly notable. Boys of 13 average 60 to 68 inches in height; by 16, they average 64 to 72 inches. This indicates a change of as much as a foot in growth within 3 years. Girls grow rapidly but not so extensively. At 13, girls average 60 to 66 inches and by 16, they average 60 to 68 inches. In fact, many girls have reached their mature height prior to entering their teenage years.

Weight changes accompany the change in height. The average for both boys and girls as they enter their teens is around 110 pounds. By age 16, boys average 150 pounds and girls average 134 pounds. Thus, on average, boys will grow an additional foot of height and gain 40 pounds in weight, while girls will grow some 8 inches taller and gain 25 pounds. Needless to say, the range of possible combinations of height and weight is enormous. Many will fret about being too skinny or too chubby, too tall or too short, and many other seemingly uncontrollable body configurations. Good nutrition is essential during these rapid growth years, but management of proper diet is often difficult. Grabbing snacks, eating fast food, and skipping meals so as not to miss exciting activities of the peer group are all too common. Eating disorders of a psycho-emotional origin may appear.

By this age, specific athletic abilities are surfacing. The drive to excel in physical sports is recognized among boys, and expertise in gymnastics for females reaches its peak. Parent and community support tend to add to the value of athletic proficiency, as evidenced from intramural sports competitions and seasonal tournament play in secondary schools. Likewise, body shape is a critical factor in determining whether the teenager can expect to continue in chosen activities such as ballet, football, or basketball.

Cognition. Members of this age group are approaching a dramatic moment when they will gain both the right and the responsibility to make a decision that may change their lives. Upon reaching the 16th birthday, individual students have the legal right to choose to remain in school or to withdraw. A variety of school settings and curricula are chosen by teenagers who have displayed special talents as in arts or mechanical and physical skills. While students are encouraged to take college preparatory liberal arts courses in secondary schools, such a program does not suit the makeup of all enrollees.

During these early teenage years, differentiation by scholastic ability becomes apparent; some master the academic program, some are minimally successful, and some fail in that setting. Unfortunately, social structure in the U.S. tends to denigrate all who do not fit the system. Even with the advent of special classes and recognition of special needs for special students, little has been done to create a system of educational tracks that can accommodate the life planning needs of the middle school and early secondary school student. With multiple alternatives available, the liberal arts curriculum is still considered the preferred track. Those who enroll in other curricula are considered to be following a second-choice program. An alternative that has gained considerable respect is participation, and even stardom, in athletics. However, these slots are limited in number and are generally dominated by males.

In general, the majority of concerned parents are conscious of grades on school work and standardized test performance, with an eye toward the future potential of their children. Parents may know little of the day-to-day discipline exercised by their sons and daughters. They tend to use teachers' judgments of their children for comparison with impressions of children of friends and acquaintances. It is also the case that many of these not-quite-adults put unwarranted pressures on themselves to demonstrate their worth and potential. Those who achieve some version of success tend to follow the mainstream. Those who perceive themselves as performing below expectations experience frustration and disappointment.

In homes where parental influence is ineffective or nonexistent, teenagers muddle their way through these years of internal and external upheaval. Intelligent, talented, and ordinary children who have developed a special yet undefined determination are often seen to break out of social class patterns of even the worst ghettos. Some are able to realize their potential and to achieve enviable goals. Others tend to join groups and imitate available role models. Teenagers from poverty-level communities are most frequently members of minority groups. Their families may be migrant workers or unskilled refugees from war-torn countries. Many parents have little schooling and do not have sufficient command of English to secure a job. Illiteracy in any language is a common problem. The uneducated are often exploited by employers who take advantage of the poverty and ignorance found in such strong young bodies.

During these very important decision-making years, previously undiagnosed learning problems such as language-learning disorders and dyslexia may overwhelm the student. In earlier years, the child's compensatory coping strategies may have covered up the disability. The sophistication of assessment batteries and the skill levels of examiners are not always sufficient to identify those problems in the preschool or elementary school child. It is both hurtful and disappointing for the teenager and the family to find such a disorder at this late stage. Often, they discover there are no satisfactory available community resources to address this newly found but long-standing problem.

Psycho-social Adaptation.   Much of the interest in socialization continues as it has progressed prior to this age. Differences in focuses of energy are related to combinations of physical growth, skill, and peer regard, which lead to recognition and inclusion in groups. Belonging is highly desired by young teens and has been described in developmental and social psychology.

Teenagers expand their relationship base by joining friends to form groups, teams, and clubs. While the wish to affiliate with others exists from birth, belonging becomes a powerful drive for identity during adolescence. Affiliation with others reduces fear and uncertainty and increases the ability to take risks and to test one's limits. Erikson (1963) referred to the conflict that can grow out of risk-taking versus conformity as the crisis of this stage of development. Social psychologists have identified six important resources provided by social relationships.

1. Attachment (security and comfort)
2. Social integration (shared interests and points of view)
3. Reassurance of worth (affirmation of self-esteem)
4. Sense of reliable alliance (trust and support)
5. Obtaining of guidance (counseling, positive leadership)
6. Opportunity to nurture others (feeling of being needed)

Relationships of trust, understanding and testing of others grow from successful affiliation. Each experience with successful affiliation forms a building block on which to establish the next relationship. As these affiliations increase in number, some will become closer relationships than others. Close, intimate interpersonal relationships of sensitivity, understanding, and interdependence begin to develop during these early teenage years. Teenagers who are unable to form such close relationships may experience loneliness and alienation as possible alternatives. Loneliness results from a gap between one's actual social role and desired social role. Alienation is the result of a deliberate estrangement from society, although it may be instigated by subconscious causes.

Environment. Other changes in the individual greatly influence the environment. Physical size alone dictates whether the space and its furnishings enhance or impede work and play of the teenager. For most teenagers, school and home are the dominant environments. Some teenagers also have part-time employment of necessity or for spending money. Some visit relatives or travel to foreign countries. Many go to specialized summer programs that are organized around an interest, talent, sport, or hobby and provide intensive learning experiences or simply an opportunity to get away from home.

Involvement with new acquaintances leads to expression of independence and self sufficiency. Although young teens continue to live at home, those homes and families tend to be mobile. New communities, neighbors, and peers comprise changing environments. With flux manifest in many aspects of the life of the rapidly changing child, it may be expected that conflict will arise. Of course, as with all traits and behaviors, a teen's individuality influences the management style used to cope with the flux:

1. Mature management at home/away from home;
2. Conflict at home/mature management away from home;
3. Conflict at home/conflict away from home; or
4. Mature management at home/conflict away from home.

Personal traits such as intelligence, temperament, and maturity affect the ways teenagers cope with simultaneous social pressures to conform and be an individual.

Of course, discussion of this period would be incomplete without mentioning the long-awaited acquisition of a driver's license at age 16 in most states. This is a particularly motivating force in pre-teens and teenagers. Ability to drive and access to the use of a motor vehicle are essential to carrying out the individuation struggle where public transportation is inadequate or unavailable. The freedom and independence allowed by driving oneself are unequaled. The responsibility concurrent with that freedom and independence is rarely credited with the overwhelming nature it actually commands. Recently, state legislatures have examined the relationship between teenage driving and high school dropout rates. One outcome of that research is that some states have instituted laws that revoke licenses of school dropouts. That is, to maintain a valid driving license, the teenage driver must be able to present proof of school enrollment or completion.

❧ ❧ ❧

COUNSELING CONSIDERATIONS

Washington "Bo" Johnson is 15 years old. He has been in therapy for fluency for 6 years. He says that therapy doesn't help his speech, but it has helped get him out of school and is an excuse for not belonging to clubs. However, he runs for the school's cross country team and hopes to make the high school varsity squad before graduating. He will get his learner's permit for driving next week. He says that maybe his mother will let him drive her car when he gets a license.

1. How do you feel about the apparent attitude of this student?
2. What do you think he feels and thinks about you and your profession?
3. What complicating and even contradictory factors are apparent in the client's remarks about himself?
4. What counseling skills will you utilize to involve this client in productive therapy?
5. Are there other people you would need to involve in team treatment of this client's communication disorder? If so, identify them and suggest the role each would play in influencing the behavior and attitude of this client.

3.2 Late Teenage Years—16 to 20 Years

During this stage, development differs dramatically in each individual. During this brief period, some boys and girls remain much as they were earlier. Others continue the developmental pattern that began toward the end of their early teen years. Still others progress rapidly to and through their young adult stage of maturity.

Biology.   Continued growth, usually in spurts, yields additional height and mass, especially in males. Voice changes accompany hormone activities, laryngeal enlargement, and increased protrusion of the Adam's apple. Forward thrust of mandibular growth further elongates the features and enlarges the face. Permanent dentition has fully erupted except for the wisdom teeth, which some individuals never produce. Strength of skeletal muscle is approaching its peak, and total body coordination is at or near its maximum efficiency. Late teenagers are fully able to care for themselves and their bodies and possessions. They are ready to be independent.

Psychiatrists have identified biological traits or needs in some early and late teens who utilize high levels of excitement to achieve physiological satisfaction. In a sense, these individuals get a physiological "high" from sustained thrills and danger. These tend to be disruptive, anti-social, sometimes violent and criminal young men and women. Biological strength and body size of the late teens contribute to success in sustaining antisocial behavior through aggressive habits and satisfaction with outcomes of destructive behavior.

Other late teens are honing their skills, learning to control emotionality and compete in higher education, athletics, performance arts, and the business world. High levels of energy and reasonable schedules of rest, diet, and exercise are a way of life.

Cognition.   Both boys and girls anticipate their 16th birthdays for the reason of getting a driver's license. To achieve this tremendous step in responsibility, the teenager must learn to manage an expensive machine, recognize the rules of the highway, obey laws pertaining to management of a motor vehicle, and contribute to the mainstream of society by acting courteously to other drivers. To do all that is required, the driver must have a vehicle to drive. Often this is the family car or truck, or sometimes a parent-owned motorcycle or motorbike.

Cognitive activities in late teenage years are noted in the way individuals occupy themselves and organize current endeavors and future expectations. The choices are many. They range from secondary and post-secondary education and professional training, vocational training, and skilled and unskilled labor, to loafing, delinquency, and crime. The choices that include study and training demand intellectual ability, approval by the system, patience, endurance, and often strenuous mental effort. Teens who have left secondary school without graduating or who graduate but demonstrate no special ability may find job placement in unskilled work starting at a minimum wage rate. Employment of this type sometimes does little to motivate workers to better themselves socio-culturally or economically. Teenagers who turn all their natural energy to loafing generally live at the monetary and emotional expense of family or friends, and may be much loved, but they are also considered atypical. Those who become involved in illegal activities such as selling drugs often do so for evidence of their importance and for economic gain. What individuals do with what they know reflects cognitive function within the context of the world in which they see themselves.

Psychological testing has been designed to assess intellectual maturation. The competency of an individual to learn, remember, analyze, synthesize, infer and perform some 120 other abilities identified as intelligence (Guilford, 1959) is believed to reach its peak during this stage of development. Increases in vocabulary as well as experience with complex decision-making continues throughout life. In that sense, cognitive function increases, too. On the other hand, during these late teenage years previously undiscovered language learning disabilities may exceed the compensatory coping skills of an otherwise very competent mind, and disrupt the educational plan of the individual or hope of the family. These late discoveries do not present an impossible situation, but remediation and moving forward with educational plans require rigor that is generally a new experience for both the teen and the family.

Not all students in public or private college preparatory schools fit the learning systems that have been established for their education and training. For students who excel in those settings, continued education is almost inevitable. Those who do not comply with the programmatic system can find alternatives or special schools for intellectual success, but they are scarce and expensive. Failure or less-than-required performance by any student imposes a negative valuation on self-perception (Tomblin & Liljegreen, 1985). Emotional distress often follows and that, in turn, reduces the efficacy of cognitive function.

Psycho-social Adaptation.   The possible variety of behavior based on this determiner is the broadest of all at this age level. Self-perception, self-regard, beliefs, and values are matched against peer pressures of belonging, recognition, and reward. Environmental influences are powerful. The child who has grown up in a traditional family must establish independence without disrupting strong emotional ties at home. The many teens who have had a less-than-ideal childhood have different needs and expectations at this stage. They must make choices and decisions that past generations did not face until much later in life. Mobility introduces new friends; new adventures are to be explored; curiosity and daring emphasize the need to take risks; ease of access to drugs and alcohol tempt members of the crowd; dreams unrealized may be discarded and not replaced, or forgotten.

Many of the conflicts experienced mildly in earlier years seem to arise more often and more intensely. For example, there are differences in opportunity depending upon gender. Some areas of study, such as engineering, medicine, law, and science, are dominated primarily by males; other areas, such as nursing, teaching, and office management, are dominated primarily by females. Community and civic roles available to young adults vary with the region of the country, but rarely is the 16- to 19-year-old found in a position of authority or responsibility. Affordable housing is more and more scarce for low-income employees; a good job with a living wage may depend as much on who the family knows as on the ability of the teen; and employment certainly relates to the teen's area of residence and mobility. For many, it seems that having moved from the realm of childhood, the older teenager is in another sort of suspension. Both wisdom and foolishness are practiced in making liaisons and commitments, and it is difficult to maintain firmly one's values and principles as they are tested.

Struggle for individuation may lead to affiliation with groups who utilize modern escape methods of chemical and sexual extravagance. Such involvements distort the normal physiological state of the body and have long-lasting effects on normalization of the homeostatic condition. Disruption of ideals, whether realistic or unrealistic, of the teenager has resulted in large numbers of teen suicides. While suicidal tendencies are considered a psychological problem, certainly suicidal attempts are detrimental to the body and are concerns that need psychiatric and counseling intervention.

Many 16- to 19-year-olds become parents themselves and renew the cycle of sharing the world as they know it with the next generation. Some of these form family constellations; others, primarily females, become single parents. Many teenage marriages, which may or may not produce children, end in divorce. Results of these socially accepted variances from the traditional family or home structure may leave the single mother or divorced ex-wife and children in a poverty-level economic position. These women and children depend on public welfare or the charity of their families or others to survive. This is especially true of teenagers who have dropped out of school due to unplanned pregnancies. They have not acquired marketable skills or high school diplomas to attest to their ability to learn.

Environment. External and internal environmental factors influence feelings, attitudes, decisions, and behavior. Houses, rooms, chairs, and other objects comprise the stimulation to which the senses respond. Inner workings of contentment/anger, happiness/dejection, ambition/despair, hope/hopelessness, elation/depression are a more immediate environmental concern. Although modern advantages like mobility and electronic media expand the individual's knowable world, the same advantages can occupy time and energy, and may impose limits or distractions from the inner resolve necessary to take risks for achievement of dreams. More of this turmoil is discussed in relation to young adulthood.

❦ ❦ ❦

COUNSELING CONSIDERATIONS

Jonathan Leroy Barker III is 17 years old. He is 5 feet 3 inches tall and weighs 107 pounds. He is very blond, fair-complexioned, and wears glasses and orthodontic appliances or braces. Jonathan asked his mother, and she agreed that he could see you because he is being teased at school about his pitch breaks that occur whenever he speaks. During your first interview session, he indicates that he has grown a couple of inches since his last birthday, but not nearly enough, and during that time the voice squeakiness started. To him, the squeak sounds awful and he knows that his face turns red when it happens.

Jonathan's father and brother are dark-complexioned and have black hair. They are athletic and large in stature. Jonathan looks like his maternal grandfather, a small, slender man, who reads a great deal. Jonathan wants to quit "squeaking and squawking" every time he opens his mouth. He wants to be big and strong and rid of glasses and braces.

1. What more do you need to know about Jonathan to interact with him appropriately?
2. What feelings has the client expressed verbally? nonverbally?
3. What inferences can you make from the information that has been provided?
4. Compose a script of the dialogue between you and Jonathan.
5. Review your script with the class.
6. Review your script with an experienced clinician.
7. Report the differences of the shared reviews in 6 and 7.

4.1 Young Adulthood—20 to 35 Years

Treatment of communication disorders in this age group generally involves clients who realize the presence of a handicapping condition. Because clients themselves are usually seeking treatment of a speech, language, or hearing problem, they recognize a need for help beyond what they can provide for themselves. To some, asking for help is admission of self-insufficiency (Allen, 1975; Fisher & Nadler, 1974, 1976; Leavitt, 1951). The clinician must be aware of the client's feelings and attitudes toward the disorder, its treatment, and prognosis. Protocols for diagnosis of the disorder and the sequence of habilitative treatments must be tempered with strategies for the client to use as coping skills. The client must cope with feelings and attitudes toward the self, the disorder, and perceived reactions of others, and with the arduous work required to remediate or manage the disorder.

The current most commonly diagnosed communication disorders in young adults are related to closed head injuries. Disorders include loss of language, totally or in part, from brain damage sustained in motor vehicle accidents or from gunshot wounds.

Biology.   Young adults typically demonstrate high energy levels and continue the high hormone output that was obvious in late teenage years. The cultural ideal of having a strong, coordinated body is popular, as evidenced by the concentration of news media reports on sports, body building, and athletics. Many of this age group continually undergo new stress patterns in organizing their lives within industrial and corporate society. Physiological reaction to stress is a major etiological factor for destructive changes in the human body. Those who succeed in work, interpersonal relationships, and recreational activities during this transitional period usually reflect intact intrapersonal management. The ability to cope with expected and unexpected pressures encountered in the many settings that comprise the young adult's environment draws heavily on psycho-social adaptive traits and habits.

The able, pliable young adult body has reached its maximum ability to function as an integrated unit. The responsibility to maintain the regimen of exercise, nutrition, and immunological care formerly built into recreational activities, home, and school now lies with the individual (Frost, 1947). Immersion in work, post-graduate school, or professional training often detracts from attention to biological well-being. Neglect of biological homeostasis is also influenced by the limited income and increased expenses of most young workers and students.

In fact, in individuals whose daily lives are stressful in extraordinary ways, biological needs are often the first to be neglected. This applies especially to those who recognize a personal deficit such as a communication disorder for the first time. Young adults trying to prove their self-sufficiency, to make it on their own, may reduce their expenditures for food as the most readily visible means to increase other budgets.

Environmental bombardment may lead to attentional overload (Kort, Ypma, & Toppen, 1975). The need to escape stress of daily living or to acquire extra money quickly can introduce the modern young adult to a chemical dependency problem or even to selling illicit substances for ready cash. Recreational drugs and widespread alcohol abuse are not uncommon in all social classes among young and mature adults. Sexually transmitted diseases create havoc with the bodies of young men and women pursuing their identities through affiliation with social partners or groups that accommodate their sensual desires. Also, during the 1970s and 1980s young adult women began to utilize their legal right to abortions to help manage their lives. These interruptions of the natural endocrinological changes of pregnancy and any psychological distress that accompanies the unplanned pregnancy and abortion have dramatic effects on the female body. Another by-product of the sexual revolution is an increase in pregnancies in which the mother is addicted to drugs or alcohol. Long-lasting neurobiological problems are transmitted to the baby in utero.

Biological damage to the young adult may be caused by disease or injury. Some congenital diseases do not begin to show symptoms until adulthood, for example, amyotrophic lateral sclerosis (ALS). Other body changes are caused by infectious agents contacted in daily routines. The effects of diseases from the common cold to cancer are spread across all possible degrees of tissue and organ damage. Typically, the diseases and traumas that involve neurological or neuromotor deficits or surgical removal of damaged tissue comprise the etiologies of conditions seen by the communication disorders professionals. These clients may be seen in hospitals, nursing homes, or in rehabilitation centers. Interdisciplinary teams are required to manage the overall care program for these patients.

Cognition.   The range of cognitive ability found among normally developing young adults is a continuation of what was present in earlier years. In fact, activity in daily life among this age group is tied closely to cognitive abilities and the settings into which those abilities thrust the possessor (Williams, 1958). The ability to apply cognitive skills depends on opportunities of the young adults to find reasonable job placement, occupational fit, and an adequate social niche. Although many in this age group continue in formal training programs, the majority have entered the work force and are applying their cognitive abilities to jobs, families, recreation, social group or work group activities, and church or religious affiliation groups.

Young adults apply cognitive abilities to the management of everyday life. They confront the immediate need to adjust their dreams and ambitions in the "cold light of reality." They may need to revise their goals, pursue new or alternate endeavors, and prepare to meet unanticipated challenges. As many experience the beginning of this maturational struggle, they soon settle for less than what was indicated as their potential by earlier assessments. By now, the need for security and belonging may override the desire for adventure, the thrill of risk-taking, and the pride of individuality.

Complexity of industry, its machines and devices as well as the dominance of managerial control, appears to reduce the inventiveness of ordinary people (Langer, 1978). Research controls, employer's patent rights, and time and energy demands of the job are more than sufficient to restrict opportunities for creative individuals to construct innovative gadgets. Individuals who succeed in significant independent inventiveness must be clever and quick enough to protect themselves and their products legally and financially. Such culturally indigenous stresses and conflicts are restrictive to individuality and creative inventiveness.

Away from school, and no longer legal minors, those between 20 and 35 years of age must make their own opportunities to enhance their intellectual functioning. One example of the constraints on talented young adults is the pursuit of a career in the creative arts, especially considering the lack of social and cultural support. Throughout history, many societies have realized the vital role of all forms of art in creating and sustaining civilization. While there are increasing numbers of private foundations and some public funds, artists must produce work that is recognized, that is, favored by influential sources, before their ability is rewarded with resources and support. In fact, the custom has long been that the artist's work increases in value posthumously. The artistic concept, performance, production, and the product itself require not only talent, skill, and creativity, but also sufficient financial and environmental security to allow artists to nurture their abilities. All too often poverty or near poverty continues to be the milieu of talented young adults. Some tenaciously survive to continue their art form. Others abandon their talents and enter the more economically substantive work world.

Psycho-social Adaptation.   During this stage, the young adults have to make many adjustments (Piaget, 1972). Reality replaces fantasies as circumstances dictate. Environmental determiners greatly affect and interact with psycho-social adaptive abilities. Dreams and expectations from childhood may take on a humorous tone as they become particularly impossible (Shaw & Skolnick, 1973). Dreams that are more within reach but not achievable may arouse disappointment or even bitterness at apparent failure. Such disappointments force a reassessment of self-worth and adjustments in self-perceptions that must be fit into the many other aspects of hectic young adult life (Festinger, 1957). Some individuals find compensatory actions or alternate achievements that satisfactorily replace disappointments and diminish the injury to self-esteem. In individuals with little or no flexibility to accept alternatives to long-held expectations, frustration and anger are fairly certain to appear.

Even in flexible individuals, management of change is recognized as the most difficult of human endeavors. Some types of change become easier as security increases toward the later years of young adulthood. Frequently, the need for change in one or many aspects of life can be overwhelming or denied. Yet, by and large, the adventure of finding one's niche and surviving in a competitive society is an integral part of the western world's work ethic. Even individuals who are disappointed in themselves and their lot tend to survive. In later life, many people spin tales about the dreams and hopes of youth that were and were not realized, and how chance intervened to shape careers, affiliations, and liaisons.

Within this psycho-social determiner of behavior, a major influence that often goes unaddressed is the set of values held by the individual young adult. Values acquired throughout childhood and adolescence affect each act and decision, even in those unaware of their influence. Decision-making may test and try the integrity, beliefs, and ethics of the decider. Flexibility and tolerance are essential for survival in social contexts, but the ethical individual must guard against the use of those traits as excuses. When coupled with the firm commitment to responsibility, as in "The buck stops here," tolerance of circumstances and behaviors that one cannot change is the only sensible recourse. Success in survival can be described as the ability to change what must be changed, to leave alone what cannot be changed, and the wisdom to know the difference.

In the modern industrialized world, young adults approaching mature adulthood are expected to be settled into an occupation, content in doing that task, and anticipating continuing success. Labor unions have improved the lives of many working-class Americans, while unskilled laborers often continue to struggle for daily survival. Many employed women can take temporary leaves of absence to have and/or raise children; others use maternity leave to regain post-delivery strength and settle the new infant into nursery care. In some social groups, upward mobility is a part of the dream of lower and middle socioeconomic classes. That mobility is intimately linked to annual income and real holdings, and success is measured primarily by material wealth. In other social groups, success is measured by position, title, respect, authority, and other evidence less tangible than material possessions. In still other communities, success is measured in terms of power and control over objects, actions, and people. The popular term for this sort of power is *influence*.

During the young adult years, ambition and reality often compete or knock heads, so to speak. Having ability is essential to achieve any ambition; having the right connections is often essential, too. An old axiom that continues to survive says, "It is who you know as well as what you know that counts." Certainly a correct or workable fit of all elements leads inevitably to success. A mismatch necessarily modifies the outcome in a negative direction.

Environment. Early in the 1990s arenas of war or hotspots of aggression and armed conflict found around the world urged reasonable governments to struggle toward negotiated non-conflict settlements of differences and to reduce armament. The successful Desert Storm campaign and internal turmoil in the Soviet Union caused conflict among third world countries to seem remote. Televised incidents of ongoing conflict, oppression, and terrorism among citizens in Africa, Asia, Central and South America, Ireland, or the Middle East shock but do not greatly alter the daily life of most young adults. The hope for world order through the United Nations seems more nearly possible than for many decades past, and the effect is increased access to personal options without continual threats of a war which would involve most of the world.

Although television and radio continually remind international audiences of inequities and brutalities all over the globe, young adults in the free world seem to perceive themselves to be at a distance from imminent danger.

Immediate environments of young adults depend largely on the community in which they are involved for work, study, or play. Most energies are directed toward achieving success. Popular involvements like spas, sports, exercise programs such as aerobics and body building, weight control programs, and jogging serve dual purposes for the participants. In addition to providing biological exercise and stimulation, they function as opportunities for social contact. In such settings, participants can compare themselves with others and study many aspects of the self that could use or need modification or that exceed the group norm. Likewise, participants can observe and assess others, make acquaintances, and promote common interests.

Just as individuals are people-watchers in social settings, so are they at work, at home, in the marketplace, and elsewhere. Such observation and the resulting interactions play a large part in self-perceptions and in conscientious efforts toward career moves, especially for white males in the corporate, industrial, and military domains (Kiesler & Kiesler, 1969). Similar control of job advancement has not been traditional or assured for females or for males of minority races.

For most young adults, mobility is no longer restricted to neighborhoods and communities, but often extends to national and even international travel. Wherever they go, these young adults see social conditions that underscore their values, whether they include achievement of goals, avoidance of economic failure, or escape from social responsibilities. Home ownership, long the ideal of many and the basis of roots in a community, has given way to rentals and leases of apartments in multiple housing units which dominate much of urbanized society. As city centers deteriorate, urban populations there tend to become transient. Rural life has greatly changed, also. While some small family farms still exist as cores of home and tradition, huge tracts of land are managed for maximum production by agri-businesses. Increased numbers of displaced, homeless people of all ages and races are seen on cities' streets and roaming the highway systems.

Cost of living in any stratum of society requires acquisition of and knowledge about money. While poverty-level citizens struggle with needs for survival, directors of corporations, megacorporations, and conglomerates struggle to retain international economic stability. The economic forces which cross national and cultural boundaries are reflected in stock markets that stretch from Tokyo and Hong Kong to Geneva, London, and New York. In that way, the influence of monetary forces never ceases, for it follows the natural progression of the earth around the sun. Despite all the recognized wealth and the increased numbers of millionaires and billionaires, the numbers of poor and very poor continue to rise, both nationally and internationally. The young adult may be desperate to establish an economic security for now and the future so as to ward off the feared poverty and loneliness that are observed in daily life.

The environment into which young adults emerge is influenced by phenomena from around the world and decisions often made by people unknown to them. Survival of the individual, or the completion of the life span, is essential to maintain social structure. By itself, survival through time is not enough. Aristotle said that time is the measure of change or motion according to before and after. Change is inevitable, perhaps stressful, and often contrary to individual preferences. Without contributions from each generation to better the human condition, the only change would be social destruction. Young adults must recognize that survival serves as the conduit for responsibility to self and to the species.

❦ ❦ ❦

COUNSELING CONSIDERATIONS

Rosa Manuela Ramirez, a 23-year-old first-generation Mexican American, has completed her Bachelor of Arts degree in accounting at the University of New Mexico. She has been offered a scholarship to attend law school at Harvard University. She very much wants to accept and use the scholarship. Her dream has long been to practice law in human civil rights; however, she speaks English with a strong Spanish accent. To be successful in her desired career field, she has been advised to eliminate evidence of dialect and to habituate Standard English. Ms. Ramirez is emotionally torn by the conflict she feels between her potential for good in the legal profession and the constraints imposed upon her from the outside world, that is, that of the racial or ethnic majority. She is placed in the position of moving one more step away from her origins by removing evidence of her native language from her oral expression of language.

1. List the decisions Ms. Ramirez must make. Consider her education, career plans, academic history, family background and loyalty, and personal identity with cultural and social custom.
2. What environmental and cultural influences are tugging at Ms. Ramirez? Consider the risks of alienation that Ms. Ramirez must take.
3. What part does counseling play in the initial interview with this client?
4. Is there a need to involve others in treatment of this client?
5. How may the clinician's values influence interaction with this client?

Note: It may be helpful to read *Hunger of Memory: The Education of Richard Rodriguez,* a book listed in Appendix C of this chapter.

4.2 Mature Adulthood—35 to 50 Years

During this stage of life, presbycusis, presbyopia, slowness in learning new material, and reduced memory for details may be initially noted in some clients. However, many individuals, whose circumstances continue to demand quick responses and sharp decisions, can be expected to perform those skills through this stage and well past it (Sheehy, 1976).

Biology. By age 35, changes in cellular function are dramatic (Schneider & Rowe, 1989). It is estimated that daily loss of some 10,000 brain cells per day commences about this time. In other types of tissue, cell loss continues at the normal pace, but cell reproduction slows down. Because of change in the microscopic units, the overall effect is observed as a reduction in muscle mass and an increase in adipose tissue. During these years, many individuals seem to thrive as they realize success in their jobs or careers and satisfaction in their personal lives. Their health tends to be stable, and except for minor illnesses such as flu and colds caused by viruses, the mature adult population coasts along as intact biological specimens.

Endocrine secretory function is decreased, and the female body loses its reproductive abilities during this stage. With this chemical change, women tend to gain weight through increased adipose tissue. Distribution of fat deposits in the female body is determined by genetic code. There is a tendency for fat to accumulate in the buttocks, hips, and thighs. However, different women show individual patterns of change in body contour. Weight control may be a problem for many because they have not changed their eating habits to match the altered chemistry of their bodies. Education in these matters has become an important focus of public and family health.

Along with stresses of work, family, and social situations, biological changes tend to occur more rapidly than previously. Mature adults with children watch them grow up, and they endure the pleasures and displeasures of living with pre-pubescent and adolescent youngsters. Death of parents and maturation of children frequently leave mature adults alone. Many cannot readily adjust to the new home situation and develop feelings of no longer being needed that may initiate depression. While these feelings appear in both men and women, historically, it is the mother of the family who experiences the greater loss, known as the *empty-nest syndrome*.

Some men start to lose their scalp hair and develop a paunch because of accumulation of abdominal adipose. It is believed that this type of fat deposit increases the risk for cardiovascular disease more than fat deposited in other parts of the body.

Heart attacks are considered a major risk among both genders in this age group, and cancer is a threat to some. Reduced use of tobacco is expected to decrease the incidence of lung cancer, emphysema, and other respiratory diseases (Saxon & Etten, 1987). During this stage of life, autoimmune deficiency syndrome (AIDS) is a also a threat. Life styles of many have unknowingly or carelessly spread the human immunodeficiency virus (HIV) which invites death through subsequent failure to resist infectious disease. Associated with the disease process, the abuse of alcohol, cocaine, crack cocaine, and other addictive substances must be included among biological threats to mature adult life. Easily accessed, these substances are often used as excuses to cope with stress, but chemical abuse affects the biological system in destructive ways.

Trauma also disrupts the easy coasting of normal biological function during this stage. Automobile accidents are the major cause of broken bodies. Gunshot wounds are frequent, and tend to increase in areas where illegal drugs are known to be sold and used.

Cognition.   Except for the onset of genetic diseases of the nervous system, as in the previous stage of life, there is little dramatic change in the cognitive function of the mature adult. Increased vocabulary and experience with communication among different types of social contexts cause the mature adult to appear to be "smarter" than when younger. However, cognitive power becomes the foot soldier of wisdom. In daily life, whether at work or at leisure, the ability to deal with multiple intellectual tasks impinges on mature adults. Priorities, selective attention to details, and caution about plunging into uncharted adventures escalate appearances of cognitive functioning.

Intelligence levels of mature adults are believed to be the same or nearly the same as in their youth. Their power of intellect often seems to exceed their previous efforts because of the assortment of experiences, problems, and situations that they have resolved or endured (Butler, 1983). Kohlberg (1984) suggested that cognitive development follows a sequence: hope, will, purpose, competence, fidelity, love, care, and wisdom. Mature adults (across a 15-year span) fall into that developmental sequence. The author's experience suggests that some mature adults remain at or near the beginning of Kohlberg's cognitive development sequence, and few have attained the last stage, wisdom.

Psycho-social Adaptation.   Many men and women in this period of life find that their thoughts turn to reevaluation of self and purpose. They recognize this as the approximate half-way mark of their lives and because of that idea, many become involved in changes of attitudes toward that which is significant and that which is trivial. Erikson (1963) assigned the conflict between generativity and ego stagnation to these years. Contrary forces arise between the desire to do something worthwhile or to leave a legacy, and the ease and security found in adhering to that which is familiar or maintaining status quo. Patterns of behavior and responses to feedback from others are well established by this age and very difficult to alter.

The establishment of economic security for later years becomes a major interest at this stage. Retirement funds and investments are popular among wage-earners and those who are self-employed. Quite often, the attention of this group is more intensely focused on political decision-making and politics than previously. Whereas young adults may declare their interests through group actions, mature adults are more likely to engage in individual actions. They might run for public office, address civic associations, or actively campaign or lobby for votes or legislative support of an interest.

Personal traits apparent in earlier years tend to be more pronounced during mature adulthood. Both pro-social and anti-social behaviors tend to become more apparent as individuals assert themselves and look toward the second half of the life span. Commonly recognized interactive behaviors are listed in Table 3.3. Like other personal characteristics, these are found in mixtures in most people. A dominance of pro-social behaviors is desired and expected. Anti-social behaviors are sometimes indicative of illness or may be overt evidence of a transient affective state (Zusman, 1966). These behaviors may be witnessed during intense emotional distress such as fear, anger, or grief.

Environment.   Environments established earlier tend to extend into this stage. Some will continue stable environments; others will create unstable environments as in the past. These conditions reflect differences in personal traits, interpersonal skills, managerial talents, actions taken on advice, and the success of those actions. Some believe that luck is a major factor in the extent and richness of environment by the time one reaches mature adulthood. Others believe that individuals make their own luck. Such myths, legends, and superstitions contribute to behavioral outcomes and determine limits on individuals' physical and psychological spaces.

Home and work environments correlate with the type of work done and interact with interpersonal behaviors. Some occupations provide luxurious work space and commodious homes, schools, and recreational facilities, as well as the opportunity to travel. In other occupations, fatigue and monotony are chronic; strikes and layoffs threaten workers' already frugal existence. Environment reflects success as measured by whatever standards or values one holds. In this sense, the significance of a physical space and the objects that fill it is the extension of values, attitudes, and expectations of the people who occupy that space.

For this age group, some are initiating a second career. For some who have completed 20 or 30 years in one occupation, and are entering a new occupation, their savings or retirement funds from the first occupation may provide a measure of financial security.

Table 3.3
Pro- and anti-social behaviors

Pro-social Behaviors	Anti-social Behaviors
Affiliation/loyalty	Abuse
Assertiveness	Accusing/blaming
Assistance	Aggression
Caring	Deceit
Charity/generosity	Deprivation
Consideration	Destructiveness
Cooperation	Deviousness
Creativity	Disinhibition
Helping	Disrespect
Humor	Hypocrisy
Modeling	Prejudice
Productivity	Provocation
Recognition	Rejection/denial
Reinforcement	Thievery
Support	Violence
Tact	Vulgarity

❦ ❦ ❦

COUNSELING CONSIDERATIONS

Pauline Crosley is a 46-year-old woman diagnosed as having spastic dysphonia and a mild to moderate hearing loss in her right ear. She wears bifocal eyeglasses. She has come to your clinic with a referral from her former communication disorders specialists in Akron, Ohio. There, medical examination found no organic defect in laryngeal tissue and the SLP had initiated voice therapy to increase sustained vocalization.

During your intake interview, you learn that Pauline has moved to your community following the death of her husband. Her two grown children and their families live here, and she has rented a small apartment, planning to support herself for several months while looking for work. She was a court reporter before her children were born and then became a full-time housewife and mother. As you continue your interview and discussion of her new apartment and her family, you notice tremor of the jaw and of both arms when they are extended to point out various photographs.

1. List Pauline's problems as she describes them.
2. Indicate what information you will need in addition to that contained in the case folder she brought with her.
3. Consider the possibility of creating team treatment for this client. What types of professionals would you want on that team?
4. In what ways will you utilize counseling in dealing with the client, her voice disorder, and her new situation? Note: You may wish to consult

information resources, texts or experienced clinicians, to gain insight into the impact of currently noted symptoms on immediate and future interaction with this client.

5.0 Middle Age—50 to 65 Years

The definition of *middle age* in terms of years varies with the perspective of the author and the discipline (Cowgill, 1972). As life expectancy extends, the definition of middle age has changed to include later and later years. There are no guarantees for long life, but genetic makeup probably is more influential in determining potential life span than any other scientifically known factor today. Examination of ancestral life spans may give a reasonable estimate of the life span expectations of individuals (Sokolovsky, 1990). However, those estimates should be viewed with caution, since a lack of records for two or more generations can lead to false conclusions. Also, previous generations have dealt with entirely different patterns of stress in daily living. Those differences may have had profound influence on aging and deterioration of physical and mental health.

Biology. The most readily apparent changes in the middle-aged population are those of the body. Biological changes noted during these years initiate the closing down of body systems (Jacobs-Condit & Ortenzo, 1985; Schneider & Rowe, 1989). This process continues for the remainder of life, eventually resulting in the natural death of the body. Study of the aging process has been confounded by the likelihood that disease or trauma will interfere with normal aging. Such interferences modify the rate and degree of loss of parts and functions.

Many scientists and a large segment of industry have contributed to better health through the development of modern devices to reduce strain on the body and improved mechanisms to facilitate work and play. While 65 is still considered the age of retirement, and the age around which the Social Security Act was built, retirement is no longer merely a term for incapacity or infirmity due to age. Perhaps the greatest contributions to longer life spans are the development of vaccines that prevent childhood diseases and antibiotics that intervene early in infections. Another major contribution to successful aging comes from the increased awareness and availability of appropriate nutrition in daily diets. Discovery of the need for vitamins and minerals in foods has enabled the aging population to maximize body capacities for longer times.

By age 50, all the organ systems of the human body have begun to slow down their functions at the cellular level. Cytochemistry involves anabolism and catabolism. A brief overview of biological systems seems the most straightforward method of approaching this massive bank of information about aging in the absence of disease.

The skin or integumentary system is the largest organ of the body. The skin loses firmness and elasticity, and overexposure to the sun will age the skin even faster, causing it to become leathery and deeply wrinkled. Normal wrinkling and dryness increase from the 50s onward, as subcutaneous fatty deposits decrease or shift placement. In the face, the skin tends to sag and fold. Brown pigmented spots or lentigo senilis may appear. Minute capillaries in the thinning skin may erupt, causing occasional discoloration; these are hemorrhages that form red blotches or bruises. Cartilaginous supports of the ears and nose appear to enlarge, especially in males. Hair, a product of the skin, loses its pigment and turns gray and/or white. Scalp hair becomes coarser and much thinner, especially in males. Finger- and toe-nails become tougher and may be brittle. There is a risk of developing ingrown toenails with improperly fitted shoes. Although these changes in appearance are not life-threatening, they do contribute to changes in self-perception.

The skeleton and skeletal muscles interact continually and therefore affect one another increasingly as the body ages. Decreases in the number of cells lessen the mass and strength of both bone and muscle. Elasticity of muscle decreases and lessens flexibility or ease of contraction across joints of long bones and the vertebrae. Changes in bony mass, or osteoporosis, apparently result from the inability of aging bones to retain sufficient calcium in the presence of reduced amounts of vitamin D. Bones become brittle and easily broken. Small unnoticed fractures, especially of vertebrae, may result from a sneeze or cough. Roundness of the shoulders is not unusual in aging women or in people of both genders whose long-time careers have imposed upper body flexion. Relative changes in bone and muscle tissue result in changes of body contour, height, and strength. Prevention or slowing of these changes has been far more successful than later treatment for reversing the process.

Other tissues and organs, such as cartilage, tendon, and ligament, and cardiac and smooth or visceral muscle are also found to show changes after the age of 50. While a properly exercised and cared-for body can retain its strength well into the 90s, poorly maintained health can lead to the breakdown of any or all of these organ systems during middle age.

The nervous system and its function are affected by changes in receptors, peripheral nerves carrying impulses to and from the brain and spinal cord, the brain, and the spinal cord. Dramatic changes in functions of the eyes and ears reduce the proficiency of their response to stimuli. In turn, if those peripheral organs are not aided with prostheses, the sensory nerves (CN II and CN VIII) lose function and transmit fewer and faulty impulses to the cortex. Other sensory organs decrease in acuteness of function, such as taste, smell, balance, and proprioception.

Since approximately 35 years of age, the brain has lost millions of cells and a large amount of water. By age 50 and thereafter, the rate of cell loss gradually increases and the chemistry of the brain matrix changes, as does that of the rest of the body. The autonomic or reflexive nerves, which maintain regulated control of cardiovascular, respiratory, and digestive systems, become more susceptible to disruption of impulse flow. Changes occur in hunger, sleep, and secretory functions, affecting homeostasis. In the central nervous system, cells and pathways change by cell loss, alteration of cell shape and size, and collection of pigmented deposits, or lipofuscin. Radical changes in body fluids and chemical composition of the blood and lymph may decrease nerve firing rate and distribution due to insufficient generation of neurotransmitters. Additionally, nervous system function is dramatically affected by the impact of aging on other systems such as circulation, respiration, digestion, and excretion.

Results of all these changes in cellular and organ structure and function can be observed in alterations in behavior (Duffy & MacDonald, 1990). Needless to say, changes observed in some 50-year-old men and women will not have been developed in others who are 70 years old. Interaction with middle-aged and older men and women must be based on the ability of the individual, not on a scale or gradation according to age.

Cognition. Along with the inevitable biological changes, cognitive function undergoes change. This change is more dramatic in some individuals than in others. The difference is believed to be related to genetics and influenced by environment and habits, both past and present. For example, consider the variety of "input" information resources available today. Individuals who have developed a love for reading continue to absorb information of current interest through the medium of print. They form mental images and opinions, which incorporate and draw from previous experience and which they may or may not discuss with family, friends, and acquaintances. Those who do not read or cannot read well may utilize electronic media for most of their information and entertainment. They, too, gain ideas and impressions, which can be discussed with people in their daily environments. McLuhan (1967) proposed that print and electronic media generate different messages to the receiver, and the media modify the message that is perceived. The argument for and against intellectual benefits of each medium continues as television selects program materials for its audience and provides broader spectra of visual images than print, reducing the viewer's opportunity to generate independent visual imaginings.

By this time of life, astute minds are at their peaks. Others, which have weathered storms from this and other determiners of behavior, especially physical and mental health, may be less keen than they could be or were in the past. Also, socio-cultural values placed on cognitive functions greatly influence the tenacity of the middle-aged individual to pursue cognitive endeavors (Levinson, 1978). There is little difference in cognitive competence between mature adult, middle-aged, and aging populations. Instead, there is apparent difference in performance levels, which decrease with age. The most noticeable change is the slowing down of function, and this may not be discernible in middle age.

In the middle-aged population, there is also the tendency for long-held practices of thinking and feeling to become more pronounced. While this is intimately associated with abilities addressed in the psycho-social determiner, it also depends on the strength and ability of cognitive abilities. Some, who are very busy with daily chores or commitments to other people, find that they set aside learning or creative activities with a notion of making room for them in the future (Brody, 1981; Gelfand, 1982). This group includes *spinners,* people who need to rehearse, verbally or otherwise, the scenario of each experience or anticipated involvement. This psycho-social adaptive device seems to justify the business of the moment, forgive the failure to accomplish other things, and rationalize hope that all will be well tomorrow, while staving off the need to act by talking at length about it.

Another identifiable group consists of people who have devoted much of their energies to the care and concerns of others (Brody, 1981). At this stage, these people are most noticeably different when they turn their current energies to the fulfillment of personal ambitions. Some enroll in higher education, some travel, some develop hobbies, and some become involved in social or civic organizations.

Psycho-social Adaptation. For the majority of this population, struggles of early job security and satisfaction are completed by this time. Family constellations are established and function as interactive support units. Social recognition and rewards are realized, or the desire for them abandoned. Dreams and expectations are modified by reality, and socioeconomic class and potential for upward mobility are determined. Middle-aged adults may seem set in their ways, and their habits firmly in place. Even in the highly mobile world of today, once settled into home, work, and social group, many middle-aged individuals and married couples move around in only a limited arena. They spend energy on few and small increments of change while they maintain advantages already acquired. They are content and even happy with their current arrangements. Into these circumstances, the sudden death of a spouse can introduce devastating psycho-social distress for the survivor.

Research has documented the relationship between the availability of social supporters and such intangibles as happiness, mental health, physical health, coping strategies, and use of resources. The Gray Panthers and the American Association For Retired Persons (AARP) are examples of middle- and older-aged populations banding together to form advocacy groups, mutual support systems, and politically influential bodies. For those without accessible resources or satisfactory support systems, daily living is quite different. Growing older is a source of stress, and depression often results from an inability to cope with the stress. These emotional and psychological responses are aggravated by biological changes, recognized loss of control, and feelings of vulnerability (Walker, Sechrist, & Pender, 1987). The range of psycho-social adaptive abilities covers the continuum from well-adjusted, mature management of daily changes as they occur to inadequate coping and distress in people who need mental health services.

Environment. Health, cognition, the internal biophysiological environment, socio-economic class, race, and ethnic group combine to designate the external environments available to the middle-aged person in the modern world (Saxon & Etten, 1984). Poverty, with all it entails, continues to be the most devastating limit to available resources for physical and mental well-being. Multiple constraints on economically depressed people restrict their access to security, freedom, and the courage to escape poverty. The very poor find it virtually impossible to avoid the grasping manipulation of people and systems that converge to keep them poor.

Expansion and variation of physical and psychological environments may occur in personal, civic, religious, political, or educational domains through experience and contacts with others. Decline of some sensory and mental abilities may reduce mobility, daring, curiosity, and even interest in surroundings. However, alert, healthy, middle-aged people become valuable resources to others.

❧ ❧ ❧

COUNSELING CONSIDERATIONS

Herman Folitz is 62 years old, a retired brigadier general. He claims that his wife of 41 years mumbles and gets worse as she gets older, and he suggests that something is wrong with her larynx. During an annual physical examination, both General and Mrs. Folitz agree with their physicians to have complete visual and auditory evaluations. They are scheduled to be seen at your office for the hearing tests.

You find that Mrs. Folitz has good hearing bilaterally with no threshold in the speech range greater than 25dB. General Folitz's audiogram shows bilateral hearing loss. The left ear is his better ear with thresholds of 45 to 60dB across the speech range. The right ear's thresholds trace a descending curve from 40dB at 250 Hz to 90dB at 3K Hz and above. There is a 15dB air-bone gap in the right ear at 250, 500, and 1K Hz.

1. List the health care problems that the hearing tests seem to have identified.
2. Determine how you will introduce your findings to General and Mrs. Folitz.
3. Anticipate their individual reactions to your disclosure.

4. What must you accomplish during this single interaction? What are your professional goals?
5. How will you proceed? What counseling skills will you need?

6.1, 6.2, and 6.3. Old Age—65 Years and Older

Also known as *the aging population,* this age group is expanding rapidly in number and in upper limits of age (Curtin, 1972; Jackson, 1980; Reichel, 1989). Observation and empirical research have shown reason to divide this group into three substages: young old (65–75), old (75–90), and very old (over 90). Increases in the aging population have accelerated since the 1950s, and the group is expected to make up one third of the total population by 2020. The Census Bureau of the Social Security Administration has projected that more than 36,251,000 people will be 65 or older by the year 2000. That number is expected to double before the middle of the 21st century. Such projections are awesome considering the present infancy of knowledge, occupation, services, and care of the independent and dependent aging population.

Sociocultural attitudes in America have long held expectations of feebleness, illness, and incompetence as perceived traits of old age. Admittedly, the age and wisdom that are revered in some societies are not necessarily a universally matched pair (Palmore, 1991). However, until recently, those past the magical number of 65 years of age have been generally regarded as unproductive members of a society that honors the work ethic. In fact, the ongoing basis of research in this stage of life is men and women who are members of various residential plans. Some are ill and some are healthy, but all have chosen to participate in a community of their peers, not a traditional home (Kimmel, 1990). Because this closing stage of the life span holds such unexplored challenges to the professional in communication disorders, Appendix E presents some special considerations on counseling perspectives.

Biology.   Aspects of body change indicated for the middle-aged population continue and accelerate as age increases (Duffy & MacDonald, 1990; Schneider & Rowe, 1989). Dramatic cytochemical alterations are noted in accumulation of lipofuscin believed to be cellular waste. Water, the most abundant compound in the body that is normally present in the tissues, is gradually reduced through time. This affects the concentration of chemical solutions and suspensions in body fluids and the efficiency of the excretory system. Connective tissues change; bone loses calcium; cartilage of the nose, ears, larynx, and ribs becomes dense, more fibrous, and less pliable. These changes affect appearance, voice quality, and respiratory function. In the very old, respiration becomes more and more reliant on the diaphragm as the rib cage becomes more rigidly fixed.

As muscles atrophy, their cellular mass is replaced by fibers that further inhibit contraction. Endocrine changes contribute to tissue changes and may help explain the fact that one in five women age 80 and older has had a broken hip. Blood supply is adequate in amount and function so long as blood volume is not lost, but replenishing the supply is inefficient. The healthy heart changes very little due to age alone. Vascular changes include exchange of muscle for fiber and reduction of elasticity, which decreases diastolic blood pressure and competence of venous valves. Poor circulation may reduce the availability of oxygen, which is disastrous to tissue health.

Normal neurological changes reduce sensation, prolong reaction time, introduce tremor, and slow the gait to a shuffle. Neuron action potential and secretory functions for neurotransmitters diminish. Loss of appetite is normal. While overall calorie requirements taper off, protein, vitamin, and mineral requirements call for a balanced diet and good oral, especially dental, and esophageal health.

Cognition. In the healthy aging, changes in cognitive abilities are less common than changes in performance (Cowley, 1980). Learning is slower, as is the rate of stimulus pattern recognition. Sensory thresholds change, selective attention lessens, and the ability to divide attention between two simultaneous events diminishes. Unlike episodic memory, generic memory is little affected.

Psychiatric disorders can and often do disrupt normal cognitive function among the aging population. Early identification and appropriate intervention can control some illnesses and biological deficits that interfere with cognitive function (Costa & McCrae, 1980). There is a great need for ongoing research on aging-without-illness to aid with early identification of symptoms of negative change in health and behavior.

Psycho-social Adaptation. With increasing years, the survivor finds fewer and fewer remaining chronological peers. This loss of social contacts who have common memories of shared experiences tends to isolate the survivor. There is also no assurance that younger generations of family and friends will continue to be available for social interaction (Bumagin & Hirn, 1990). Unresolved internal conflicts, loss of affection, and the relinquishing of authority or control often lead to depression, which further interferes with mental and physical health.

Psycho-social adaptive abilities are profoundly affected by individual personality traits, health and vigor, environment, whether institutional or not, life style, and interactive capabilities (Atchley, 1980; Nahemow, McCluskey-Fawcett, & McGhee, 1986). Changes in the social context of the aging impose reduced responsibilities for the individual within a group structure, and further isolate the individual. Many theories have evolved concerning the change and breakdown of socialization (Cox, 1984). While each theory has merits, gerontologists continue to pursue explanations for this phenomenon among the aging. Meanwhile, various intervention strategies have been devised and applied through social service agencies and by individual health care practitioners (Newman, Rice, & Struyk, 1988; Soldo, 1983). There are no definitive answers to questions of care management of the aging population. One movement called *congregate living* contributes to active participation in a shared environment with chronological peers that allows full or minimally limited independent self care. In settings that provide care for the aging population, the most important element for maximum benefit is recognizing the need for individuals to maintain control over their lives as far as is feasible (Regnier & Rynoos, 1987; Struck & Kalsura, 1988). This is important information for the practitioner in communication disorders to keep in mind to achieve maximum beneficial treatment outcomes.

Aging individuals, their families, and friends find that coping with the realities of life is made more difficult by reduced economic status, physical changes, loss of meaningful associates, and inaccessibility of beloved activities. Gerontophobia in the general societal milieu is fed by observations of the old by the young and the surety that old age is the destiny of those fortunate enough to survive the trials of youth and middle age. Fears and dreads, myths and superstitions tend to isolate the aged and the idea of aging as a remote issue. With that attitude, many of the young and middle-aged population develop poor and unrealistic plans for their own futures.

Environment.   As indicated previously, the environment differs with each aging man or woman. Internal environment inevitably changes by a slowing of body functions. External environment varies from no significant change to the total disruption of all known spaces, objects, and persons (Knight & Lower-Walker, 1985; Regnier & Rynoos, 1987; Walker, Sechrist, & Pender, 1987). Health remains the most significant factor in where and how members of the aging population thrive. Economic resources determine the amount of services available. Public social services sometimes provide more for the very poor than for the less poor but independent elderly person. Coping abilities and knowledgeable demands for adequate access to available resources are the ingredients that garner help from the maximum expertise currently available.

❦ ❦ ❦

CLINICAL CONSIDERATIONS

Below are three situational descriptions, one for each of the identified substages of the *old age* stage.

6.1 The Young Old

Mr. Peter Quinn is 72 years old. He has moderate presbycusis for which he has used amplification for about 8 years; he is recovering from a cerebral hemorrhage (CVA), which occurred 16 days ago. The treating neurologist has indicated that his medical condition has stabilized. He has right hemiplegia and cannot recall the names of people or objects. This is your first visit with the Quinn family. The patient apparently recognizes his wife, son, and oldest grandchild, but he cannot name them. He cries because he feels frustrated by this evidence of his own feebleness. His wife left his room yesterday and today because she was going to cry, too, and didn't want her husband to see her in tears. Mrs. Quinn tells you that he has always been fiercely independent and will hate his infirmity. She dreads to think of the future. Her son and grandson must return home the day after tomorrow.

In addition to assessment of the communication abilities of the patient and planning for his treatment, the situation calls on your counseling skills to interact with the patient, wife, son, and grandson.

1. List the considerations that comprise part of your context for each family member.
2. Write a dialogue between Mr. Quinn and yourself.
3. Write a dialogue between Mrs. Quinn and yourself.
4. Write a dialogue among yourself, the son, and grandson.
5. Review the three scripts you have written. Identify helping or counseling skills you used during the conversations.
6. Compare your dialogues with those of your classmates.
7. Ask two classmates to role-play the scenario you have created.
8. With videotaping facilities, review the interaction for verbal and nonverbal helping behaviors.

6.2 The Old

Mollie Rae Richards is 81 years old. She lives in a congregate home with seven other senior citizens who are mostly independent, but they have a housemother who cooks for them and tidies up their common rooms. Mollie Rae is a strong-willed woman who takes excellent care of herself. Every year, she has a complete physical, including eyes, ears, speech, and language, and then she spends several hours bragging about how tough she is for several days. This is interwoven with her memory of being one of the world's first women pilots. Her attitude is, "So what if I need reading glasses and a hearing aid now? It's time I had a little help." She is in your office now, waiting for your report on recent testing, which she expects will be favorable.

1. Write a dialogue between Mollie Rae and yourself as you share the test results.
2. How does your attitude toward this patient differ from that toward the Quinn family?
3. How do your behaviors with this patient differ from those you used with the Quinns?
4. Explore those differences and try to explain why they exist.
5. As you explore differences in yourself, review your values and Mollie Rae's values. Make comments on these values.

6.3 The Very Old

Martha Barrett Wallace lives at Colonial Manor Retirement Center, where you are director of the Communication Center. Miss Wallace is 97 years old, a former schoolteacher of 54 years and the author of seven books of stories for adolescent boys. She is in good health, but she uses a wheelchair for long distances, such as going to the dining room. Miss Wallace had her lower denture relined last Thursday, and she is experiencing some discomfort in her left lower alveolar ridge. That soreness in her mouth makes talking quite difficult, and trying to eat with the denture in has proven to be very painful. Yesterday and again today, she removed the relined denture from her mouth and carried it in her jacket pocket. This afternoon, following a light lunch, Miss Wallace meets you in the hallway and tells you that her ears hurt. She believes that she has caught a cold and wants you to get her some medicine to ward off the worst symptoms.

1. How do you react to Miss Wallace's story and request?
2. What is the appearance of her face with the lower denture missing?
3. What is the effect of the missing denture on her speech articulation?
4. Do you inquire about the denture? If so, how?
5. Write a dialogue of, or role-play, your interaction with Miss Wallace in the hallway.
6. List the possible arenas of inquiry or referral that you may need to make to resolve Miss Wallace's painful condition. As you identify these resources, verbalize your inferential reasoning and discuss probabilities with classmates and colleagues.

EXERCISES

1. This chapter contains 12 brief introductions to client cases. The disorders vary, as do the ages and family constellations of the clients. These cases can be used to identify and practice counseling skills.

a. Enlist the assistance of a classmate in role-playing the client or significant other in one of the client cases while you play the role of counselor. You are not expected to solve a client problem. Instead, you should use your interpersonal communication skills to elicit sufficient information to guide the client in analyzing the problems and posing rational solutions.

b. If you have access to a closed-circuit television system, use it to videotape your interaction. If no video equipment is available, find a third classmate to act as the monitor or camera to record your use of the counseling behaviors described in chapter 2.

c. Regardless of the recording method, sustain the interaction for 5 minutes. This is not a social conversation. The counselor's role is rigorously devoted to getting an understanding of the thought and affective status of the client/caregiver, accepting that situation, and helping the client/caregiver identify one or more possible alternative actions, behaviors, or solutions.

d. Upon completion of the 5-minute interaction, carefully review the tape or the recorder's notes. Observe your own interactive skills, whether you were the counselor or the client. It is helpful to use a tally sheet to count the incidences of those behaviors. Describe the type of behaviors used, the information gained in each exchange, and possible alternate directions that the interaction could have taken if the exchange had been altered.

Note: If this is done as an in-class exercise, dyads or triads are then encouraged to compare experiences. Remember that in role-playing, your ability to move into the other character is being challenged. Some of your behaviors will be acting, but some of the acting will reflect yourself. This is important for the counselor, in that full comprehension of a client's message always requires that the counselor perceive that message from the perspective of the client. That is, the counselor must move into the world of the client and understand the situation from the perspective of the client.

2. Create a character and disorder for a client who could be expected to remember some of the phenomena or affairs from the past half-century. Draft a biographical sketch of that client and include probable family members, two or three associates or friends, and two or three items the client would purchase in local stores.

When you have completed the biographical sketch, begin to draw word pictures of the family members and associates you identified and the merchants who supply the items you listed as needed. Draw these word pictures from the perspective of the client whom you originally introduced in the biographical sketch. Make use of the age-related information in this chapter to elaborate the depiction of the client, family, and friends you are creating.

Note: A variation on this exercise is to agree with another classmate about the age, gender, and region of origin of the client, and then complete the exercise independently. If this creation is a collaborative endeavor among two or three classmates, be careful not to confuse cultural, regional, or religious differences in a single person.

Regardless of the way in which this exercise is undertaken and completed, discuss the products and the characters in class. Modify their descriptions as the observations of others help clarify the personalities, behaviors, and abilities.

3. Following the completion of exercise 2, the frame of reference for the client will be fairly complete. It will now be possible for individuals in the class to portray this character while others role-play the counselor as treatment of the communication disorder gets underway. While it would be ideal to address the disorder at this time, the reader's level of information in speech-language pathology and audiology must regulate that portion of the exercise. The intended focus here is to move forward in the counseling relationship, which is established as part of the treatment, and not to apply specific treatment techniques to the disorder that is habilitated.

4. Review three of the supplementary readings listed in Appendix C. Contrast and compare the different life perspectives found in those sources and your own reactions to similar situations or circumstances.

REFERENCES

Allen, V. L. (1975). Social support for nonconformity. In L. Berkowitz (Ed.), *Advances in experimental social psychology* (p. 8). New York: Academic Press.

Atchley, R. (1980). *Social forces in later life.* (3rd ed.). Belmont, CA: Wadsworth.

Bayley, N. (1969). *Manual for the Bayley scales of infant development.* New York: The Psychological Corporation.

Behrman, R. E., & Vaughn, V. C., III. (1986). *Nelson textbook of pediatrics.* (13th ed.). Philadelphia: W. B. Saunders.

Brazelton, T. B. (1973). *Brazelton neonatal behavioral assessment scale.* Philadelphia: Lippincott.

Brody, E. M. (1981). Women in the middle and family help to older people. *The Gerontologist, 21*(5), 471–480.

Brophy, J. E., & Good, T. L. (1974). *Teacher-student relationships.* New York: Holt.

Bumagin, V. E., & Hirn, K. F. (1990). *Helping the aging family*. New York: Springer.

Butler, R. N. (1983). The life review: An interpretation of reminiscence in the aged. *Psychiatry, 26,* 65–75.

Carey, W. B . (1981). The importance of temperament-environment interaction for child health and development. In M. Lewis & L. Rosenblum (Eds.), *The uncommon child*. New York: Plenum Press.

Cattell, P. (1947). *The measurement of intelligence in infants and young children*. Baltimore, MD: Penguin.

Chess, S. (1967). Temperament in the normal infant. In J. Hellmuth (Ed.), *Exceptional infant: Vol. 1,* pp. 143–162. Seattle: Straub and Hellmuth.

Costa, P. T., & McCrae, R. R. (1980). Still stable after all these years: Personality as a key to some issues in adulthood and old age. In P. B. Baltes & O. G. Brim, Jr. (Eds.), *Life span development and behavior: Vol. 3* (pp. 65–103). New York: Academic Press.

Cowgill, D. C. (1972). A theory of aging in cross-cultural perspective. In D. O. Cowgill & L. D. Holmes (Eds.), *Aging and modernization*. New York: Appleton-Century-Crofts.

Cowley, M. (1980). *The view from 80*. New York: Penguin.

Cox, H. (1984). *Later life: The realities of aging*. Englewood Cliffs, NJ: Prentice-Hall.

Curtin, S. (1972). Aging in the land of the young. *Atlantic Monthly, 230,* 68.

Duffy, M. E., & MacDonald, E. (1990). Determinants of functional health of older persons. *The Gerontologist, 30*(4), 503–509.

Erikson, E. H. (1963). *Child and society*. New York: Norton.

Festinger, L. (1957). *A theory of cognitive dissonance*. Stanford, CA: Stanford University Press.

Fisher, J. D., & Nadler, A. (1974). The effect of similarity between donor and recipient on recipient's reaction to aid. *Journal of Applied Social Psychology, 4,* 128–148.

Fisher, J. D., & Nadler, A. (1976). Effect of donor resources on recipient self-esteem and self-help. *Journal of Experimental Social Psychology, 12,* 139–150.

Frost, R. (1947). Mending wall. In R. Frost, *Complete works of Robert Frost* (pp. 940–941). New York: Holt, Rinehart, and Winston.

Gelfand, D. E. (1982). *Aging: The ethnic factor*. Boston: Little, Brown.

Greenfield, P. (1966). On culture and conservation. In J. S. Bruner et al. (Eds.), *Studies in cognitive growth* (pp. 43–76). New York: Wiley.

Greenspan, S. I. (1983). Parenting in infancy and early childhood: A developmental structuralist approach to detailing adaptive and maladaptive patterns. In V. J. Sasserath & R. A. Hoekelman (Eds.), *Minimizing high risk parenting* (pp. 79–91). New Brunswick, NJ: Johnson and Johnson.

Guilford, J. P. (1959). Three faces of intellect. *American Psychology, 14,* 469–479.

Jackson, J. J. (1980). *Minorities and aging.* Belmont, CA: Wadsworth.

Jacobs-Condit, L., & Ortenzo, M. L. (1985). Physical change in aging. In L. Jacobs-Condit (Ed.), *Gerontology and communication disorders* (pp. 26–72). Rockville, MD: American Speech, Language, and Hearing Association.

Kiesler, C. A., & Kiesler, S. BV. (1969). *Conformity.* Reading, MA: Addison-Wesley.

Kimmel, D. (1990). *Adulthood and Aging.* New York: John Wiley and Sons.

Knight, B. G., & Lower-Walker, D. L. (1985). Toward a definition of alternatives to the institutionalization for the frail elderly. *The Gerontologist, 25,* 358–363.

Kohlberg, L. (1964). The development of moral character and moral ideology. In M. Hoffman & L. Hoffman (Eds.), *Review of child development research: Vol. 1.* New York: Russell Sage.

Kohlberg, L. (1969). *The stages of development of moral thought and action.* New York: Holt, Rinehart, and Winston.

Kohlberg, L. (1984). *The psychology of moral development: The nature and validity of moral stages.* San Francisco: Harper and Row.

Kort, C., Ypma, I., & Toppen, A. (1975). Helplessness in Dutch society as a function of urbanization and environmental level. *Journal of Personality and Social Psychology, 32,* 996–1003.

Langer, E. J. (1978). The psychology of chance. *Journal for the Theory of Social Behavior, 7,* 185–207.

Leavitt, H. J. (1951). Some effects of communication patterns on group performance. *Journal of Abnormal and Social Psychology, 46,* 38–50.

Levinson, D. J. (1978). *The seasons of man's life.* New York: Knopf.

McLuhan, M. (1967). *The media is the message.* New York: Random House.

Nahemow, L., McCluskey-Fawcett, K. A., & McGhee, P. E. (1986). *Humor and aging.* San Diego: Academic Press.

Newman, S., Rice, M., & Struyk, R. (1988). *Overwhelming odds: Caregiving and the risk of institutionalization* (Urban Institute Project Report 3691-01). Washington, DC: The Urban Institute.

Palmore, E. (1991). *Ageism, negative and positive.* New York: Springer.

Parten, M. (1932). Social play among preschool children. *Journal of Abnormal and Social Psychology, 27,* 243–269.

Piaget, J. (1951). *Plays, dreams, and imitation* (C. Gattagno & F. M. Hodgson, Trans.). New York: Norton.

Piaget, J. (1952). *The origin of intelligence in children.* New York: International University Press.

Piaget, J. (1955). *The moral judgment of the child.* New York: MacMillan.

Piaget, J. (1972). Intellectual evolution from adolescence to adulthood. *Human Development, 15,* 1–12.

Regnier, V., & Rynoos, J. (Eds.). (1987). *Housing the aged: Design directives and policy considerations.* New York: Elsevier.

Reichel, W. (Ed.). (1989). *Clinical aspects of aging.* Baltimore, MD: Williams and Wilkins.

Ripich, D. N., & Spinelli, F. M. (1985). Some conclusions about school talk. In D. N. Ripich & F. M. Spinelli (Eds.), *School discourse problems.* San Diego, CA: College Hill Press.

Saxon, S. V., & Etten, M. J. (1984). *Psychosocial rehabilitative programs for older adults.* Springfield, IL: Charles C. Thomas.

Saxon, S. V., & Etten, M. J. (1987). *Physical change and aging.* New York: The Tiresias Press.

Scheuerle, J. (1989). Stimulating language development in infants and toddlers with cleft palate. In K. R. Bzoch (Ed.), *Communicative disorders related to cleft lip and palate* (3rd ed.), Boston: College Hill Press.

Schneider, E. L., & Rowe, J. W. (Eds.). (1989). *Handbook of the biology of aging,* San Diego, CA: Academic Press.

Serunian, S., & Broman, S. (1975). Relationship of APGAR scores and Bayley mental and motor scores. *Child Development, 46,* 696–700.

Shaie, I. W., & Willis, S. L. (1986). *Adult development and aging* (2nd ed.). Boston: Little, Brown.

Shaw, J. I., & Skolnick, P. (1973). An investigation of relative preference for consistency motivation. *European Journal of Social Psychology, 3,* 271–280.

Sheehy, G. (1976). *Passages: Predictable crises in adult life.* New York: Dutton.

Sokolovsky, J. (Ed.). (1990). *The cultural context of aging: Worldwide perspectives.* New York: Bergin and Garvey.

Soldo, B. (1983). *The elderly home care population: National prevalence rates, select characteristics, and alternative sources of assistance, Vol. 3.* (Urban Institute Final Report 1466). Washington, DC: The Urban Institute.

Struck, R. J., & Kalsura, H. M. (1988). Aging at home: How the elderly adjust their housing without moving. *Journal of Housing for the Elderly, 4,* 1–192.

Thomas, A., Chess, S., Birch, H. G., Hertzig, M. E., & Korn, S. (1963). *Behavioral individuality in early childhood.* New York: New York University Press.

Tomblin, J. B., & Liljegreen, S. J. (1985). The identification of socially significant communication needs in older language-impaired children: A case example. In D. N. Ripich & F. M. Spinelli (Eds.), *School discourse problems.* San Diego, CA: College Hill Press.

Walker, S. N., Sechrist, K. R., & Pender, N. J. (1987). The health-promoting lifestyle profile: Development of psychometric characteristics. *Nursing Research, 36,* 76–81.

Williams, D. (1958). Attracting topflight scientists and engineers. *Personnel, 34,*(6), 79–81.

Zusman, J. (1966). Some explanations of the changing appearances of psychologic patients; Antecedents of the social breakdown syndrome concept. *The Milbank Memorial Fund Quarterly, 64,* 2.

CHAPTER FOUR

❦ ❦ ❦

Serving Clients Across Disorders

Issues

❦ *Clients/caregivers who seek services for speech, language, or hearing share common pre-treatment experiences and characteristics in relation to their communication disorders.*

❦ *During the transition time between request for services and scheduling treatment, the clinician can infer the counseling needs of clients and caregivers from responses to case history forms, intake interviews, and/or client records.*

❦ *Counseling in the treatment of speech, language, and hearing disorders is profoundly influenced by ideas, expectations, and feelings of the client/caregiver who is faced with a problem that is preventable, remediable, modifiable, or irreversible.*

❦ *Clients and caregivers recognize the communication disorder as a loss of something that was expected or desired and may or may not be replaceable.*

❦ ❦ ❦

COMMON CHARACTERISTICS AMONG CLIENTS AND CAREGIVERS

Communication disorders are often grouped into five distinguishable categories: articulation, fluency, hearing, language, and voice. Each category includes many specific communicative impairments, each of which may result from one or many etiologies. Etiology, age of onset, degree of severity, and the history of the disorder and its management all profoundly influence the status of the disorder and the client's communicative ability at any given time. The state of the disorder and its effect on the daily life of the client and the family contribute to their decision to seek professional help. In preparation for a clinical practice that is open to clients from the total spectrum of human experience, it is important to consider what characteristics are common among clients and families seeking treatment.

Studies of counseling needs across the categories of communication disorders indicate that a client and/or caregiver may exhibit anxiety, guilt, anger, depression, denial, rejection, hostility, isolation, oversolicitousness, psychosomatic symptoms, or unrealistic expectations (Ainsworth, 1981; Leith, 1984; Luterman,1984; Rollin, 1987; Shadden, 1988). Feelings, attitudes, and communicative behaviors commingle in infinitely varying proportions. Reports of case studies describing treatment of communicative disorders note that quite different personal traits often emerge as the treatment process moves toward resolution or reduction of the handicapping problem. With improved communication abilities and/or acquired coping skills, clients and caregivers exhibit calmness, reality orientation, self-control, tolerance, self-acceptance, and assertiveness (Ling-Phillips, 1981, 1987; Moses, 1985; Saxon & Etten, 1984).

It seems appropriate to approach any given client, potential client, or caregiver with the expectation that any of these success-related traits may also be part of the personal makeup of that individual. However, the clinician cannot anticipate which of the possible array of traits will be found dominant in a single client at the initial meeting. Factors such as the disorder itself or the age, geographical region, ethnic group, or educational background of the client cannot predict the presence or absence of these traits.

A professional practice in communication disorders may have a designated specialization according to its parent institution (e.g., a public school or veterans' hospital), the expertise of the clinicians (e.g., a developmental disabilities or cochlear implant center), a staff preference for clients of a certain age (e.g., a pediatric or geriatric practice), or for those who exhibit specific types of disorders (e.g., a closed head injury or cerebral palsy clinic). Such specialization does not mean that clients or their communication disorders are identical or that working with them is routine. Each potential client brings to the treatment setting personally unique aspects of the disorder influenced by life experiences. On the other hand, even in the most diverse caseload, the insightful clinician finds common experiences and needs for counseling among clients regardless of their communication disorders.

This chapter explores some aspects of pre-treatment experiences and configurations of communication disorders that evoke the role of counselor in the speech-language pathologist and audiologist. The clinician can find reassurance in those common experiences and needs. Confidence in meeting and dealing with clients and their problems grows with clinical experience and conscientious research into clients' backgrounds as well as with continuing study of emerging techniques in remediation. Specifically, the client/caregiver environments that have major impacts on their relationships with the clinician include pre-treatment experiences (recognition of a handicapping communication disorder), clinical intake (becoming a client), and treatment phases.

❦ ❦ ❦

PRETREATMENT EXPERIENCES AMONG CLIENTS ACROSS DISORDERS

Identification of a communication problem may be based on a global, nonspecific, or vague impression of need for change in the potential client's communicative interaction with others. This impression may be the result of the potential client's own discomfort or frustration in interpersonal discourse or in some other form of verbal or nonverbal exchange. Family members may notice the communicative impediment because of their concern for the well-being of a relative, whether child, adolescent, or adult. A caregiver may want or need better communication with the potential client or hope for a respite from painful observations of the potential client's struggle or failure to communicate with others. Regardless of the motivation, the act of seeking professional intervention suggests the recognition of the communication disorder as a condition that is unacceptable and perhaps no longer tolerable.

Long before the initial appointment with a specialist in communication disorders, potential clients or caregivers have typically progressed through five stages of experience:

1. They have become consciously aware that a behavioral problem exists and that behavior involves aspects of communication.
2. They have decided that the communication problem interferes with daily activities and is severe enough that something must be done about it. That is, it cannot be ignored, and it will not go away by itself.
3. They have recognized the limits of their own abilities to resolve the problem unaided.
4. They have expressed their concerns and need for help in a manner and place that has resulted in access or referral to appropriate resources for help.
5. They have applied for professional help to resolve the acknowledged communication problem.

A closer look at each of these five steps provides insight into the behaviors of potential clients and their caregivers. Consideration of pre-treatment experiences of potential clients also enables the clinician to identify common concerns which must be addressed or resolved through counseling during the initial interview and subsequent therapy sessions.

I. Conscious Awareness of a Behavioral Problem

All rehabilitation of communication disorders has a common basis in awareness that the exhibited behavioral difference interferes with intra- or interpersonal communication. Relatives, caregivers, and associates react to the difference and consider it a behavioral problem. The potential client or others in the realm of daily activity need to change the current situation. The individual's communication problem does not exist in isolation; the behavior is crucially shaped by others in the environment. The problem behavior influences perceptions, reactions, modes of interaction, styles of communication, and expectations of those who observe it, just as their behavior selectively reinforces the person who exhibits the differences.

Of particular interest to the professional in communication disorders are elements and influences in the home environment that may continue to place a client at risk for failure of rehabilitation. Identification of such influences early in the treatment relationship allows timely introduction of family behavior-modification into the treatment plan. In some cases, consultation with a psychiatric social worker or other colleague may be necessary to facilitate communication rehabilitation.

Parent/Caregiver Report. During an initial interview with a family and potential client, the clinician often hears remarks that reveal the interviewee's reaction to the communication problem. In addition to the particulars of the communication disorder, the interviewee or reporter may be relied upon to provide information about the home communication environment. The reporter may present such information without conscious awareness of the revelation. The following statements are examples heard from parents, grandparents, spouses, and adult children of communicatively disordered individuals.

Mother of a pre-adolescent: When she was 2 or 3 years old, it was cute. But it's not cute any longer. She's too big to act the way she does.

Father of a pre-schooler: He just grunts and mumbles. We've got to do something. People will think he's retarded.

Son of an aging parent: I've done everything I know how to do. I've run out of tricks and patience.

Grandparent: She's just like her sister, except she won't talk. I never could stand a stubborn child.

Middle-aged wife: He doesn't pay any attention unless I yell at him.

Mother of boy in kindergarten: There's something wrong. He's never still . . . never rests . . . up all day and night. I'm exhausted just trying to keep him from getting hurt or getting into trouble.

Mother of a third-grader: We thought that the way she looks at us was just Jessie's way. But Dr. Rice thinks there's more to it.

Spouse of octogenarian: John tells the same stories over and over again. Sometimes he forgets names and places . . . and he always gets in the way.

Although these statements may seem straightforward and clear, there are multiple facets of meaning in each. To identify the full meaning of each statement, the counselor must respond to the verbal and nonverbal messages and spend enough time on the topic to assure that listener impressions are well-founded. What can the counselor infer from a first reading of each statement about the home communication environment and the communicative relationship between the speaker and the potential client? How does the speaker seem to feel? What does the speaker appear to want? What does the speaker expect, hope, fear? Can those inferences be modified by shifting the emphasis or pause structure in the second reading of the statement? Upon hearing such statements, the counselor can pursue the ramifications of meanings embedded in each. The clinician must verify inferences through dialogue designed to help the speaker clarify the intended and delivered messages and to prevent the counselor from retaining misinformation or biased impressions. Helping skills described in chapter 2 offer practical means to accomplish this.

Each of the statements above reflects the speaker's perception of a remembered unacceptable behavior and reaction to it. The statements also reveal strong feelings experienced by those around the affected individual and their concern, or even worry, that the problem will not diminish on its own over time. Since feelings and attitudes shape behaviors (Galvin & Book, 1975), the progress of treatment necessitates that the clinician appraise the role of the reporter's current relationship with the potential client as a contributing factor to the disorder and its remediation.

Checking Out Caregiver Report. Caregivers report observations that reflect their expectations, which have resulted from watching the behavior of others in similar circumstances or from personal history. Some impressions may be based on guidelines from medical and educational literature popularized by modern media. During an initial interview, the clinician must elicit enough information to discern clearly to what extent the reporter's descriptions are based in fact or represent a biased view. It is important to learn early in the relationship if the reported severity of the disorder is objective and realistic. This is typically done by evaluation of the potential client's communicative abilities. An honest report by a concerned caregiver reflects that person's value system and tolerance level. It may be possible for the interviewer to identify interactive influences in the home environment that have contributed to poor communicative interaction. The careful counselor may recognize the possibility that the communication problem belongs to or is shared by the individual who is reporting. For example, if one spouse insists that the other mumbles, a wise clinician suspects that there are two sides to the story and introduces a need to interact with both partners in a variety of assessments of their communicative practices.

Social psychology literature provides additional insights into family communication networks and family environments that generate and perpetuate distorted communicative networks. Satir (1967) and others have contributed greatly to modern understanding of how family units work, interact, communicate, and influence one another's behavior in both positive and negative ways (Bailey & Simeonsson, 1984, 1988; Beckman-Bell, 1981; Lynch, 1986; McCubbin & Patterson, 1983; Murrell & Stachowiak, 1967; Shadden, 1988; Shaw, 1964, 1978; Stachowiak, 1968; Stordtbeck, 1951).

II. Recognition of the Need for Help

Differentiation is a cognitive skill that is critically necessary to survival and maturation. The practice of noticing differences among individuals in a family or peer group is common in everyday social settings across cultures and ethnic groups (Benedict, 1989). An identified interpersonal communication difference that is dramatic, recurs often, and endures over time becomes important enough to be considered a problem and warrant special attention. That attention typically leads to a decision that something must be done to modify the difference. Actually *making that decision* is the second experience which is common among those who become speech, language, and hearing clients. For some, the decision-making may be encouraged by comments or suggestions from relatives or neighbors. Often a trusted confidant such as a family physician, minister, public health nurse, or teacher may volunteer a suggestion that help is needed or at least begin to verbalize the family's previously unspoken thoughts and fears. In such cases, caregivers and potential clients tend to be receptive to a suggestion from a respected and knowledgeable adult who knows the community in which they live. Sometimes, however, even the most carefully orchestrated suggestion to seek help may be rebuffed by individuals who deny that the problem exists. On the other hand, many well-meaning people, including professionals, will advise concerned caregivers simply to be patient and wait. Typically, the basis for such advice is an expectation that the problem will dissipate and the needed skill will develop naturally. Only through knowing and educating the community can the communication specialist help to assure appropriate and timely referrals.

Among the informed public, socio-cultural attitudes about disabilities and differences are slowly moving toward a more realistic acceptance and away from the stigma traditionally associated with a disability or disorder. However, the cautious and sensitive clinician remains aware that potential clients and caregivers perceive their own status from a personal perspective on the social value system in which they function (Bateson, 1989).

The potential client's ability to make the decision that interactive behavior is not normal and that the communication behavior must be changed reflects the attitudes and practices of society at large and local culture in particular. Mead (1989) defined *culture* as "the systematic body of learned behavior which is transmitted from parents to children." Readiness to accept the diagnosis and treatment of a disability are found in many facets of the community. The health and education professions have made the most visible strides in the advancement of efforts to maximize the potential of the general population.

Health. During the last decades of the 20th century federal interest focused American national attention on wellness. Scientific advances led to the prevention of infectious disease and decreases in the incidence of heart disease and cancer, and interest focused on the terrifying auto-immunodeficiency syndrome (AIDS). With accelerated access to information and acknowledgement of the extension of the human life span, federal resources and local interests turned to concerns for normalization of development from prenatal life through the gerontological years.

Daily exposure to mass media informs viewers in all socio-economic strata that social and corporate institutions sanction practices for the promotion of wellness and good health and the reduction of handicapping agents and environmental conditions. Examples of decisions that help reduce the prevalence of communication handicaps are regulations to control industrial noise levels; require seatbelts in cars, helmets for bikers, administration of the measles vaccine; and restrict the use of ototoxic drugs. Elementary school programs in sex education and drug abuse, nutrition programs, deaf service centers, and community-based support groups provide further examples. Constituent interests have influenced political leaders to target the worth, responsibilities, and rights of the individual. Resources have emerged and continue to support the betterment of daily life and the reduction of disabling conditions. These and other efforts to realize the potential of each individual have had ripple effects into even the smallest communities and the most private homes. The move toward universal wellness appears to have become widespread in urban and rural America.

Education. Public education is a broad base for aid to the disabled. The now-famous P.L. 94–142 and subsequent legislation were brought about through organized efforts of citizens to reduce handicapping conditions of physical, cognitive, and behavioral dysfunction among children. Through federal laws and billions of federal dollars, public education from preschool to post-secondary school became a place where "wellness of learning" is a goal. There parents are encouraged to believe that non-traditional ways of teaching and learning continue to be developed, monitored, and encouraged for students who have differences that interfere dramatically with their progress through academic programs.

Societal and professional interest in and support of individuals whose differences were formerly considered handicapping continues to elicit responsible choices among parents and other caregivers. They seem better able to acknowledge evidence of not-normal behavior in someone they love or whose care they manage. Acknowledgement that the potential client has a problem is not an admission or implication of the caregiver's inadequacy or an imposition of guilt upon the caregiver. Instead, acknowledgement implies a perception that it is acceptable to identify the communication problem and to admit that the disorder exists.

Identification of a communication problem is for many a straightforward and realistic attempt to differentiate the actual developmental progress of the individual from hopes, desires, and expectations. This is especially true in communities wherein recognized services for such disabilities are a matter of record and where caregivers can identify evidence of a strong possibility for normalization.

Ongoing Counseling Needs of Caregivers. Rational acknowledgement of a non-normal or non-acceptable behavior in a potential client does not automatically circumvent emotional distress in the caregiver. During the initial interview and subsequent treatment sessions, the clinician must observe verbal and nonverbal behaviors to assess the feelings and attitudes of the caregiver and the client and to determine the influence of those traits on interactions with each other as well as with the clinician. A few minutes of conversation at the beginning or end of each treatment session may be judiciously used to assess the progress of change in the home communication environment that prevailed at the time of application for help. Some clinicians consider that these frequent and informal exchanges are sufficient to accommodate parents' needs for counseling concerning changes in the daily experience of the client. Others directly involve caregivers in the therapeutic process from the time of the initial appointment. They use specially scheduled interviews and discussions to help generate changes in the home environment that are necessary to expedite rehabilitation. The successful carry-over of acquired communication skills requires adaptation in the home environment as well as the client. To facilitate the client's treatment progress, the feelings, attitudes, and behaviors of caregivers must contribute to the effort rather than detract from its success. Just as the problem behavior will not go away unaided, it may persist or even return if the home environment lacks appropriately paced acceptance and supportiveness for the changed behavior.

III. Admission of the Need for Help

A third common experience found among clients and families is the recognition that they are unable to resolve the problem and achieve the desired communicative outcomes on their own. The ease with which they can accept the need for help relates to the internal workings of the individuals and the family constellation. Their degree of comfort, security, and experience in handling problems relates to how the individual members of the family feel about themselves and their place in the community. In the absence of training in caregiving, family expectations for the potential client are influenced by information and attitudes found in daily encounters. Acquaintances and strangers share their feelings, thoughts, and beliefs about a handicapping condition, the availability and success of rehabilitation services, and their cost in time and money.

Caregivers inexperienced in dealing with behavioral disorders tend to try a variety of home-made interventions to reduce the impact of the communication disorder. Some may be effective, but many are not. Families hear and heed implications and suggestions of friends, relatives, and neighbors. Unsolicited curiosity, concern, empathy, derision, and pity are forthcoming in everyday settings. The caregiver's inability to modify the potential client's undesired behavior or to cope with its multiple ramifications often leads to feelings of helplessness, which generate a variety of reactions. Underlying those reactions is the perception that the biological or behavioral difference has denied them the perfect baby, the normal child or adult, or the wise and nurturing elder. Life experience has changed from the routine and expected to an unwelcome and alien situation.

Most people seeking professional services for communication disorders have recognized the alien situation as beyond their coping abilities. In seeking help, they tend to be compliant, realistic, and objective about the specific diagnosis of the problem and accept the proposed treatment regimen. However, the self-acknowledged need for help can lead to the expression of feelings and attitudes which, if left unmodified, will dilute and defeat outcomes of the best possible therapies.

Other Caregiver Concerns. Families deal with the *recognition of their own limits* in various ways. Some will experience intense feelings of inadequacy and guilt. Others may focus blame on a certain member of the household. The introduction of an outsider, the professional who understands the problem, may be a threat to the family's privacy and social integrity. On the other hand, they may gain relief from learning that the acknowledged disability is treatable within the expertise of a recognized discipline, that help is available. Learning that professionals have identified similar communication disorders can help the client and the family regain self-esteem and recover from feeling alone in their difference.

Knowing that others in the community exhibit similar communicative traits can be highly beneficial, so the introduction of a support group may be appropriate early in the clinical relationship.

Another important client/caregiver consideration is the dollar value of outside help and the economic status of the client. The decision to seek professional help must address the cost of those services in dollars, transportation, time, including taking time off from work, and other commitments on the part of the caregivers. Treatments that are purchased by third party insurance payment usually require medical orders to activate the insurer's payment schedule. In some settings, direct payment on a sliding scale is available to a large number of clients. Public schools maintain tax-supported treatment programs with no additional cost for school-age children who meet specified criteria. Typically, these programs allow for a two-year delay or gap between expected and actual performance levels. Admission of the need for help implies that the client and caregiver are able to coordinate multiple resources to support resolution of the communication problem.

Clients who refer themselves for treatment of a communicative disorder may represent a slightly different configuration of attitudes. These self-referrals may express a long-held desire to remove or reduce an acknowledged or secret communicative problem. Such clients usually express a high level of interest and industry in improving skills as rapidly as possible. The steadfast clinician must often exercise caution to avoid unwarranted acceleration of treatment. Careful data collection and records are helpful in maintaining an objective clinical view of the communication disorder. Treatment of self-referred clients may bring accompanying deep-seated feelings to the surface that they will freely, if not eagerly, share with the clinician. Earnest discussions of the ramifications of the communication disorder may introduce the need for simultaneous co-therapy with another professional or a referral for counseling for change in career, direction of interests, and emphasis on abilities. All these factors present a readily recognizable role for counseling as a part of the therapeutic process.

IV. Making the Request for Help

In their search for help with a communication disorder, potential clients and caregivers must *express their need* in such a way that help is forthcoming. Responsible persons must identify a resource, the specialists, who can provide needed help, gain access to the specialized services, and present the potential client to the clinician at the appropriate time and place. The facility with which these seemingly simple measures are accomplished depends on many factors. As indicated, the internal workings of the client and family play a dominant role in obtaining diagnosis and treatment for the identified problem. Formulating and expressing a request for help require complex intra- and extra-personal action on the part of responsible individuals. Their influences at home and in the community interact to facilitate or impede the search for appropriate professional intervention for the communication disorder.

Additionally, other external factors influence the ease and success with which potential clients actually obtain the needed services. External situational influences on the acquisition of services include location of the potential client, availability of services, proximity and association of multiple interrelated disciplines, and financial support. The following paragraphs suggest to the reader some of the external situational forces which modify the potential client's activities in the search for clinical services.

Underserved Populations. Particular external restraints are imposed on the acquisition of rehabilitative services if the potential client belongs to any of the underserved communicatively handicapped populations (Flower, 1985). Such groups include populations that are linguistic minorities, economically disadvantaged, rural or remote, or institutionalized. The supply of clinicians with the interest and training to serve these populations adequately is apparently insufficient. Also, the employment mechanism for placement of qualified clinicians within access of these populations is limited.

Health-related Communication Problems. An outgrowth of the wellness concept is the evidence of referral for communication services within health care facilities. This was instigated by increased visibility of the speech, language, and hearing profession, improved third-party funding, both public and private, for rehabilitative services, and growing awareness within the medical community of enhanced recovery among patients through a variety of therapies. The growth of interdisciplinary patient care management in hospitals and other health care facilities includes potential clients whose communicative disorders result from a birth defect, trauma, or disease. Medical referrals to in-house or itinerant professional personnel or specialized rehabilitation centers such as Easter Seals rehabilitation centers, cerebral palsy centers, deaf service centers, and nursing homes help the potential client and caregiver access the appropriate communicative rehabilitative diagnosis and treatment.

Relationships between physicians and their patients often open the door for either party to introduce a discussion of suspected communication disorders. Informed physicians are ideal community resources for helping caregivers gain access to appropriate services. In some communities, however, controversy persists as to the appropriateness of speech, language, or hearing intervention in some areas of patient care. In addition, not all health care experts are experts in behavioral phenomena. While it is becoming more commmon to encounter physicians who are empathic with communication needs, some health care personnel still believe that biological health is the end goal of all therapies. Those professionals may advise an inquiring caregiver simply to wait and be patient or accept the noticed differences in behavior as unfortunate quirks of the affected person. Controversies among professionals concerning their perspectives on treatment procedures may be resolved over time with persistent education, sharing of information, and careful documentation of outcomes of treatments provided to patients of health care professionals.

Educational Settings. Educational facilities employ nearly half of all speech, language, and hearing clinicians (American Speech-Language-Hearing Association, August, 1988). These clinicians screen and test children and adolescents (1–21 years of age) for evidence of speech, language, and hearing problems and offer services as dictated by federal law. Any student who meets the selection criteria is automatically offered therapeutic intervention for the identified communication disorder. For those students, access to treatment is facilitated by the situation in which the child routinely is placed. Once the child is identified by school personnel as a candidate for therapy, parents finalize access to treatment by agreeing with the diagnostic findings and the individual educational program (IEP).

In spite of the proficiency of most public school systems in serving children with communication disorders, three external situational influences may impede a child's access to speech, language, and hearing services. First, some parents fail to sign the authorization to commence therapies. This failure to act may result from denial, resistance, or carelessness, but occasionally a parent believes an error has been made in regard to the child. In such cases, the desire for access to appropriate treatment can be pursued through a legal procedure with a hearing officer of the courts making the final summary and recommendations for the family and the school. A second external factor that impedes enrollment in appropriate therapy lies in the lack of definitive methods of testing for all possible types and combinations of communicative disorders. For unusual or unrecognized conditions, practices such as trial placement in inappropriate classrooms or a wait-and-observe protocol may postpone getting treatment. A third impediment exists for those who exhibit communication disorders that are not severe enough to warrant placement in a treatment program. Often, help for these potential clients must be sought in the private community-based sector.

Private Practice Services. Success in the private practice of service delivery to the communicatively disordered is well-founded in the need of the population-at-large for such services (American Speech-Language-Hearing Association, January, 1988). However, the cost of therapy often exceeds the personal budgets of clients, thus inhibiting their access to private services. Insurance funding supports diagnostic and treatment costs for designated periods of private therapy, and some public agencies and social organizations reimburse consultants who serve the communicatively handicapped. Typical target populations for these funds are the poor and the de-institutionalized.

Battin and Fox (1978) described a less well-recognized situational impediment to achieving appropriate treatment in the private practice domain as the unrefined expertise of the generalist. The particular need of a specific client may require expertise not acquired by the independent practitioner.

There are ways to circumvent these and most other external situational impediments and obtain help for a client with a speech, language, or hearing disorder. To succeed in overcoming obstacles, clients and families usually need the advocacy of a knowledgeable, concerned professional or interaction with a support group.

V. Expectations of the Potential Client and Caregiver

People seeking help with communication problems have *expectations* of what treatment involves and what outcomes will result from getting that treatment. Following the traditional medical perception of therapy as a progression from diagnosis to treatment to cure, clients bestow their trust and loyalty upon professional practitioners of speech, language, and hearing therapies. However, differences between anticipated and actual progress toward goals of treatment may disappoint even the most loyal client. The clinician is wise to identify client expectations of treatment results early in the relationship and incorporate reality orientation into the therapy plan, especially in this age of frequent malpractice claims. Communication therapy is not an instant cure and the length of treatment varies from client to client. It is essential that clients and caregivers understand the significance of habilitation through behavior change.

The request for help incorporates underlying hopes and fears of what a specialist's diagnosis will find, what must be done, and what the outcomes will be, that is, what the future holds. Imaginings of potential clients may or may not be realistic. Ideas and expectations may incorporate facts, myths, or superstitions gathered through a lifetime. Beliefs may be based entirely on referral from a trusted, experienced professional.

Different clients may exhibit communication disorders that are equally severe by standardized testing, but the impact of those disorders on speakers and listeners may vary greatly. Values, beliefs, feelings, and attitudes relate directly to the motivations and behaviors of clinicians and clients alike. The following definitions borrowed from social psychology apply to these terms in the communication disorders setting:

> *values:* broad abstract goals or standards. Values serve as criteria for judgments through which an individual may develop specific beliefs and attitudes (Rokeach, 1973).

beliefs: concepts or ideas that a person holds. Beliefs may or may not be founded in fact and are held separate from considerations of liking or disliking the referent (Fishbein & Ajzen, 1972).

feelings: emotional experiences that are dependent on both cognitive (naming and describing labels) and physiological (autonomic and endocrine reactions) factors (Schachter, 1964).

attitudes: essentially evaluative predispositions to liking or disliking behavior. Attitudes involve biases; prejudices, as in racial or religious discrimination; and preferences, as in literary or gustatory selection (Ajzen & Fishbein, 1977).

Caregivers and potential clients conceptualize the role of the professional in a limitless variety of ways. For some, the role of the communication disorders specialist is much like that of a physician who treats a disease with a fast-acting miracle drug, expecting treatment to consist of diagnosis and explicit prescription for a quick, curative regimen. Others may think of the clinician as an artist who paints a portrait, expecting the clinician to analyze and synthesize the client's traits and behaviors and then to create or restore an ideal or normal individual.

The specialist is expected to assume responsibility for treatment and guidance of the client through a process. While that may seem a straightforward expectation, the manner in which it is internalized makes a dramatic difference in the actual role and job of the clinician. To clarify this idea, four different client/caregiver perspectives are designated: objective, nonparticipatory, depressed, and resigned.

Objective clients and caregivers gather information, identify steps to be taken, and initiate participation in the course outlined by the clinician. Such clients and caregivers ask questions and share ideas and experiences. They show their understanding and appreciation of their own and their combined progress in acquiring the minute steps of the treatment of the communication disorder. Clients who enjoy this type of environment make substantial progress according to their actual abilities.

The *nonparticipant* delivers the client to the clinical setting, steps back, literally or figuratively, and waits for the professional to do the necessary work and return the finished product. The nonparticipant may be either the caregiver or the client. The essential message of such behavior is, "We trust you, the expert, to resolve this communication problem, because you have the solution and know how to apply your skills to our needs." Some nonparticipants even feel that they are paying dearly for professional care and therefore interpret their expectations into unreasonable demands on the clinician as well as on themselves. In so doing, they anticipate removal of the problem and return to normal daily life, while they remain distant from the problem, its treatment, and its resolution. The clinician must make choices in dealing with such situations. When the distancing phenomenon is observed in the caregiver, the essential choice is whether to modify the caregiver's behavior or incorporate into the client's treatment scheme the necessary coping skills to facilitate dealing with the unyielding attitude and consequent behavior of the caregiver. When the distancing phenomenon is found in the client, treatment must incorporate methods for reducing the denial of involvement.

Depressed clients and caregivers often present an anxious, saddened, euphoric, or confused demeanor, compensating for feelings of embarrassment, inadequacy, or distress. Having discovered a behavior problem beyond their own resolution, they often believe that they are less than they should be. While they have accepted the need for professional help with a recognized problem, these clients and caregivers continue to grieve for the loss of the ideal infant, child, friend, spouse, or parent for whom they seek help. Verbal and nonverbal behaviors noted in these individuals may reflect feelings of denial, anger, and sadness, all of which affect the problem that the clinician is expected to resolve. Reassurance and objectivity are two critical ingredients that the clinician must add to the bank of treatments provided for these clients and caregivers.

Resigned attitudes found among clients and caregivers indicate acceptance of a belief that they are no more than they should be. They view the communication disorder as further evidence of their failure to belong in the normative plane of society. They think of the problem as one more notice of their low status, or they see the need for additional help as symbolic of the hopelessness with which they face all aspects of their lives. Their attitude says, "We are here because we must be here; we will comply with the demands this service imposes upon us." This attitude is often associated with many generations of poverty, psychological and physical abuse, or a notion of being perceived as societal outcasts. Such self-negation may also be associated with psychiatric illnesses such as severe depression, paranoia, or dementia.

Recording Observations. Table 4.1 presents a generic checklist that has been found useful for recording observations of client or caregiver behaviors. While this is not a scale to assess or rate behaviors, it gives the observer a method of noting and monitoring characteristics of interactive behaviors. Behaviors that are observed to interfere with communication can be incorporated into therapy by the use of counseling techniques. The client/caregiver behavior checklist also provides a mechanism for the clinician to compare observations and impressions with those of supervisors and colleagues.

To use the checklist, the observer circles the number of an item under each subheading which seems to describe best the individual observed. Recording observed behaviors and impressions in this way will often help clinicians plan for and work with the observed individuals. Also, clinicians with heavy caseloads and who see some clients infrequently can quickly review a checklist completed during a previous session to refresh their

Table 4.1
Client/caregiver behavior checklist

I. Approach to situation
1. Cooperative and friendly
2. Tense and anxious
3. Lack of interest and involvement
4. Willing, but poor comprehension/ability
5. Resistant, suspicious, distrustful
6. Does not apply

II. Affect/attitude
1. Competent/centric, realistic, coping
2. Happy, pleased
3. External center of focus
4. Unhappy
5. Indifferent, apathetic
6. Distressed

III. Information level
1. Appropriate for circumstances/accurate
2. Seeks/requests/asks for more
3. Generally uninformed/needs information
4. Misinformed
5. Does not want information
6. Does not apply

IV. Appearance and grooming
1. Looks healthy/well
2. Appropriate/comfortable
3. Unkempt/shabby
4. Looks tired
5. Appears to be ill
6. Does not apply

V. Style of interaction/communication
1. Open give-and-take
2. Deliberate, orderly, self-correcting
3. Random, careless
4. Inconsistent (combination of 2 & 3)
5. Apparent lack of interest/motivation
6. Does not apply

VI. Speech of responding
1. Maintains conversational rhythm and pace
2. Apparent pre-visit preparation
3. Reflective and thoughtful
4. Impulsive and rapid
5. Slow/apparently careless
6. Does not apply

Table 4.1 (continued)
Client/caregiver behavior checklist

VII. Involvement level
    1. Realistic/managing situation
    2. Above average
    3. Average
    4. Below average
    5. Indifferent
    6. Does not apply
VIII. Communication and language skills
    1. Reflects cognitive and affective information
    2. Fluent, spontaneous, mature
    3. Not spontaneous, brief, unelaborated
    4. Quiet/restrained/hesitant
    5. Apparent disorder/difference
    6. Does not apply
IX. Response to instruction/suggestions
    1. Follows successfully/no apparent problems
    2. Requests repetition
    3. Needs clarification
    4. Attends but shows no comprehension
    5. Appears confused
    6. Does not apply
X. Reaction to new ideas
    1. Provides suggestions
    2. Adapts readily and easily
    3. Has difficulty adjusting to new task
    4. Confusion and perseveration noted
    5. Rejects anything new/different
    6. Does not apply
XI. Response to difficulty/frustration
    1. Recognition of difficulty
    2. Tolerance/patience
    3. Consistent effort to respond/interact
    4. Adequate effort – willing to take risks
    5. Disregard for the difficulty/problem
    6. Does not apply
XII. Estimated validity and reliability of interview
    1. Complete
    2. Valid and reliable
    3. Not valid or reliable
    4. Incomplete information available
    5. Interview interrupted by other
    6. Does not apply

---

memory about observed behaviors. A brief review of impressions of client characteristics allows the clinician to enter the therapy room better prepared to meet the counseling needs of the client. In other situations, recurrent and consistent notations on a behavior checklist can be used as evidence of need for referral for additional medical or psychological treatment of the client. Those who find the checklist useful may want to modify it to serve the counseling needs of their clients more effectively. The checklist can be useful during intake and assessment as well as throughout treatment.

Ideally, the caregiver and potential client exhibit none of the extreme perspectives suggested. With guidance and counseling, the client and caregiver establish realistic perspectives on the disorder, its prognosis, and the work to be done. Through understanding and acceptance of shared responsibilities in accomplishing the best outcomes, they commit their own energies and resources to the rehabilitation process. The clinician guides the treatment with knowledge and empathy. Whatever perspective the client brings to the therapy setting, the clinician accepts it and adjusts procedures to accommodate and enhance those traits which are expected to be conducive to rehabilitation.

❧ ❧ ❧

BECOMING A CLIENT: A TRANSITION PERIOD

Potential clients enter communication treatment settings from many different backgrounds, each containing its own unique external situational factors. As Backus (1960) predicted, the discipline of communication disorders has grown rapidly and technically. In highly technical human services disciplines, efforts toward efficiency and professionalism often seem to take precedence over the personal aspects of clients and the relationship between clinicians and clients. Intensive professional identification of the communication disorders discipline with the medical sciences has come about through interdisciplinary treatment of health-related communication disorders. Among the many outcomes of those collaborative efforts has been the adoption of medicine's prioritization of problem-oriented treatment.

Problem-oriented Treatment. Clients referred by other professionals often present a folder of records to the communication disorders clinician. Problem-oriented records contain data and notes that focus on professional considerations of clinical problem-solving (American Speech, Language, Hearing Association, 1984; Frattali, 1986; Kent & Chabon, 1980; Weed, 1969). The receiving clinician may elect to accept that content of such documentation as sufficient, deciding not to undertake completion of an independent case history of the client or an extensive assessment of the designated disorder. Immediate and brief assessment of the client's communicative condition may be followed quickly with the initiation of treatment. Treatment may be structured, following a formula or program. A different therapy mode sometimes applied in the referral situation follows the diagnostic therapy scheme. Based on data in hand, the clinician begins at the point of probable deficit and cautiously applies treatment, observation, and diagnosis techniques to discern the most efficient way of reducing the communication handicap. From this point, careful recording of plans and progress notes ensure that therapy is having a positive effect on the problem being treated. These and similar procedures are often found in hospital and health care facilities where in-house referrals are routine. Such procedures place the speech, language, and hearing clinician in the situation recognized in health care disciplines (Scheuerle, Olsen, Guilford, Redding, & Habal, 1984). In the absence of training in counseling and the presence of institutional restraints on holistic therapies, each clinician is left to apply personal beliefs, values, and causally developed interactive skills to the management of client needs for counseling.

An inherent risk in the problem-oriented method of intake, assessment, and treatment is that the disorder remains the focus of the interaction while the client as a whole becomes secondary (Flower, 1984; Scheuerle et al., 1984). Additionally, the increasing paperwork associated with speech-language pathology and audiology in the educational setting may have a similar effect of reducing the significance of holistic treatment, even though creation and administration of the Individual Education Plan was designed to avoid just that.

Client-Centered Intake. A different perspective on client, caregiver, and clinician interaction, which Backus (1960) called the *I-Thou relationship,* can be found in the works of Emerik and Hatten (1979) and Darley and Spriestersbach (1978). These authors consider the initial interview to be the essence of client intake and assessment. The client remains central in this approach, and work on resolution of the problem is the target of both client and clinician. The focus of this intake method aligns itself with the counseling paradigm more satisfactorily than does the problem-oriented method. The initial interview provides the climate to establish rapport, dispense information, and confirm and augment information derived from the client's records. Likewise, the interaction is a ready-made opportunity to observe behavior, gather data about the client, and formulate initial impressions of the appropriateness of recommendations for therapy or referral. Table 4.2 contains a list of clinical observations that can be made informally and that greatly aid the counselor.

Intake: Questionnaires and Interviews

Some speech, language, and hearing clinics facilitate the intake process with the use of mail-in case history questionnaires. Samples of client

Table 4.2
Informal clinical observations

Physical appearance and motor behavior
1. Size – height, weight (relative to family)
2. Coloring – hair, eyes, pallor, flushed
3. Grooming and dress
4. Facial appearance – asymmetries, mouth breathing, allergic "shiners," teeth, facial expression
5. Physical anomalies – facial features, hands, head shape, visible scars, discolorations
6. Gait
7. Balance – especially when moving, changing from sitting to walking
8. Hand preference – difficulty in tool manipulation, tremor upon extension
9. Tension release behaviors – hair twisting, foot jiggling, finger scratching, cheek chewing, wiggling, rising from seat
10. Drooling – when does it occur?
11. Thumb sucking, nail chewing
12. Facial grimaces, tics
13. Eye blinking, winking
14. Oculomotor problems – movement, bilateral incoordination
15. Visual acuity, attention, attention span
16. Auditory acuity, attention, attention span
17. Posture – body, head, facial aversion
18. Atypical tonus – hypotonic, hypertonic, tremor, jerky movements (limbs, head and neck, chin, lips and oral structures)
19. Activity level – appropriate for age
20. Vocal characteristics – appropriate for age and size
21. Acoustic evidence of vocal tract control and coordination

records and case history forms can be found in a variety of texts on diagnostic methods in speech-language pathology and audiology. The completion and return of the case history form by potential clients and caregivers constitute an application for evaluation and treatment of a communication disorder. The completed forms initiate the process of scheduling intake sessions as they are received by the clinic. In other settings, practitioners of speech-language pathology and audiology indicate that such questionnaires are cumbersome and time-consuming. They find that responses are unreliable and information must be checked against the client's records. Some practitioners add that, in practices open to the public, initial appointments often result from walk-in clients and telephone contacts, precluding the opportunity to complete elaborate written forms. However, many clinicians find that completed case history questionnaires are valuable guides for preparing for the initial interview with new clients and caregivers.

Table 4.2 (continued)
Informal clinical observations

Personal-social behaviors
  1. Interaction between client and caregiver – proxemics, conversation, social skills, observation
      • Is play aimless and random?
      • Is play stereotyped, creative, imaginative?
  2. Affect – friendly, shy, relaxed, tense, comfortable, anxious, passive, crisis behavior
  3. Caregiver-client interaction – degree of dependency versus independence; amount of control or direction by caregiver; nature of caregiver's verbal and nonverbal messages; separate easily or not
  4. Clinician-client interaction – client reaction to stranger, tactile defensiveness

Communicative/attentional behaviors
  1. Client nonverbal, nonvocal behaviors – gestures: elaborate or abstract, ratio of gesture/verbal communication; eye contact and facial scanning; turn-taking patterns
  2. Response to stimulation – across various sensory modalities
  3. Distractibility – response to multiple simultaneous stimulation; scanning ability; response lag time; effect of unexpected incidental stimuli
  4. Attention span – quality of attention; need for special cues to alert client to new task
  5. Verbal patterns – jargon, prosodic features, voice, echolalia, mumbling, length of utterances, articulation (intelligible), sentence fragments, correct syntax, appropriate semantics (stays on topic); age-appropriate vocabulary, comprehension and expression of language; fluency
  6. Caregiver communication – amount, level, complexity, appropriate for condition of the client

The beginning clinician, or one adapting to a new community or professional setting, may have difficulty developing techniques of interviewing and feeling at ease in the interview situation. Discomfort on the part of the clinician affects the progress of the interview, the client's perception of the clinician as a professional, and outcomes of the initial session for the client-clinician relationship. When used appropriately, the information gathered in a case history questionnaire and records from referral sources can provide helpful, reassuring tools to organize the clinician's thoughts and materials in preparation for the initial interview.

A Word of Caution. The clinician must always take great care to avoid misinterpretation by *guessing* at a respondent's meaning or prejudging the person completing the form or the potential client. The clinician should strive to extract pertinent facts from the perspective of the parties who submitted the information. It is helpful to remember that the clinician is interpreting responses to another person's interpretation of the questions.

The entering client or caregiver presents the clinician with the identified or suspected problem, a communication disorder, and unidentified problematical conditions. Regardless of the accuracy or completeness of questionnaire responses, the counselor should accept them as a contribution by a person interested in rehabilitation. During the initial dialogue, reviewing the questionnaire items and the client/caregiver's responses to clarify, expand, and update information gives an organizational structure to the communication. This procedure places both parties on common ground, reducing the risk often inherent in surprise questions.

The counselor should keep in mind that the request for help often signals a below-normal self-perception on the part of the client or caregiver. The clinician must exercise caution in the identification and approach to non-specified but suspected problems that may evoke strong feelings. The client may or may not have experience in handling those feelings by talking about them. Feelings that have never been addressed verbally are often difficult to acknowledge and discuss. As indicated in chapter 2, clients often reveal unrecognized and unacknowledged concerns or feelings nonverbally. Counselors frequently find that the simple act of naming a nonverbally expressed feeling or concern enables the client to grasp the experience and begin to deal with it in a positive way.

An insightful clinician may infer many of the client's or caregiver's concerns that are not verbalized. The clinician's world view, set of values, professional knowledge, and skill serve as the starting point for any such inferences. By gathering data from records, the intake interview, and observations, the clinician can discern those aspects of client or caregiver behavior, both verbal and nonverbal, that comprise the topic of concern. The counselor may identify and reflect a topic verbally in a way that names the concern without judging its importance. This counseling behavior constitutes an invitation to the client or caregiver to agree or disagree with the clinician, to accept or reject the clinician's observation and statement, and to join or not to join in the discussion of the named concern. Thus, even the most experienced clinician must test inferences through discussion and clarification with the client.

Intake: Preparation for Treatment

To prepare for a first interaction with an applicant from an unfamiliar socio-cultural background, the clinician should include research on the community environment and daily-life experience of the client. In addition to selecting nonbiased and culture-free tests and therapy materials, the clinician must exhibit a professional behavior that represents an attitude congruent with those same principles. Reviewing records of clients from the same or similar geographical environments can be a tremendous resource for understanding holistic client needs. An appreciation of the subtleties that influence the client's behavior, and therefore the progress through treatment, assists in anticipating the clinician's counseling role. Together, these elements contribute to the formulation of prognostic statements early in the relationship.

For example, consider Earnest, a 9-year-old Zuni Indian boy, who was referred for language assessment by his teacher at the Consolidated Zuni School. The reason for the referral was his academic difficulties in the third grade. The astute clinician recognizes that Earnest is a member of a population identified as underserved by speech-language pathologists and audiologists. The counselor further knows that Earnest's life and that of his family are profoundly influenced by cultural traditions (Benedict, 1989; Brugge, Brogan, & Quam, 1972; Camazine, 1980; Lasiloo, Lewis, & Gray, 1975; Osborne, 1989; Smith & Roberts, 1954; and Vinje, 1982). The counselor must approach Earnest and his parents in a way that will be meaningful and acceptable to them and be sensitive to their perspective that the agency that has identified the child's potential problem is foreign to their tribal community.

The counselor realizes that Zuni ideals and institutions are rigorous and committed to precedent and tradition (Benedict, 1989). For this family, influences such as individualism or "being different" are contrary to tradition, uncongenial, and to be avoided. Among other things, the counselor must discern whether Earnest's apparent need for help identifies him as too much of an individual for the Zuni perspective. Can this request for a language evaluation be seen as part of the child's regular educational experience and not as a threat to Earnest's tribal position? Questions that the counselor must consider before meeting Earnest include: What place has this request for help come to hold in the life of the child and family? What degree of comfort do family members feel with the decision to keep the appointment? Will the child and family accept and comply with the clinician's recommendations as part of the natural flow of Earnest's life? Will each parent continue to accept the child as formerly if he needs special rehabilitative attention? Will these parents be able to discuss their concerns about the matter with the counselor, who is a stranger?

Before formulating a counseling plan, the clinician will need information about the manner in which Earnest's difference is displayed, how others react to it, and his management of that feedback within the environments that comprise his home and school. The counselor can gather this information through direct interaction with the client and family .

In fact, some experienced clinicians prefer to interview the client without bias introduced by reading records. Nevertheless, the counselor who is familiar with the socio-cultural background of the client can gain a great deal of insight into the client's problem behavior by learning about, interacting with, and observing the client and family. Further, the impact of the family communication network on the client's interactive behavior can be identified for discussion during treatment or noted for further investigation.

Intake Counseling Goals. The goal of the initial session is to gather and clarify enough information to rule out and rule in areas of professional concern. Throughout the session, the counselor is alert to provide information to the client and caregiver according to their readiness to receive it. Questions that demand answers and unfamiliar ideas that require clarification may arise. By assimilating all available information, the clinician formulates recommendations for treatment or referral to another resource and presents and discusses these plans with the client/caregiver. Prior to the close of the initial session, the clinician should arrange appointments for recommended follow-up testing or treatment. Through verbal and nonverbal communication skills, the counselor enables the client and family to understand and accept information derived from their initial session together. The clinician who takes care to offer explanations that are clear and acceptable to the client and caregiver is likely to meet with the greatest cooperation. Goals for the initial session are most readily accomplished when the clinician incorporates the entire family's concerns and priorities into overall planning.

An experienced clinician may experience tension in meeting a new client from an unfamiliar background. Such anticipation of diagnosis, prognosis, and planning for the new client is expected and stimulates professional excitement. Meeting and serving each new client provide the counselor both challenges and rewards.

❦ ❦ ❦

COUNSELING IN TREATMENT OF COMMUNICATION DISORDERS

The four distinguished categories of communication disorders are derived from dysfunctions of the normal communication process. Risks to the normal communication process are associated with the four determiners of communication skills. Biological risks to normal communicative function are found in the genetics, pre- and postnatal development, wellness, maintenance, and aging of the body, particularly the brain. Cognitive risks involve genetic and prenatal influences as well as stimulation-response interactions within the postnatal environment. Risks to psycho-social adaptation lie in the ability of the individual to adjust the self or to modify the environment. Risks in the environment depend on whether it supplies sufficient communicative experiences and rewards.

The complex overlapping matrix of influences on and risks to acquiring and maintaining appropriate communicative skills may seem to imply an infinite and unmanageable number of ways that the communicative process is molded and modified for each individual. For the purpose of exploring the role of counseling in treatment of clients and caregivers, we will set aside the numerous professional categories of specific disorders and approach the problem more appropriately from a perspective like that of the client or caregiver. Clients and caregivers often indicate interest in knowing what is the matter, what caused it, whether they did something wrong, and what can be done to fix it. They frequently introduce these questions to communications specialists because those professionals are easy to talk to and have shown concern for the client or caregiver. To address such questions, we can utilize arbitrary categories of congenital and postnatal adventitious dysfunctions. Both these categories include genetic and environmental factors, but birth is the most dramatic delineation of the usual stages in the life span. Birth inaugurates a specific, dated reference point for the life of the client and provides a starting place for exploring the onset of the communicative condition and the interpersonal relationships built around it or in spite of it.

Counseling needs across disorders and throughout the treatment of communication problems depend on clients' and caregivers' characteristics. Those characteristics include individual and shared integrity and cohesiveness; customs, competencies, and experiences in maintaining focus on a specific task; management of alterations to routines; capacities to comprehend findings concerning the communication disorder; and mutual valuation of the client's acquisition of proficient communicative skills. Accordingly, regardless of the specific disorder, counseling needs during treatment can be considered in terms of the magnitude of the problem and the ability of clients and caregivers to handle the demands it imposes on their daily lives. To look at these counseling needs, we can consider a sampling of disorders from the perspective of four prognostic categories: preventable, remediable, modifiable, and irreversible.

I. Prevention

Prevention suggests elimination of the causes of communication disorders ("Prevention '89/'90", 1990). That is, the communication disorder is averted when the potential condition is known, its etiology understood, and the risk eliminated. However, the concept of prevention held by the American Speech-Language-Hearing Association (ASHA) has been influenced by federal policies and terminologies. In the mid-1970s the U.S. Department of Health, Education, and Welfare placed national emphasis on wellness. That agency identified several levels of care: Preventive, Primary, Secondary, Tertiary, Restorative, and Long-term. Preventive Care was described primarily as education and prevention through community health services. Shortly thereafter, medical and nursing disciplines adopted terminology descriptive of three levels of care:

1. Primary Care—the point of entry of the patient into the health system for care oriented toward prevention of disease and treatment of common, uncomplicated, or chronic illnesses in an outpatient setting.
2. Secondary Care—referral of a patient for treatment of a specific condition by professionals who specialize in that type of treatment.
3. Tertiary Care—referral of a patient from primary or secondary level for treatment of complex or complicated health needs that require highly refined knowledge and skill in a clinical specialty area.

The 1983 ASHA Committee on Prevention of Speech, Language, and Hearing Problems (American Speech-Language-Hearing Association, 1984) reported need for but limited training in prevention of communication disorders. The concept of levels of care was adapted to present levels of prevention. Four years later, the Legislative Council of the national association adopted a revised position statement on the prevention of speech, language, and hearing disorders defining three levels of prevention of communication disorders (American Speech-Language-Hearing Association, 1988):

1. Primary Prevention—the elimination or inhibition of the onset and development of a communication disorder by altering susceptibility or reducing exposure for susceptible persons.
2. Secondary Prevention—the early detection and treatment of communication disorders. Early detection and treatment may lead to the elimination of the disorder or the retardation of the disorder's progress, thereby preventing further complications.
3. Tertiary Prevention—the reduction of a disability by attempting to restore effective functioning. The major approach is *rehabilitation* of the disabled individual who has realized some residual problem as a result of the disorder. (p. 90)

The discussion of prevention will be limited to the consideration of those conditions that ASHA defines as primary prevention. Secondary and tertiary prevention as defined by ASHA will be discussed more appropriately in later sections of this chapter under the topics of remediation and modification of communication disorders.

A lack of communication is one of the chief barriers to dynamic forward movement toward the prevention of communication disorders. Common language is needed among disciplines to enable collective intervention in the many facets of prevention of communication disorders.

Marge (1984) discussed a prevention matrix of strategies and community resource personnel. He suggested strategies to reduce the incidence of handicapping conditions derived from health, education, and welfare. Preventive measures include the decrease of disease and dysfunction, increase of wellness, extension of developmental monitoring across the age span, and elimination of poverty in all urban and rural areas. The immensity of the task is overwhelming. The large majority of communication specialists expend their energies on intervention in forms of identification, diagnosis, and treatment of existing disorders.

Chezik, Pratt, Stewart, and Deal (1989) described family intervention for the prevention of communication disorders in high-risk children. One reason for the slow development of prevention as a specialty of speech pathology and audiology may have to do with the scarcity of positions that provide a livelihood. As a result, some speech pathologists and audiologists with a professional interest in prevention of communication disorders have added a specialization that is recognized in a second field of influence. For an example, Sylvia O. Richardson, M.D., started work in speech pathology that led her to advanced training in pediatric medicine and a successful career dedicated to reducing the language and learning needs of children in the United States and abroad. Other communication disorders specialists have undertaken doctoral work in the field of public health (Communication Disorders Prevention and Epidemiology Study Group, 1989). In that field, they perceive the opportunity to initiate much-needed epidemiological research, as suggested by Davis and Sancho (1988), to establish a causal model for the prevention of communication disorders.

Systematic training in the prevention of communication disorders is not yet available to the clinical student in speech-language pathology or audiology. Additionally, there is no organized resource for information about the experiences of clinicians who work with populations that need the service of prevention of conditions causing communication disorders. In the absence of such training or resources, examples of common preventive practices that apply to congenital and postnatal or adventitious communications disorders may be helpful.

Congenital Conditions and Prevention of Related Communication Disorders. Prevention of communication disorders dominates the role of speech-language pathologists and audiologists who serve on high-risk infant care, neural-tube defects, genetic anomalies, or craniofacial teams. These multidisciplinary professional groups collaborate to share knowledge and experience in the management of handicapping conditions among patients from birth through the developmental years. In these settings, parents of an existing patient need and want counseling for themselves as well as for the patient. Parental understanding and acceptance of the patient's condition, care requirements, and prognosis invariably elicit questions about future pregnancies and the risk of having another baby with the same or similar congenital defects or dysfunctions.

Treatment Knowledge Base. To participate effectively in an interaction with these parents, the audiologist and speech pathologist must be knowledgeable of syndromes, anomalads, intra-uterine environmental teratogens, and sporadic birth defects. The clinician must understand dominant and recessive genetic traits, accidents of timing in fetal development and trans-placental passage of agents due to maternal exposure to viruses, drugs, alcohol, and environmental contaminants. Information concerning these matters in relation to speech, language, or hearing problems is covered in specialized courses in university training programs. The clinician must also be aware that physical abuse during pregnancy, like accidental trauma, can inflict damage to the unborn fetus. Low birth weight, premature delivery, and fetal malnutrition are hazards to the normal development of body systems, which are the foundation for normal speech, language, and hearing. Prenatal development problems that are precursors to communication disorders include neurological damage, head and face dysmorphologies, muscle tone deficits, and perceptual defects, especially congenital deafness.

A team geneticist or genetics counselor is an immediate primary resource for probability data about the recurrence of each inheritable condition expressed in the current patient and potential conditions that are possible or probable in additional children. At some institutions, teams also have access to fetologists, radiologists, and obstetricians who collaborate on monitoring prenatal development. Whether or not the communication specialist has access to those types of expertise, it is helpful to maintain a reference shelf of factual and probability data to counsel parents struggling with decisions about having more children and the future of their families. Table 4.3 provides a list of resources for information about prenatal conditions that cause communication disorders.

Parent Reactions and Concerns. Parents with a disabled child are usually dealing with the loss of their ideal/perfect child and the many unanticipated anxieties and demands brought about by having a different child. As they ponder and investigate their own ability to be normal parents to a normal second child, some parents will have heard of in-utero tests such as amniocentesis and sonography to aid in the early identification of chemical, genetic, and visible fetal defects. Typically, parents will be informed of these and other scientific resources by other members of the team. Their motivation to discuss such medical information with the speech pathologist or audiologist is more likely to request counseling than to seek additional technical information.

The counselor is expected to assist the parents through identification, discussion, and exploration of the risks involved in having additional natural children. The clinician has a variety of options to introduce, ranging from no alteration in sexual practices to implementation of birth control, sterilization of one or both parents, or abortion in the case of an existing embryo. These intimate thoughts and decisions have obvious implications for and are influenced by religious or ethical beliefs and moral values of the individuals involved or even their immediate and extended families.

Table 4.3
Resources for information about prenatal conditions that cause communication disorders

---

Galjaard, H. (1980). *Genetic metabolic diseases*. Amsterdam: Elsevier North Holland.

Goodman, R., & Gorlin, R. (1977). *Atlas of the face in genetic disorders*. St. Louis: C. V. Mosby.

Gorlin, R., & Pindburg, J. (1964). *Syndromes of the head and neck*. New York: McGraw-Hill.

Jaffe, B. F. (Ed.) (1977). *Hearing loss in children: A comprehensive text*. Baltimore: University Park Press.

Jung, J. H. (1989). *Genetic syndromes in communication disorders*. Boston: Little, Brown.

Konigsmark, B. W., & Gorlin, R. J. (1976). *Genetic and metabolic deafness*. Philadelphia: W. B. Saunders.

McKusick, V. A. (1972). *Heritable disorders of connective tissue* (4th ed.). St. Louis: C. V. Mosby.

McKusick, V. A. (1986). *Mendelian inheritance in man* (7th ed.). Baltimore: Johns Hopkins University Press.

Northern, J. L., & Downs, M. P. (1984). *Hearing in children* (3rd ed.). Baltimore: Williams and Wilkins.

Smith, D. W. (1982). *Recognizable patterns of human malformation: Genetic embryologic and clinical aspects* (3rd ed.). Philadelphia: W. B. Saunders.

Sparks, S. (1984). *Birth defects and speech and language disorders*. San Diego: College-Hill Press.

Taybi, H., & Lachman, R. S. (1989). *Radiology of syndromes, metabolic disorders, and skeletal dysplasias* (3rd ed.). Chicago: Year Book Medical Publishing.

Likewise, discussions of this nature involve the beliefs and commitment of the counselor.

Realistically, the risks of having another affected baby include the drain on time and energy of the parents, as well as reduction of time and attention now given to their first child alone. Reduced interaction with the affected child will modify the home language environment of the child. Also, the additional demands for parental involvement with two affected children may overload the parents in physical, emotional, and economic ways and increase stress on the relationship between the parents. The disruption of marital stress on a family dramatically changes the home communication environment of the child. On the other hand, the probability of having a normal second child is very high in families whose child's congenital problems were caused by a foreign agent, such as a prescribed medication taken during pregnancy or exposure of the mother to the rubella virus during the first trimester of pregnancy. The family may benefit greatly in many ways from the birth of a non-affected second child, and the siblings can become a life-long mutual support system. Parents who love children and want to have a larger family face a dilemma. Their fear of imposing similar handicapping conditions on another child is in direct conflict with their plans, dreams, and earlier expectations.

Clinician/Counselor Constraints.   In discussions of any thoughts and feelings with families, the counselor must refrain from imposing biases on the decisions of the parents. At the same time, the counselor must accept and confirm ideas and feelings that are founded in fact and give honest, informed opinions if asked, and when appropriate. A beginning clinician may be uneasy about giving opinions to clients even when it seems the only acceptable, humane, and informed thing to do. Different recommendations from various professionals may be misconstrued as one opinion being right and the other wrong. All too often, unexplained differences of opinion among professionals can lead hurt, distressed, or confused parents to a decision that they and their child have been victims of malpractice. The dilemma of how to give an opinion when appropriate without jeopardizing ethical practice can be resolved. Stating a professional or personal opinion is legal and ethical when it is presented in a form that clearly indicates the statement is an opinion, neither advice nor recommendation (L. Stein, personal communication, 1979). Further, the practice of any human services discipline is not an exact science, so the individual expertise of the practitioner determines the quality of service rendered. Based on these concepts, clinicians are encouraged to give professional and personal opinions with caution and to introduce the opinion with appropriate language. For example, when a professional gives an opinion that incorporates consideration of the family situation, the magnitude of the congenital problem, and the likelihood of recurrence of the problem, the clinician can say:

My opinion is that . . .
or
In my professional opinion . . .
or
If I were making this decision for my family, I'd opt for . . .
or
If I had to make the decision, I would . . .
or
If it were I, I would choose . . .

Any of these or comparable clauses indicates that the remainder of the statement applies to the world of the speaker only and not to the world of the client or caregiver. That is, the clinician is not telling the client or caregiver what to do. Any one of those statements would be followed by a second statement, such as:

> You have the right to make your own decision and to live by your beliefs. Whatever you decide, our team is here to work with you and your family.
> *or*
> There is no right or wrong decision. You must decide for yourselves. You have some hard choices to make. I can help you with information and opinion, but ultimately the decision is yours.
> *or*
> Now that I have given you my opinion, you may want to seek a second opinion as you are working on this decision. I can suggest other professionals who have experience working with clients who have similar conditions.

With open and honest discussion, the counselor shares and elicits ideas and helps the parents find words to express their own thoughts, that is, to wrap language around covert internal wanderings. Feelings and attitudes that have been hidden, unnamed aspects of turmoil generating fear and doubt become recognizable entities that the clinician can address in a forthright manner through the use of simple, everyday vocabulary. The outcomes of such discussions are as varied as the parents. The specialist can inform and educate families in measures of prevention of congenital causes of communication disorders, but ultimately must abide by the decision and behavior of the parents or the caregivers of the client.

Prevention of Adventitious Communication Disorders. Many aspects of adventitious communication disorders generate differences in the magnitude of the problem created for the client or caregiver. Age of onset and severity are commonly considered two remarkable factors in determining the necessary management of the resulting communicative abilities. Prevention of adventitious communication disorders involves the diverse framework of society, including home, community, industry, and government. Individuals develop throughout the life span among these settings. The influences on communication abilities that may enter those settings over a lifetime include development/maturation, home environment, disease, trauma-injury, and daily living experience.

Development/Maturation. The concepts of development and maturation are often misconstrued as referring only to the early years of life. In fact, normal development traces an ongoing sequence of changes and modulations throughout the life span in every simple and complex mode of existence. Developmental progress can be impeded in ways that are not predictable. In children, for example, autism is considered a developmental condition believed to be related to brain dysfunction (Springer & Deutsch, 1985), for which the cause is unknown. Prevention of autism is therefore one of many keenly interesting topics for which research is needed to understand the condition, its incidence, and etiology. In the aging population, unpredictable development often leads to the onset of dementia (Schow, Christensen, Hutchinson, & Nerbonne, 1978), which continues to challenge the best of modern medical scientists to explain causes or prevent cognitive deterioration. Some types of dementia may be familial, but there is a lack of consistency even in the scarce research available. Why some aging individuals suffer this malady and others do not remains a mystery. Many members of the aging population retain their cognitive powers and communicative abilities (Butler & Lewis, 1986). Mental facility can be readily observed in the enthusiastic activities of the American Association of Retired Persons (AARP).

Some genetic conditions are precursors to physiological changes that are not evident until adulthood or middle age. Examples of these conditions are some types of inherited hearing loss and select neurological degenerative diseases. Another example, Huntington's disease, typically occurs in middle age (Butler & Lewis, 1986; Hogg, Massey, & Schoenberg, 1979). Since these late-developing conditions are not preventable or curable, they will be included in a later section on counseling for clients with irreversible communication disorders.

In addition, some communication disorders appear to be developmental problems that are manifested and aggravated through interaction with agents in the environment. Two such communication disorders are childhood stuttering (Bjerkan, 1980; Dickson, 1971; Van Riper & Emerick, 1990) and chronic conductive hearing loss in childhood due to otitis media with effusion (Brandes & Ehinger, 1981; Davis, 1986; Klein, 1986; Todd, 1986). Because these conditions are typically found in childhood, their management usually involves the parents, who must modify their interaction with the child and change or adapt the child's communication environment.

Home Environment. For a child who is experiencing dysfluency, environmental changes needed include the reduction of environmental stress and the child's reaction to it, as well as parental support of the normal communication abilities of the child. A child with conductive hearing loss may need to use low gain amplification or hearing aids, with frequent hearing tests to assure proper instrument fit. Timely and age-appropriate language stimulation by the parent is essential, and medical or surgical intervention may be required. While the clinician is dedicated to the care of the child, it is the parent who is responsible for orchestrating the environmental changes that will be reflected in the communicative proficiency of the child.

Counseling of parents in these cases involves helping them to perceive the problem as subordinate and to recognize the dominant place of the whole child in family relationships. Together, the clinician and the parents will explore the child's experiences, behaviors, reactions, and feelings. The parents may discover aspects of the child or themselves that they do not like. The parents' feelings of anxiety, guilt, anger, hostility, or fear can interfere with their work with the child. The clinician can often bring out these feelings in the open discourse of counseling sessions. During counseling sessions, self-discoveries or self-disclosures often serve as moments of enlightenment that help the parents make sense of obscure remembered happenings. However, when these discoveries surface and begin to interfere with the progress of treatment for the dysfluent or hearing-impaired client, the speech-language pathologist or audiologist may wish to refer the parent or family for psychotherapy. In many instances, such referrals are essential for satisfactory, lasting resolution of the child's communication problem. However, referrals to psychotherapy are often rejected or ignored by needful parents and clients. The clinician who perceives the need for such a referral must spend sufficient time, perhaps even several counseling sessions, preparing the parent or client for reception of and appropriate follow-through on the referral.

When making referrals to colleagues within an institution or a community, the clinician is well advised to know the professional strengths of the colleague and to be aware of the match between personalities and philosophies of the professional and the family being referred for treatment. This suggestion is based on two disparate reasons. On the one hand, the referring clinician has an ethical responsibility to see that clients receive the best possible care. On the other hand, the client is being referred for a specific mode of treatment that does not preclude the need for further treatment of the communication disorder. With a successful referral, the communication clinician is assured that the family's interfering developmental or maturational problems are being treated while continuing communication therapies can move forward simultaneously. Neither problem area should be treated to the exclusion of the other.

Disease.   In preventing communication disorders caused by disease, clinicians join other professionals in the human services fields to encourage wellness. Wellness is necessary to maximize the potential of each individual. There are many types of diseases—some are infectious, some tumorous, involving uncontrolled cellular growth, some degenerative. Preventive measures currently include an array of medical interventions such as inoculations, surgery, radiation, and nutritional supplements. Certainly wherever appropriate, the communication disorders discipline concurs with and encourages the use of all these measures. The eradication of smallpox, like the control of rubella, pertussis, and polio, has improved the chances for normal communicative abilities in thousands of individuals. Communicable diseases that are not currently prevented or controlled by medical means range from the common cold to acquired immune deficiency syndrome (AIDS). Both these extremes of viral diseases are seen in the communications disorders field. Chronic middle-ear infections with effusion affect the hearing of thousands of children and adolescents. Vocal abuse occurs during bouts of laryngitis. Postnasal drip, which may be initiated by allergies, can cause chronic vocal fold irritation and voice quality disorders. If untreated, permanent damage to the middle-ear space, the larynx, or the throat can result. Infection with the human immunodeficiency virus (HIV) destroys the body's recuperative power from any secondary infection. Children born with AIDS have very short lives and suffer distress of the nervous system accompanied by great pain. Those born HIV-positive have developed AIDS within 5 to 7 years. While medical research pursues intervention vaccines and medications, communication disorders personnel can become involved with socialization and the verbal and nonverbal communication skills of the child (American Speech-Language-Hearing Association, February, 1990).

Each clinician should set an example of wellness and good health, be careful to obtain up-to-date inoculations, and stay current on research to prevent diseases that cause communication disorders. Clinicians should encourage clients and their families to participate in community immunization programs or other timely preventive medical treatments. Parents and adult clients are often unaware of such programs, especially as they get busy in daily routines that include getting to weekly treatment sessions for existing speech, language, and hearing problems. Informational counseling is beneficial, and most people appreciate assistance in arranging access to immunization programs. Encourage clients and caregivers to maintain a log of the types and dates of inoculations, as different vaccines protect the recipient for varying lengths of time.

In cases of tumorous diseases, the suggestion of cancer often introduces an element of fear. However, many tumors are benign and only obstructive. Removal or reduction in size of an obstructive benign tumor may be the recommended treatment to facilitate use of the impaired body part, such as an ear, tongue, or lip. Through counseling, the patient is able to express the feelings that accompany the condition and its proposed or completed treatment. Acceptance of the expressed feelings by a trusted clinician not only decreases the impact of the feelings, but also assures the client that having those feelings is acceptable and not unexpected.

In some cases, the progress of degenerative disease may be retarded, or a remission may occur at unexpected times and for unexplained reasons. Counseling the patient or caregiver to continue a self-care regimen, while maintaining records of experiences and procedures followed, may help give some structure to a daily routine. The clinician should note the patient's endurance level for discomfort and pain. The client's need for reassurance, acceptance, and contentment may be satisfied through the experience of sharing the frustrations of minutia with a knowledgeable, willing listener who is an interested conversational partner.

Trauma-Injury. Trauma that results in communication disorders occurs in many forms, three of which are abuse, accident, and armed conflict. Traumatic experience in any of these forms may result in physical and/or psychological injury or dysfunction. Likewise, all can lead to loss or diminution of communication abilities.

In society, the abused are found in three intrafamily positions: child, spouse, and parent (Commission on the Status of Women, 1988; Gelles & Cornell, 1985; Helfer & Kempe, 1987; Moore and Thompson, 1987; Nelson, 1984). Concussions and intracranial hemorrhages that produce brain damage are not unusual as the result of an uncontrolled assault on one family member by another. Such brain damage often involves the perceptive cortex cognition and language centers. Additionally, emotional trauma through abuse can lead to psychological etiologies for voice, fluency, articulation, hearing, and language problems. While treatment of the recipient of abuse often falls to the speech pathologist and audiologist, resolution of the abuse problem more often lies in the domains of psychology, social work, and law. In the process of treating the communication disorder, the clinician will meet and work with family members as well as other professionals. It is essential during these family encounters that the clinician accept the person, but not the act or result of the abuse. Ongoing collaboration among professional colleagues and careful sharing of information concerning the individuals and their interrelationships are essential to gaining or regaining communication skills.

It is not unexpected that the target of abuse may have had a pre-existing communication problem. It is also not unusual that the abuser has a current or past communication problem. The clinician may be placed in the position of becoming a bridge between the communicative deficits of the client, the communicative problems of the abuser, and the team of professionals involved in working with distressed family members. In this situation, where a professional team of experts work together, the speech-language pathologist and audiologist may be called on to perform only the specialized tasks of their individual disciplines. However, it is not uncommon for clients or family members to perceive and seek to utilize the speech-language pathologist or audiologist as an empathic counselor. In that role, the clinician can enhance therapeutic progress by cooperating and directing the energies of family members continually toward improving the communication network within the family. Through cooperation with other members of the treatment team, open and free discussion of the team's collective decisions will derive the best overall program of treatment for the family. Before inviting this sort of open discussion, however, it is strongly recommended that the communication disorders clinician consult with the psychologist or psychiatrist on the team. This con-

sultation will more nearly ensure that any dialogue the clinician introduces in the communication treatment setting will be within acceptable
bounds for the progress of the client and family in all dimensions of the
multifaceted treatment. The consultation will alert the clinician to subject
areas that should not be discussed with the client or family either at a
given time or in the absence of the mental health specialist. Young teams
and beginning clinicians often find such collaborative efforts quite time
consuming in terms of organization and planning. After working together
for some time, however, team participants tend to become quite proficient
in closing the informational gaps between specializations without dupli-
cating work efforts or confusing patients.

The best way to prevent abuse before it occurs is to ensure that the
communication network of all concerned parties is at its optimum proficiency. Preventive measures must include educating people to participate
in open, honest, and appropriate communication with family, friends, and
acquaintances. Each participant in the communication process must
understand that the abilities of others, like their needs, change over time.
Such educational endeavors are a part of the prevention ideal of ASHA
(American Speech-Language-Hearing Association, March, 1988). Settings
that are appropriate for such activities include schools and church groups
and professional, social, and work-related groups in local and national service clubs.

The most common types of accidents that result in communication disorders are motor-vehicle accidents and gunshot wounds. The most frequent victims are young men, and alcohol consumption is often cited as
the cause of the accident. The types of injuries that typically result from
these accidents are open or closed head injuries or loss of function in
peripheral organs. In head injuries, brain damage to the linguistic and
cognitive functions may be devastating. Full recovery of function is rare,
and a whole new way of life often becomes necessary for the patient.
Dysfunction of peripheral organs affects the client and caregiver in pro-
portion to the site of trauma, normal utility of the damaged body part
(e.g., hands, legs, trunk, face), the degree of loss of function (e.g., paralysis
or paresis), and the effect the loss has on previous lifestyle and abilities.
In any case, the condition of the accident victim exhibits a diminished
capability in comparison to the premorbid status.

Counseling may have little place in the prevention of communication
disorders that result from accidents. However, clinicians may want to support laws that address motor vehicle operation and consumption of alcoholic beverages. Sharing information about the results of accidents with
the age groups at greatest risk can become a powerful weapon in the ongoing battle against their destructive effects on adolescents and young
adults.

As a visiting teacher, a clinician might ask a class to deliberately
refrain from talking for two hours to experience the effects of the loss of

speech. Another way to allow students to experience a communication disorder is to ask them to use cotton or commercial ear plugs during ordinary daily activities. Still another experience to bring home the trials of restricted communication abilities is assigning students to speak in phrases of three or fewer words, using only nouns, for a selected period of time.

The results of traumatic injury due to domestic quarrels and armed conflict such as drug and gang wars or military action are similar to those resulting from other types of trauma. However, some of these circumstances involve a major difference: the present or past use of addictive drugs and their effects on the body, especially the nervous system. In addition to systemic disruption of the body, a chemically disturbed nervous system presents symptoms of distractibility and reduced adaptability. Communications disorders specialists may not see such patients until they are no longer actively taking the pre-injury drug. The behavior of a client may in part reflect the former addiction or unfocused resentment and anger that the injury occurred. Some clients will express anger toward any staff member assigned to the case. Others exhibit symptoms of depression and withdrawal from the treatment process.

Counseling for prevention of trauma-caused communication disorders, whether or not they are complicated by chemical abuse, may lead the clinician to become involved in programs outside the clinic itself, often working as a volunteer in the community. Interacting with the staff in educational facilities can add critically needed community energies and information. For example, clinicians can provide training in the parenting of young children or caregiving to the elderly. They can be effective in teaching pre-teens and teenagers about the dangers of unsafe sex and drug abuse as well as the value of respecting the power of motor vehicles. Clinicians can contribute to interpersonal communication facilitation, demystification of normal life-span development through aging, and education of the public concerning the reality of being a victim. Such topics are appropriate for the clinician who wants to keep a community safe or make it safer. Increased awareness of safety will help reduce the incidence of communication disorders that result from disease or trauma.

Daily Living Experience. Adaptability of the environment has been mentioned in concert with the adaptability of the individual. In many instances, mutually cooperative efforts can prevent the onset of a communication disorder. Additionally, the environment presents external influences that can cause communication disorders in normal members of the community. Some of these environmental problems are being addressed by national and international groups. Industry and entertainment both contribute irritants to the human environment. Common sources of noise pollution are industry, entertainment, and traffic on streets and highways, in the air, and on the water. Industrial dumping of chemical wastes pollutes the atmosphere, water, and land. Chemical pollution occurs around landfill sites, where human waste and untreated solid or liquid waste from industry are buried. Other common pollutants include lead in old paint found in houses that have long needed to be replaced or refurbished, asbestos in residential, public, and industrial insulation, and radon from electric cables. Such pollutants, often innocently consumed, endanger the development and function of the body's organ systems in exposed human beings. Additionally, some food additives are believed to be carcinogens. Combinations of foods, eating habits, and sedentary lifestyles are known to be destructive to body function.

Poverty continues to be the most devastating of all the environmental factors. Some of its effects are deprivation, ignorance, prejudice, illiteracy, hopelessness, malnutrition, inadequate shelter, and lack of clothing or human companionship. Prevention of all of these influences would demand superhuman effort. The prevention of environmental conditions that cause speech, language, and hearing disorders may be achieved most effectively through organized political influence. Clinicians may accomplish this through state, national, and international organizations that represent a large special-interest block of voters and taxpayers. The seriously committed communication specialist should use the opportunity to participate in community efforts to prevent environmental destruction of all sorts.

The needs of neglected children and aging dependents for the services of communicologists must be accommodated. Many of these individuals are victims of poverty who live in remote areas, away from regular service systems. Creative new programs to prevent their many problems are making inroads into their territories and experiences. An example of such a program is PARENTS AS TEACHERS NATIONAL CENTER, Marillac Hall, University of Missouri - St. Louis, 8001 Natural Bridge Road, St. Louis, Missouri 63121-4499. This program began in 1981 as an innovative model project to study the impact of a home-and-school partnership beginning at birth on a child's development and learning. Since that time, Parents as Teachers has become a state-supported program that provides education in child development and care to new parents (birth to 4 years of age), early developmental screening for children (birth to 4 years of age), and parent-child programs for developmentally delayed 3- and 4-year-olds. Studies have found children who participate in the program to be advanced in language, problem-solving, and social development (Parents as Teachers, 1987).

II. Remediation

Clinicians tend to spend a major portion of their time and energies in the remediation of communication disorders. In remediable disorders, the symptoms and effects of a speech, language, or hearing difference can be reduced to the point of eradication of noticeability and/or interference with normal transmission of ideas among the concerned individuals and others with whom they speak. Remediable disorders are non-progressive; many are functional-habitual, but some are temporary or transitional following an unusual experience such as a mini-stroke, fitting of an intra-oral prosthesis, grafting a tympanic membrane. Through diagnosis and therapy, clinicians intervene to reduce the symptoms of the communicative disorder and help the client communicate in normal ways, not distinguishable from those of others in their homes and communities. Across the four categories of disorders, the possibility of remediation depends on the severity of the problem, the age of the client at the onset of the disorder, and, in some moderate to severe cases, an unnamed ingredient that elicits the strength and determination to communicate normally.

Remediation of a communication disorder may involve obtaining intervention from a colleague in an allied health field. For example, a conductive hearing loss may be remediated through removal of cerumen from the external ear canal; the positioning of the tongue may be facilitated by removal of the tonsils (whole or in part); intensity of the voice may be enhanced through habituation of stronger, more regulated respiratory patterns such as those acquired in running or swimming. Other therapies for remediable communication disorders consist largely of teaching the client to identify a particular element of behavior that needs to be changed and how to perform an alternate skill, utilize perceptive judgment of that performance, and recognize the acceptableness of the skill.

Sometimes, remediation involves the client in clinical work that consists largely of a demonstration for caregivers to practice at home. The clinician facilitates the client's adaptation to the new or altered method of communication. At the same time, the clinician instructs the caregiver as to the technique necessary to reduce the symptomatic speech, language, or hearing disorder, essentially changing the home communication environment of the client. Another type of therapy addresses the sensitivity of the client to perceptions of ridicule for a communication disorder that is not evident to the speaker, such as mild to moderate hearing loss or regional dialect. Desensitization of the client may or may not involve the participation of caregivers. The goal of therapy is to toughen the easily bruised feelings of the client. Therapy helps identify what is happening in the behavior of the client and the reaction of the listener. Counseling helps the client reduce the tendency to interpret behavior of conversational partners in biased terms or lay blame or guilt on the self or on others.

Scheduled Therapy Sessions. The most common type of therapy for remediation of communication disorders occurs over time in a series of scheduled appointments. Interactions between the clinician and the client are individually programmed over a period of time to address the particular needs of the client in suitably scaled increments of progress toward normal communication abilities. Counseling during this experience is often seen as a part of the routine therapeutic procedure. Instruction, clarification, reinforcement, and summarization of the treatment session's work are certainly useful as treatment procedures, as they are components of counseling.

Client and caregiver perceptions of the progress of therapy toward specific goals usually incorporate their hopes and feelings of accomplishment. The clinician can encourage such feelings by providing treatment in appropriate increments, measuring progress in an understandable way, and summarizing the advances made during each therapy session before ending it.

Some therapy participants may view their involvement in a few sessions of treatment as an inconvenience. They may work diligently to keep the number of appointments to a minimum and achieve early or timely dismissal. Others will begin to enjoy the friendly approval they find in the therapy sessions, and the therapy that started out as a needed service becomes a pleasure to which they return for a companionable visit. In clients wanting to continue therapy after the communication problem is resolved, the clinician may need to examine aspects of the client's interpersonal communication skills in daily use. If therapy is too comfortable, the client may request that dismissal be postponed. The client may anticipate difficulty in applying learned skills to the nonclinical world. In such a case, some field-work experience with the clinician may suffice to demonstrate that the client's performance is adequate to meet the demands of other settings. In another case, a client may have developed a dependency on the clinician that is stronger than desirable. In that instance, group therapy may be helpful (Deal & Deal, 1978; Hughes, 1985; McCormick & Schiefelbusch, 1984; Yolam, 1970). Groups provide a communication setting for participants to improve their skills and gain access to information, shared hope, and recognition of the universality of their problems. Clients who are active in groups often experience altruism, emotional catharsis, and improvement of intragroup participation by developing socializing techniques, perhaps through imitative behavior. They enjoy becoming a part of a cohesive group, which is interested in the welfare of each member. In complex cases, the client may need to see a psychotherapist to resolve the problem that is being manifest as a communication disorder. Group therapy or support organizations that involve the psychotherapeutic needs of clients may be sponsored and managed jointly by a communicologist and a psychologist or psychiatrist.

During therapies for remediation, client/caregiver attitudes and feelings tend to be supportive of the work being done. Their expectations are molded by the diagnosis and prognosis made by the clinician. Therefore, in most situations, harmony develops among all parties as the work progresses. When clinicians, clients, and caregivers conscientiously share information and thoughts on progress, their expectations are synchronized with the rate of change. Together, they observe progress toward the specified goals.

Therapy Programs May Generate Discomfort in Clients. Clinicians should respond to signs of discomfort in clients or caregivers. Discomfort with the therapeutic process may be apparent when the scheduled time is tolerable, but not convenient. Practice at home may be taking time that needs to be devoted to other things. A client may be present for each arranged session, but tends to arrive in a rush, always a few minutes late. Each of these situations may be absolutely true, or each may indicate that the relative importance of the therapy has not been realistically meshed with the rest of daily demands. After noticing any degree of discomfort in the client or caregiver, the clinician should introduce a discussion of the observation in a way that invites the client or caregiver to participate honestly in the dialogue. In one case, a simple change of the scheduled time for therapy may make a dramatic improvement in the home schedule. In another, it may be that the added stress of the homework effort is more disabling than beneficial to the family. The only way to penetrate the reality of the clinician's observation is to ask for information and work together with the client or caregiver to resolve problems and conflicts. The counselor must be cognizant of the feelings and attitudes within the nonclinical environment of each client and manage the effect of that situation appropriately. Essentially, the result of therapy depends on what the client or caregiver puts into it. If changing the scheduled time or some other logistic compliance is helpful, the clinician is well advised to suggest it. However, if interference with therapy lies in the attitudes of the clients or caregivers, then the clinician must spend time helping them adjust their perceptions of the communication disorder, the method recommended for remediating it, and their roles in the process. In the event that the client or caregiver cannot or will not comply with the prescribed service, it may be best either to delay enrollment until an appropriate commitment can be made or to recommend another therapist for treatment.

Some clients or caregivers will perceive remediation of a communication disorder as more than a slight inconvenience or an interlude in their routine daily lives. They may be annoyed or distressed by the need for this extra involvement. Even when the disorder is mild, its existence and demands can loom large and ugly, as something that should not happen to them or their family. In some instances, the accompanying feelings are anger and fear. Disappointment and resentment will be apparent in nonverbal behavior. Such feelings, attitudes, and behaviors in the client or the caregiver interfere with therapeutic progress and must be considered part of the problem to be dealt with by the counselor. The starting point with each client or caregiver may differ, but the core of the problem lies in the difference between reality and the expectations of the parties involved.

Some expectations may remain unverbalized or even unacknowledged by the client. For these individuals, therapy can be a significant way to learn about themselves, especially about their strong points. As the clinician verbally points out strengths and expresses approval of the communicative accomplishments of the client and of all the right things that the caregiver has been doing, the reality of the problem or perceived problem becomes evident. As the client and caregiver learn about themselves, they also learn new and different things to do and how to do some things differently. Familiar and new communicative experiences become something to talk about as a real entity in the client's life. Becoming comfortable with themselves and each other is important to becoming comfortable with the changes in communication that therapy will produce. These experiences, and the sharing of them, ultimately lead to the acceptance of the modified communicative abilities as a part of the client, not as an add-on, but as natural, habituated skills.

Completion of Treatment. Remediation of speech, language, and hearing disorders is the ideal business of the communication disorders discipline. Most clinicians derive pleasure from the completion of treatment that results in dismissing a client with intact communication abilities and assurance to use them in daily encounters. Often dismissal from therapy is the beginning of personal friendships between former clients or caregivers and therapists. It is wise to delay the development of such friendships until after therapy is complete. The clinician who becomes too close to a client or caregiver may allow emotions to interfere with objective professional judgments and may expend unwarranted energy on the tangent ramifications of a single case. Competent clinicians, of course, care about their clients; however, retaining objectivity is essential to achieve the best treatment and a mutual appreciation of clinician, client, and caregiver roles in the therapeutic process. Objectivity underscores the opportunity of each party to carry out the responsibilities of the roles designated by the treatment.

III. Modification

Modifiable disorders are those that can be changed to increase the communicative effectiveness of the client while reducing the impediment of the communicative difference. Some examples of these disorders are sensory-neural hearing loss, adult dysfluency, cognitive dysfunction related to closed head injury, alaryngeal voice, and lingual apraxia. Most clients with these disorders will not eradicate the impediment altogether. Some may learn coping skills and not change the actual oral-aural signal production or reception. The goal of therapy is a serviceable communication modality that enables the individual to remain or become a fully functioning member of the community. To achieve this, therapy helps the client reduce the impact of the disorder. The client accepts responsibility for and management of the residual effects of the disorder. Therapy must enable the client to acquire and habituate techniques of control that utilize the maximum level of physiological and/or psychological ability.

Counseling clients and caregivers in the modification of communication disorders can be as varied as in any therapeutic encounter. The essential principle remains for the clinician to stick to reality and observe any difference that may emerge between expectations and reality on the part of clients or caregivers. Dealing with a disorder that will not go away, that cannot be completely removed or disguised, demands acceptance and adjustment by individuals with a desire to make things all right. The counselor may find elements of regret or grieving in the behavior of these clients and caregivers. They have lost an essential human quality in the dysfunction of meaningful communication. Grief will be discussed further in the context of counseling in the treatment of irreversible communication disorders.

Counseling is an integral part of therapy that seeks alternatives to current communicative practices. The counselor must study each modifiable communication problem thoroughly, evaluating the potential benefits of retaining or modifying it. A significant part of the habituation process involves appreciating small increments of advancement toward better oral-aural communication. Patience is essential for both the clinician and the client. Continually reviewing expectations versus experience helps to retain a realistic focus on progress and goals, reducing the chances of disappointment or fear of failure when the client is away from the clinical setting. Giving assurance of competencies and approval of positive changes should comprise a part of every therapy session for clients struggling to gain or regain a level of performance they know to be lost.

Acceptance of Best Communication Ability. Ultimately, clients or caregivers dealing with modifiable communication disorders must learn to accept their best communicative abilities, which are less than ideal, less than ordinary. That acceptance is based on realizing that the modification has resulted in their maximum proficiency for their current status. The following statements are examples of the conclusions that clients may reach and express in informal dialogues with clinicians.

Losing words is not bad. It's sure inconvenient. (9-year-old with language-learning disabilities)
or
I know I sound funny, but now I can talk. You just have to listen and be patient. (Young adult with cerebral palsy)
or
I tell Sue what I want. She not guess anymore. (Aging client with aphasia)

or

I'm grateful for a voice. It may sound a little like a robot, but it's precious to me and my wife. (Middle-aged alaryngeal client)

or

I-I-I-I have ways to use to help me be fluent. By thinking about letting the air carry my words, I-I-I-I-I can say whole sentences, even in stressful situations. (Teenage client with fluency disorder)

or

When I had to start on such basic things, I hated it. I felt silly. I thought I'd never do all right. It was hard to stick to doing all the detail that I had to make up. I wanted to quit many times. (Young adult client with closed head injury)

One can well imagine that each of these speakers could use nonverbal cues to signal discontent or anger while uttering these same words. However, the intent here is to suggest that the speaker's nonverbal cues correspond with the listener's expectations regarding the message being demonstrated. Contentment or acceptance is largely dependent on the adequacy of the counseling program incorporated into the therapy process. Each client requires a unique type and amount of support and guidance from the counselor.

Counseling the Client With Strong Feelings.   Some clients who present modifiable communication disorders may also possess strong emotions, which may defy rapid changing as much as the verbal communication problem itself. Different treatment techniques must be utilized with these clients, for the emotionality is a large portion of the communication problem. The clinician must first accept such clients with whatever traits they bring to the therapy room. Then, realistic assessment of all aspects of behavior must enter into the plan and prognosis for that client. Application of all the counseling skills at the command of the clinician may be called upon to identify and tame emotional components that may distort the communication ability even more than the disorder itself. As the emotional aspects of the disorder are brought out into the open and discussed, the client can begin to build a repertoire of techniques for dealing with the remnants of the communication disorder, which will remain after the best of therapy has been applied.

The clinician must remember that it is both expected and acceptable for the client to feel anger, fear, resentment, and other negative emotions. However, those feelings must be focused on the appropriate target. The target must be identified and evaluated in terms of its worthiness of such strong feelings. The clinician may find that the client exhibits negative feelings when asked to try a new and difficult task. The client may resist the task, reverting to behaviors that were addressed previously and thought to be resolved. Such resistance is most common when the tasks are difficult and the client feels discouraged by a slow rate of improvement, the length of the therapy program, the level of communication that is usable away from the clinic, or other "non-normal" experiences despised by the client.

IV. Irreversibility

Irreversible communication disorders present a somewhat different situation to the clinician or counselor. Even if a disorder consists of a minute difference in speech articulation, such as a distorted sibilant or a muted vowel, the fact that its presence is permanent and unchanging gives it an important place in the life of the possessor. Irreversible communication disorders often seem to be tied to an irremediable or progressive physical and/or psychological condition. Apraxias, dysarthrias, aphasias, aphonias, nerve-deafness, and mental retardation are examples of neurogenic communication disorders. Laryngectomy and glossectomy, which are accepted as modern medical treatments for carcinoma, present other examples of irreversible communication disorders that impose catastrophic results for the management of complex oral-aural communication. The physical conditions and the related irreversible communication disorders are not always severe; in fact, they can be very mild or moderate in intensity. As with those that are remediable or modifiable, irreversible communication disorders vary greatly in their effect on a client's overall ability to function linguistically in daily life. An additional consideration in the treatment of irreversible communication disorders is whether the underlying physical or psychological condition is progressive, that is, deteriorating.

Nonprogressive Irreversible Communication Disorders. *Mild* articulatory distortions are heard in everyday settings. Salespeople, physicians, bank tellers, professors, or television personalities find little problem with a distorted sibilant or muted vowel. Sometimes, such differences are even considered attractive or suggestive of a foreign language dialect. Mild dysfluency may be observed in public speakers without discredit to their message or their charisma. In some speakers, hesitating or apparently searching for the right word is interpreted as an effort to be accurate. Even mild aphasia is sometimes accepted in an older person, whose memory is not expected to be as good as it was years ago.

The clinician gains a quite different perspective on non-progressive communication disorders in treating a patient with a congenital cleft lip or palate. The physical condition can be corrected, but not eradicated. In the large majority of these patients, communication disorders that are commonly thought to be sequelae of the birth defect can be prevented through early intervention. Management of the birth defect, the reaction to it, and the developmental guidance of treatment can obliterate the physical manifestation except for a minimal, distracting, and sometimes telltale upper lip scar. Yet the parents may remember the shock of discovering the orofacial birth defect and may retain feelings of remorse, even after the child is a thriving adult getting on with life. Thus, mild communicative differences, which may or may not be related to an otherwise noticeable deviation from the norm, elicit reactions from the communicative environment, even if the affected person pays little attention to them.

Moderate nonprogressive communication disorders that cannot be reversed or diminished add the burden of accepting and accommodating the difference imposed by the speech, language, or hearing problem. This dimension of adaptation was mentioned in the brief discussion of modifiable communication disorders. The difference with irreversible disorders is the absence of opportunity to reduce the diagnosed disorder, requiring the client or caregiver to acquire coping strategies to deal with the unremitting total aspect of the communication problem. Management of one family member's disability demands change in the communication behavior of all the other family members. While the affected member strives to meet requirements for maximal function in society, the family must often vary routines to accommodate the single member's inherent needs. This ideal day-to-day management process involves an adaptive client in an adaptive environment. An example of such a relationship might occur in a young family, in which the client is a wife and mother who has sustained a moderate to severe sensory-neural hearing loss. Besides personalized amplification of sound, the client needs skills, devices, and techniques to allow her to interact with her family and alert her to phenomena in areas of the home that she cannot monitor visually. An amplified telephone or a teletypewriter (TTY) can provide access to social contacts in the community, emergency information, and business interests. Within the family, members learn modified methods to share their knowledge of the community with her and conscientiously assist her in outreach efforts to be an active participant in the social milieu in which they carry on daily activities. They involve her with the children's schools and teachers, playmates and their families, the husband's work, recreation and entertainment, interest groups, or civic duties. That is, the client learns through therapy to manage her existence with all the changes the hearing loss imposes on her. By changing themselves and their environment, the whole family can continue to participate fully in a continuing, adapted life.

Severe nonprogressive communication disorders might be found in clients of any age group. One instance of this problem is a child with complex mixed cerebral palsy. The child is an 11-year-old girl with normal intelligence. Although her reception and comprehension of spoken language are intact, there is complete lack of motor control. Because of this, she has always used a modified wheelchair and she has never talked, although she can make sounds. The child is nonverbal and her distorted facial features do not depict typical configurations for meaningful nonverbal communication. As a result, family members have learned to recognize her special reflexive reactions to emotional responses and verbalize them for her. She has had considerable experience with a communication board, and she is currently learning to use a computerized communication system. Her desire to communicate and the slow rate at which she is able to do so are understood by her family, who are patient and cooperative with the child as she learns. However, the parents and the child know that they must be prepared to make realistic decisions about her education, future occupation, and leisure activities. They must realistically assess her chances of living independently and becoming gainfully employed as an adult. They need to set a course that will steer her toward maximum fulfillment of her potential in the rapidly changing world.

Irreversible communication disorders that are non-progressive can come to be accepted over time. Clients and caregivers can learn to adapt to the demands of the disorder and accompanying disabilities. This adaptation process contains the hope of a culture that thinks of a future as a positive, real entity. Planning for tomorrow or next year or 10 years from now provides a target for the efforts of each day. When an irremediable communication disorder is an element necessarily involved in that planning, its static status becomes a constant focal point around which to work. Plans that are reasonable and well thought out can accommodate changes in the family, the work environment, community social relations, and civic responsibilities. To reach this degree of organization, insight, and acceptance, families often travel a torturous route from discovery of the disabling condition to stable, structured, and positive management of their collective need to change. It is the counselor's role to participate, when needed, in helping them along the way.

It is not possible to imagine the multitude of ways in which dialogues between the counselor and client or caregiver might be structured. What a family member or a client may introduce to discuss or never mention depends entirely on the people involved, their experience in life prior to the onset of the problem, and their flexibility in handling unanticipated change. The counseling role of the speech, language, or hearing specialist includes providing the best available information concerning the communication disorder and its effects on the client and the family. Counseling utilizes all the behaviors discussed in chapter 2 as well as those that have been personally specialized and proven by individual clinicians. This is especially applicable to the most challenging category of irreversible communication disorders, those that are progressive and non-reversible.

Progressive Irreversible Communication Disorders. Disorders that are both irreversible and progressive are those in which the client's condition worsens, the communicative abilities deteriorate, and the outcome of these problems is death. Like other disorders, they can occur at any age and may involve a variety of speech, language, or hearing problems. One example is the disorder of dementia. The unresolved etiology and treatment of Alzheimer's disease, which leads to degenerative dementia and eventual total disability of the body, is a major cause of concern for the increasing aging population. Another disorder, multiple sclerosis, affects both children and adults, as does AIDS. AIDS in children is an increasing and deadly malady. Communication is greatly affected in the congenital AIDS victim (American Speech-Language-Hearing Association, 1990). Appendix E summarizes some characteristics of AIDS patients, along with suggestions for speech-language pathologists and audiologists who work with them (ASHA Committee on Quality Assurance, 1989).

Loss of function, as well as impending death, signals grief, along with all the personal and familial adjustments implied for the victim, the family and close friends. It is not unusual for various individuals affected by the disability to blame others or themselves for the accident, illness, or their outcomes. The feelings generated by the disability may be focused in the victim by the family and the victim alike. The clinician may find that strong negative feelings make treatment of the communication disorder a secondary consideration, at least temporarily. For clients who are unable to retain or recall correctly performed skills from one treatment session to the next, the work is often discouraging for the clinician and the family alike. The patient may not realize the extent of memory deficit and may not understand its effect on those who observe the behavior.

Observable differences in pre- and post-onset behavior will at some time become part of the counseling dialogue between the clinician and the client or caregiver. As in other situations, the most competent counselor is careful to remain realistic and optimistic, but not to any degree that falsifies or exaggerates the promise of recovery in any patient. In patients and families who reject realistic expectations, the counselor may wish to consult a psychologist to discuss the appropriate management of this problem. Professional referral for psychological or physiatric assessment of the concerned parties may be advisable. The counselor may anticipate resistance to the suggested referral. To circumvent this problem, the counselor may present the recommendations in terms of their usefulness in clarifying maximum goals for communicative treatment or designing augmentative devices to be used in the treatment of the acknowledged communication disabilities. It helps the counselor to remember that spending time preparing clients and caregivers for their involvement in a task or experience establishes a strong foundation for what is to come. Such preparation does more than eliminate surprises and disappointments that can be the outcome of unrealistic expectations. It allows the client and caregiver to recognize that they are dealing with an honest and forthright professional who places their best interest foremost.

Multidisciplinary Treatment. In urban settings, as well as in large multidisciplinary institutions, counseling is rarely left to the speech-language pathologist or audiologist alone (Shewan, 1988; "Trends Affecting U.S. Health Care Systems," 1976). However, many clinicians practice in settings far from large urban treatment centers. Those professionals may find themselves alone, serving the counseling needs of clients in addition to therapizing their communicative problems. In the best of all possible worlds, every clinician would have a complete team of experts with whom to work. But in reality, clinicians often work without assistance from peers in complementary disciplines. Applying professional expertise within the limits of the individual clinician's training and abilities is all that can be expected. This is realistic and ethical. It does not, however, deny the availability of telephone conferences with colleagues at other or larger centers. Networking is encouraged among ASHA members (Koenigsknecht, 1990), with the National Office serving as a resource to help find desired information and contacts for individual professionals. It is also beneficial for clinicians to become acquainted with resources available in the community, the state, and the region where assistance can be gained for the best outcomes of work with each client. In the event that the needs of the client or caregiver are realistically beyond the abilities of the clinician, the clinician must say so. This may mean that a particular clinician will not accept some potential clients for treatment. Hardships caused by the absence of appropriate personnel to serve a population must be made known to community leaders, whose influence can change the situation. Public awareness that an inadequately staffed community or institution further victimizes the victim must become a part of the care management efforts of communication disorders personnel.

❦ ❦ ❦

COUNSELING CLIENTS/CAREGIVERS IN FACING A PERMANENT LOSS

The dominant need for counseling among clients and their caregivers relates to finding emotional and attitudinal balance. They are striving to find their way through the loss of a desired or expected ability as they undertake to gain new skills and cope with their ongoing lives and limitations. Reaction to recognized losses takes many forms. In some clients or caregivers, regret or mild disappointment may be the most severe reaction to a communication disorder. This is often found in families who have experienced and accepted other dramatic life experiences or other losses. An example may be found in a 3-year-old Down's syndrome child who is found to have a bilateral moderate hearing loss. While family members may want to talk about their feelings in relation to the hearing loss, their concern for its late discovery, and the influence of that loss on the child's learning and on their lives, they tend to be matter-of-fact about the circumstances with which they must deal. They are aware of possible lost language stimulation during the first 3 years of their child's life. Their questions are reasonable and appropriate for the diagnosis and treatment recommended. They are able to handle the added equipment for the child to compensate for the loss of auditory acuity. They understand the modifications to be introduced into their at-home stimulation program. The additional deficit seems to place far fewer demands on them than what they have already faced because of the child's other problems.

Unexpected Losses

The clinician may meet some clients who are experiencing unexpected communicative losses. Closed-head injury patients and their families often present this situation. The family may realize the extent of the actual loss of abilities more fully than the victim. Some families wear smiles and work hard to show the patient that everything that can be done is being done and that everything is going to be all right. The intrafamily message reflects assurance that no matter what the ultimate outcome of the trauma, the family will stick together and take care of each other. When the clinician observes this over several sessions, there may be reason to investigate the reality of the opinions and beliefs of the client and the family members. It may be the case, for example, that the client and family have truly misunderstood the long-term involvement of rehabilitation. In another case, the family may mistakenly believe that the client neither comprehends nor feels the loss of cognitive and linguistic abilities.

Often, medical records do not contain this information. If the patient has been seen by a psychologist or psychiatrist, medical chart notes may be too brief to reveal information that is important to the reality orientation of the home communication environment and clinical treatment for speech and language deficits. When this occurs, the clinician may request supporting information from the professionals involved in the case or schedule an interview session with any or all of the family members. The primary caregiver in a family may be expected to have the most direct observations of the client's actual ability and motivation. The clinician must accept that caregiver's interpretation of such observations with caution. An interview session with the primary caregiver may provide the clinician with the information needed to confirm the adequacy of the planned program, the realistic orientation of the family to the client's condition, and the communicative interaction in which the client participates outside the clinic. At the same time, an interview with the primary caregiver recognizes the significance of that individual's role in the maximum therapeutic progress of the client. This is not to say that credit or blame for progress belongs to the caregiver. Instead, the caregiver is recognized as a constant influence in the client's world.

Communication Disorders May Signal Onset of Grief

One additional perspective on loss of communicative function needs to be considered, that which is seen as loss of the individual who experiences the functional deficit. This may happen in families where the actual loss is minimal. For our purposes, consider a family whose grandmother has developed Alzheimer's disease, that is, senile dementia of the Alzheimer type. In most instances, this is a terminal disease, but its duration is long-term. During the course of the disease, the mental abilities of the patient slowly decrease. Early features of this disease include errors in judgment, decline in personal care and habits, impairment in capacity for abstract thought, and lack of interest and/or apathy. As the disease progresses, other traits appear, including depression; anxiety; irritability; hallucinations, especially at night; poor orientation to time, place, and person; confused comprehension; incoherent speech; fabrication; paranoid and manic states; and incontinence (Butler & Lewis, 1986). These changes occur slowly over years, sometimes 6 to 10 years or longer.

Reactions of the family members to the changed behavior of the grandmother develop slowly, even before they recognize that symptoms are severe enough to warrant a medical diagnosis. Those changes may be gradual, and the reactions of family members may change to follow the pattern of change in the aging relative. Shachter (1986) discusses the effects of a prolonged illness on the emotional responses of family members. The initial reaction to the aging family member's deteriorating behavior is shock and disbelief, followed closely by great anguish and emotional pain (Moore & Thompson, 1987). The anguish results from not knowing what will happen from day to day, and from being unable to help the loved one.

Although the grandmother is still present physically, she is no longer available psychologically to the family. She has become a stranger to them and to herself. Family members begin to feel the loss of the loved parent and prepare themselves through her daily care for her actual physical death.

Early in the illness, when the confirmed diagnosis is new, loneliness and anticipatory grief may be assuaged at times when the grandmother momentarily seems lucid. Her brief participation in their world soothes the family and allows a minute shift in the burden of losing her. This is more often true of dying patients, whose diseases do not destroy the mental and linguistic functions of the patient so rapidly. Feelings of anger in the patient and the caregiver may be focused at any or all of the people in the environment. Its targets are influenced by the circumstances of the moment and may change from time to time. At the same time, guilt about not doing enough or not doing the right thing or feelings about having given enough of oneself may haunt the caregiver with regrets. However, the long duration of the senile dementia often provides time to work through these feelings. These reactions are recognized to be those often related to the *grief syndrome*.

Mention of the grief syndrome is found in speech and hearing literature, especially in research related to hearing impairment, laryngectomy, and cleft lip or palate. Grief is a normal chain of human reactions to profound loss (Viorst, 1986). Most often associated with death, the ultimate loss, the same emotional and behavioral sequence has been found to apply to the loss of a body part or a behavioral capacity. Admittedly, each person grieves in an individual way, needing more or less time in each stage. In communication disorders, the counselor of a bereaved client or caregiver listens a great deal. In one case, the mother of a newborn child with Down's syndrome cried through three visits before she was able to talk about the status of her infant. In another, the wife of a recent stroke victim with mixed aphasia talked only about his garden during the initial two sessions with the clinician. The counselor must be cautious to accept the grief and the bereaved as natural and stay alert to recognize the instant that a minute shift occurs in the speaker's needs. At that moment, an equally small increment of the rehabilitation process can be introduced. With patience and insight into the needs of the client or caregiver, the clinician can facilitate the critical change from self-sorrow to renewed recognition of the outside world. Table 4.4 presents a compiled list of experiences referred to as the tasks involved in the work of grieving. It is believed that the order tends to be universal, but the duration of each stage or step varies greatly from individual to individual.

What words does the counselor use? What nonverbal communication is helpful for the grieving client or caregiver? Each counselor must choose. Marlow and Redding (1988) indicate that for the child who asks, "Am I going to die?" the appropriate response is "Yes, but we don't know when that will be." Following this exchange, the conversation typically goes on about something of importance in the current life of the child. This same open and honest response is useful with clients who ask, "Am I going to hear (or talk) again?" The response may be, "Yes, but in a way that is different from how you used to hear (or talk)." Another response may be, "No, you are going to learn to communicate in a different way, and I'm here to help you learn."

Upon receiving news of a negative prognosis or a diagnosis that is not expected or wanted, the client or caregiver may be distressed and upset. It is appropriate for the clinician to say, "That is scary news," or "That information is upsetting." This actually puts words around the unspoken but nonverbal message sent by the client or caregiver. Insightful verbalization opens the door for the recipient of the news to express the negative reaction verbally and to learn that such feelings are acceptable to the clinician.

Table 4.4
The work of grieving

Shock
Numbness – feeling of unreality
Disbelief – denial, avoidance
Emotional control – passive calm, guilt, hysteria
Altered perspectives
    intellectualization – objectifying, as an observer
    rationalization – explaining away
    humor – converting tragic to absurd
Faith – provides meaning
    facilitating acceptance – There is a purpose.
    offering help and support – Someone cares.
    promising continued relationship with family member in an afterlife
    combatting loneliness – someone shares grief
Avoidance – avoid experience, avoid feelings
Being busy – activity distracts from feelings
Passive distraction – mass media occupies attention
Involvement with others
    support from others – understanding, sympathy, sharing
    investment in others – working with people
    compensation for the loss – new acquaintances
    pets – substitutions, care and company
Expression of painful emotions – get them out of the system
Indulgence in external sources of gratification
    food – stress may stimulate hunger centers of the brain
    alcohol, tobacco, and other drugs – forms of escape
    spending money – compensation
    sex – need for closeness, intimacy
Pursuit of physical fitness – gratification, counterattack
Effects of prolonged illness on coping
    preparation for reality – put affairs in order
    preparation for psychological reality – learn new tasks, role acceptance

---

Note. Compiled from: Kubler-Ross, 1969, 1983; Miles, 1985; Morris, 1972; Rocklin, 1965; Shachter, 1986; Viorst, 1986.

EXERCISES

Read and complete the following exercises and discuss them with classmates, teachers or supervisors, and colleagues.

1. A 5-year-old child says, "Am I going to die?" Discuss the meaning and implications of the following two possible responses:

    a. "Yes, but we don't know when it will be."
    b. "Yes, but I don't know when it will happen."

You may need to state each response aloud in as many different ways as you can. Select one intonation pattern and discuss it. Also, describe the facial expression that accompanies the response statement.

2. You are completing the diagnosis of a severe communication problem, and you have just informed the primary caregiver of your findings. The caregiver responds, giving emphasis of stress and pitch elevation to the underlined word. Interpret the meaning of the verbal and nonverbal message. Try to discern the differences in effect expressed in the subtle shift of emphasis.

   a. It's just one more *thing.*
   b. It's just one *more* thing.
   c. It's just *one more* thing.

   Now, formulate an appropriate response to each of the *messages* you have identified. Remember that you are interested in the whole person, not only in assuring that he has understood what you told him about the diagnosis. For example, to which of the statements might you respond:

   a. This new diagnosis is distressing.
   b. Taking care of your wife/child/parent is very demanding.
   c. You're feeling overworked.
   d. You sometimes feel overwhelmed.

   Identify other possible verbal responses of the counselor to the caregiver. Also, describe the counselor's responsible and consistent total message to the caregiver.

3. You are the manager of a non-profit multidisciplinary rehabilitation center in a medium-sized urban community. One of your current clients was referred to you by a local otorhinolaryngologist. You have seen the client four times for diagnostic therapy. Data which you have collected indicate the presence of a condition that may be medically correctable using a radical new treatment. That treatment is reported to be available in a recognized medical research hospital that is 1,500 miles away. As the primary clinician for this client, outline the steps you would take to achieve the best possible service and outcomes for the client and the family.

4. A family secures an initial interview with you to discuss the communication handicap of their pre-adolescent son. When they arrive for the interview, the mother, father, and son are accompanied by the clinician who has been treating the child. As you interact with the group, you come to believe that the previous treatment has been inappropriate and

even harmful because it has postponed the initiation of adequate therapies.

a. Suggest a communication disorder for the client.
b. Describe the family and their socio-cultural background.
c. Describe the visiting clinician's credentials and skills.
d. Describe the previous therapy and its effects.

REFERENCES

Ainsworth, S. (1981). *Positive emotional power*. Englewood Cliffs, NJ: Prentice-Hall.

Ajzen, I., & Fishbein, M. (1977). Attitude-behavior relations: A theoretical analysis and review of empirical research. *Psychological Bulletin, 84*, 888–918.

ASHA Committee on Quality Assurance. (1989). AIDS/HIV: Implications for speech-language pathologists and audiologists. *ASHA, 31*(6–7), 33–38.

American Speech-Language-Hearing Association (1990). Martinez succumbs to AIDS [News]. *ASHA, 32*(2), 9.

American Speech-Language-Hearing Association. (1988). 1988 omnibus report. *ASHA, 30*(8), 27–30.

American Speech-Language-Hearing Association. (1984). Prevention: Challenge for the profession. *ASHA, 25*(8), 35–37.

American Speech-Language-Hearing Association. (1988). Prevention of communication disorders [Position Statement]. *ASHA, 30*(3), 90.

American Speech-Language-Hearing Association. (1988). Private practice. [Special section]. *ASHA, 30*(1), 29–47.

Backus, O. (1960). The study of psychological processes in speech therapists. In D. A. Barbara (Ed.), *Psychological and psychiatric aspects of speech and hearing.* Springfield, IL: Charles C. Thomas.

Bailey, D. B., & Simeonsson, R. J. (1984). Critical issues underlying research and intervention with families of young handicapped children. *Journal of the Division of Early Childhood, 9,* 38–48.

Bailey, D. B., & Simeonsson, R. J. (1988). *Family Assessment in Early Intervention*. Columbus, OH: Merrill.

Bateson, M. C. (1989). Foreword. In R. Benedict, *Patterns of Culture*. Boston: Houghton Mifflin. (Original work published 1934).

Battin, R. R., & Fox, D. R. (1978). Opening the doors. In R. R. Battin & D. R. Fox (Eds.), *Private practice in audiology and speech pathology*. New York: Grune and Stratton.

Beckman-Bell, P. (1981). Child-related stress in families of handicapped children. *Topics in Early Childhood Special Education, 1*(1), 45–53.

Benedict, R. (1989). *Patterns of culture*. Boston: Houghton Mifflin. (Original work published in 1934).

Bjerkan, B. (1980). Word fragmentation and repetitions in the spontaneous speech of 2- 6-year-old children. *Journal of Fluency Disorders, 5*, 137–148.

Brandes, P. & Ehinger, D. (1981). The effects of early middle ear pathology on auditory perception and academic achievement. *Journal of Speech and Hearing Disorders, 46*, 250–257.

Brugge, D. M., Brogan, R., & Quam, A. (1972). *The Zunis: Self-portrayals*. Albuquerque: University of New Mexico Press.

Butler, R. N., & Lewis, M. I. (1986). *Aging and mental health*. Columbus, OH: Merrill.

Camazine, S. M. (1980). Traditional and Western health care among the Zuni Indians of New Mexico [Social Science and Medicine, Part B]. *Medical Anthropology, 14*(2), 73–80.

Chezik, K. H., Pratt, J. E., Stewart, J. L., & Deal, V. R. (1989). Addressing service delivery in remote/rural areas. *ASHA, 31*(1), 52–55.

Commission on the Status of Women. (1988) Violence against women: Problems of rural women given priority. *U. N. Chronicle, 25*, 74.

Communication Disorders Prevention and Epidemiology Study Group. (1989, November). *Promoting health/preventing disease: Year 2000 objectives for the nation*. Unpublished discussion at the ASHA Annual Convention, St. Louis, MO.

Darley, F. L., & Spriestersbach, D. C. (1978). *Diagnostic methods in speech pathology* (2nd ed.). New York: Harper and Row.

Davis, J. (1986). Remediation of hearing, speech, and language deficits resulting from otitis media. In J. F. Kavanagh (Ed.), *Otitis media and child development* (pp. 182–191). Parkton, MD: York Press.

Deal, J. L., & Deal, L. A. (1978). Efficacy of aphasia rehabilitation: Preliminary results. In R. H. Brookshire (Ed.), *Clinical aphasiology conference proceedings*. Minneapolis: BRK.

Dickson, S. (1971). Incipient stuttering and spontaneous remission of stuttered speech. *Journal of Communication Disorders, 4*(4), 99–110.

Emerick, L. L., & Hatten, J. T. (1979). *Diagnosis and evaluation in speech pathology* (2nd ed.). Englewood Cliffs, NJ: Prentice-Hall.

Fishbein, M., & Ajzen, I. (1972). Attitudes and opinions. *Annual Review of Psychology, 23*, 487–544.

Flower, R. M. (1984). *Delivery of speech-language pathology and audiology services*. Baltimore, MD: Williams and Wilkins.

Flower, R. M. (1985). 1985 National Colloquium on Underserved Populations Report. *ASHA, 27*(3), 31–35.

Flower, W., & Sooy, C. D. (1987). AIDS: An introduction for speech-language pathologists and audiologists. *ASHA, 29*(11), 25–30.

Frattali, C. (1986). Are we reaching our goal? Developing outcomes measures. In P. Larkins (Ed.), *In search of quality assurance: What lies ahead?* [ASHA Quality Assurance Workshop Manual]. Rockville, MD: American Speech-Language-Hearing Association.

Galvin, K., & Book, C. (1975). *Person to person.* Skokie, IL: National Textbook Company.

Gelles, R. J., & Cornell, C. P. (1985). *Intimate violence in families.* Beverly Hills, CA: Sage.

Helfer, R. E., & Kempe, R. S. (Eds.). (1987). *The battered child* (4th ed.). Chicago: University of Chicago Press.

Hogg, J. E., Massey, E. W., & Schoenberg, B. S. (1979). Mortality from Huntington's Disease in the United States. *Advances in Neurology, 23*(4), 27–35.

Hughes, D. L. (1985). *Language treatment and generalization: A clinician's handbook.* San Diego, CA: College-Hill Press.

Kent, L., & Chabon, S. (1980). Problem-oriented record in a university speech and hearing clinic. *ASHA, 22*(4), 151–158.

Klein, J. O. (1986). Risk factors for otitis media in children. In J. F. Kavanagh (Ed.), *Otitis media and child development.* Parkton, MD: York Press.

Koenigsknecht, R. A. (1990). The power of networking. *ASHA, 32*(2), 27.

Kubler-Ross, E. (1969). *On death and dying.* London: Collier-Macmillan.

Kubler-Ross, E. (1983). *On children and death.* New York: Macmillan.

Lasiloo, P., Lewis, R. E., & Gray, J. (1975). Comment on reservation-based industry: A case from Zuni, New Mexico. *Human Organization, 34*(2), 217–226.

Leith, W. R. (1984). *Handbook of clinical methods in communication disorders.* San Diego, CA: College-Hill Press.

Ling-Phillips, A. H. (1981). Early habilitation: A blend of counseling and guidance. In G. T. Mencher & S. E. Gerber (Eds.), *Early management of hearing loss.* New York: Grune and Stratton.

Ling-Phillips, A. H. (1987). Working with parents: A story of personal and professional growth. *Volta Review Monographs, 89,* 131–146.

Luterman, D. (1984). *Counseling the communicatively disordered and their families.* Boston: Little, Brown.

Lynch, E. (1986). *The family of handicapped infants and young children (Family Network Series Monograph 1).* Moscow: University of Idaho, Family Involvement with At-Risk and Handicapped Infants Project.

Marge, M. (August, 1984). The prevention of communication disorders. *ASHA, 25*(8), 29–33.

Marlow, D. R., & Redding, B. A. (1988). *Pediatric nursing* (6th ed.). (1988). Philadelphia: W. B. Saunders.

McCormick, L., & Schiefelbusch, R. L. (1984). *Early language intervention: An introduction.* Columbus, OH: Merrill.

McCubbin, H. I., & Patterson, J. M. (1983). Family transitions: adaptation to stress. In H. McCubbin & C. Figley (Eds.), *Stress and the family: Vol. 1. Coping with normative transitions* (pp. 5–25). New York: Brunner/Mazel.

Mead, M. (1989). Preface. In R. Benedict, *Patterns of culture.* Boston: Houghton Mifflin. (Original work published in 1934).

Miles, M. S. (1985). Emotional symptoms and physical health in bereaved parents. *Nursing Research, 34*(6), 76.

Moore, T., & Thompson, V. (1987). Elder abuse: A review of research programs and policies. *The Social Worker, 55*(1), 115–122.

Morris, S. (1972). *Grief and how to live with it.* New York: Grosset and Dunlap.

Moses, K. (1985). Dynamic intervention with families. In E. Cherow (Ed.), *Hearing-impaired children and youth with developmental disabilities: An interdisciplinary foundation for service* (pp. 87–103). Washington, DC: Gallaudet College Press.

Murrell, S. A., & Stachowiak, J. G. (1967). Consistency, rigidity, and power in the interaction patterns of clinic and nonclinic families. *Journal of Abnormal Psychology, 61*(3), 265–272.

Nelson, B. J. (1984). *Making an issue of child abuse: Political agenda setting for social problems.* Chicago: University of Chicago Press.

Osborne, A. B. (1989). Insiders and outsiders: Cultural membership and the micropolitics of education among the Zuni. *Anthropology and Education Quarterly, 20*(1), 196–215.

Parents as Teachers. (1987). *Evaluation from model project to statewide parents as teachers program.* St. Louis, MO: University of Missouri-St. Louis Parents as Teachers National Center.

Prevention '89/'90. (1990). Washington, DC: National Health Information Center.

Rochlin, G. R. (1965). *Griefs and discontents: The forces of change.* Boston: Little, Brown.

Rokeach, M. (1973). *The nature of human values.* New York: Free Press.

Rollin, W. J. (1987). *The psychology of communication disorders in individuals and their families.* Englewood Cliffs, NJ: Prentice-Hall.

Satir, V. (1967). *Conjoint family therapy*. Palo Alto, CA: Science and Behavior Books.

Saxon, S. V., & Etten, M. J. (1984). *Psychosocial rehabilitative programs for older adults*. Springfield, IL: Charles C. Thomas.

Schachter, S. (1964). The interaction of cognition and physiological determinants of emotional state. In L. Berkowitz (Ed.), *Advances in Experimental Social Psychology* (Vol. 1, pp. 36–43). New York: Academic Press.

Scheuerle, J., Olsen, S., Guilford, A. M., Redding, B., & Habal, M. B. (1984). A survey of nursing care for parents and infants with cleft lip and palate. *Cleft Palate Journal, 21,* 110–114.

Schow, R. L., Christensen, J. M., Hutchinson, J. M., & Nerbonne, M. (1978). *Communication disorders of the aged: A guidebook for health professionals*. Baltimore: University Park Press.

Shadden, B. (1988). Interpersonal communication patterns and strategies in the elderly. In B. B. Shadden (Ed.), *Communicating behavior and aging* (pp. 182–196). Baltimore, MD: Williams and Wilkins.

Shaw, M. E. (1964). Communication networks. In L. Berkowitz (Ed.), *Advances in experimental social psychology* (Vol.1, pp. 111–147). New York: Academic Press.

Shaw, M. E. (1978). Communication networks 14 years later. In L. Berkowitz (Ed.), *Group processes* (pp. 351–361). New York: Academic Press.

Shewan, C. M. (1988). Adaptation and progress in times of change. *ASHA, 30*(8), 27–30.

Shuchter, S. R. (1986). *Dimensions of grief*. San Francisco: Jossey-Bass.

Smith, W., & Roberts, J. M. (1954). *Zuni Lay: A field of values*. Cambridge, MA: Peabody Museum.

Springer, S. P., & Deutsch, G. (1985). *Left brain, right brain* (rev. ed.). New York: W. H. Freeman.

Stachowiak, J. G. (1968). Decision-making and conflict resolution in the family group. In C. E. Larson & F. E. X. Dance (Eds.), *Perspectives on communication* (pp. 113–124). Milwaukee: University of Wisconsin Press.

Stordtbeck, F. I. (1951). Husband-wife interaction over revealed differences. *American Sociological Review*. 468–473.

Todd, N. W. (1986). High-risk populations for otitis media. In J. F. Kavanagh (Ed.), *Otitis media and child development* (pp. 52–59). Parkton, MD: York Press.

Trends affecting U.S. health care systems (DHEW Pub. No. HRA 76-14503). (1976). Washington, DC: U.S. Government Printing Office.

Van Riper, C., & Emerick, L. L. (1990). *Speech Correction* (8th ed.). Englewood Cliffs, NJ: Prentice-Hall.

Vinje, D. L. (1982). Cultural values and economic development: U.S. Indian reservations. *Social Science Journal, 19*(1), 87–100.

Viorst, J. (1986). *Necessary losses*. New York: Fawcett Gold Medal Books.

Weed, L. (1969). *Medical records, medical education, and patient care: The problem-oriented record as a basic tool*. Cleveland, OH: Case Western Reserve University.

Yolam, I. D. (1970). *The therapy and practice of group psychotherapy*. New York: Basic Books.

CHAPTER FIVE

❦ ❦ ❦

Counseling/Helping Across Treatment Settings

Issues

❦ *Clients/caregivers who are confronted with communication disorders have needs for counseling regardless of the work setting where they are seen for evaluation and treatment of the problem.*

❦ *The environment of the clinician's work setting influences the counseling role and the opportunity to utilize interactive abilities with co-workers.*

❦ *Therapeutic power lies in the communication of knowledge, skill, values, beliefs, attitudes, and ideas that the counselor expresses through interactive behavior.*

❦ *Counselors or helpers must be aware of both personal biases and communicative strengths that may influence interpersonal communications.*

❦ ❦ ❦

COUNSELING NEEDS EXIST IN ANY TREATMENT SETTING

Some clinicians may enjoy an entire career in a single work setting. Others may change practice sites every few years to experience something new, to achieve another standard of excellence, or simply to live in a different geographical location. Most clinicians will not work in all possible settings. Those who serve clients in several work settings must exhibit flexibility, competence, and self-assurance among their personal traits. The potential for limitless elements to enter a discussion of counseling/helping across treatment settings could be overwhelming. An organized approach considers three major aspects of services to communicatively handicapped clients and their families: characteristics of treatment settings, therapeutic power of the counselor, and personal values related to counseling.

❧ ❧ ❧

CHARACTERISTICS OF TREATMENT SETTINGS

Shewan (1989) reported that 75% of audiologists and speech-language pathologists are employed in direct service to clients. Work settings include schools, hospitals, clinics, universities, and private offices. Although working with clients/caregivers has many similarities regardless of the setting, the counseling role of the clinician can vary considerably from place to place and position to position in the organizational structure of each setting. Settings where clinical services are offered have been described in many ways, and the variety of sites continues to grow. As we consider the application of helping skills across settings, it will be efficient to group the settings and discuss workplaces of communication disorders professionals from two organizational foci: institutional and independent.

Institutional Settings

Institutional settings include all those which have recognized organizational structures for administration of facilities and staff and which provide services and/or products (Oyer, 1987). An institutional setting may be public or private, industrial, educational, or health-related, nonprofit or for-profit. To maintain existence and sustain economic soundness, the primary administrative purpose of a business is to stay in business. Employees of an institution must be able to effect continuity of the establishment as well as to provide services. The placement of professional services personnel in the institutional management scheme is often referred to as *front line*. The clinician meets and deals with the client, who is the consumer of the institutional product or service, while many layers of managerial backup or support positions distribute other necessary work to sustain the integrity and solvency of the institution within its legal corporate structure and the highly competitive business community. Figure 5.1 shows a scheme of an institutional management hierarchy. Policy-makers occupy the top boxes in the diagram. The more layers or strata of middle management found in an institution, the greater the distance between the chief executive officer and the front-line staff who carry out their policies. The greater this distance, the more critical is the communication network within the institution to assure the availability of needed information that is both accurate and timely. Efficient communication informs staff members of the establishment's maintenance factors such as policies, interdepartmental relations, job security, and job status and motivational factors such as achievements, recognition, advancements, work progress, growth, and change.

If the speech, language, and hearing service has a large base of clients, one or more of the clinicians may be appointed to carry out administrative duties or assume responsibility for overall function of the communication

Figure 5.1
Institutional management hierarchy

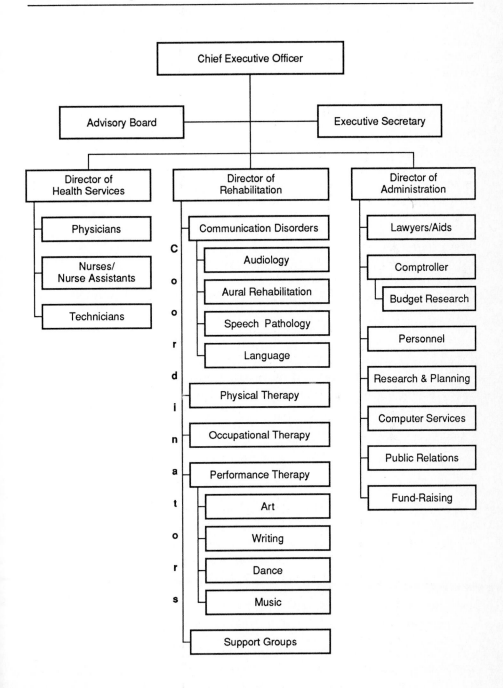

disorders clinic. Those responsibilities usually carry with them a job title of director, coordinator, or manager of comparable status. In day-to-day performance of duties, each employee affects the work setting and others within the work unit. This influence may be expressed or felt between individuals whose positions lie on a horizontal plane of the diagram, or between individuals whose relative positions in the hierarchy appear above or below each other.

The two-dimensional display shown in Figure 5.1 demonstrates the principle behind McLuhan's (1964) statement that the "media is the message." The need to represent pictorially the order of the relationships among employees in an institution has resulted in the appearance that administrative status is higher than that of front-line personnel. This concept is reinforced in the corporate atmosphere of contemporary society and reflected in differentials in pay scales and language to describe positions, such as upper-level administration or top management. While the stratification of management positions may be artificial, people who hold those positions exercise power over subordinates. This power is recognized in theory and in fact. One way this power is recognized is in the salary differentials associated with administrative positions (Guthrie, 1988). Managers exercise power through decision-making in matters that affect their subordinates. Dale (1969) identified five types of decision-makers.

1. The *ideal* decision-maker—uses capacities to the fullest; is totally productive; is fully accepted in harmonious group.
2. The *receptive* decision-maker—is happiest when a subordinate presents a summary of a problem and suggests a solution.
3. The *exploiting* decision-maker—likes and steals new ideas; cleverness exceeds performance.
4. The *hoarding* decision-maker—does not welcome ideas; resists change.
5. The *marketing* decision-maker—is opportunistic; looks for institutional (or division) advantage; wants to look good and increase share of budget.

Admittedly, any single administrator, manager, or supervisor may have traits of more than one type of decision-maker. However, each manager usually exhibits a dominant type of decision-making behavior.

In an institutional setting, the communication disorders clinician is a front-line professional staff member employed to serve other employees, residents of the institution, or clients, patients, or students. Recipients of these services may be participants in prevention programs such as industrial hearing screenings or routine health care examinations or in treatment programs such as in public schools, rehabilitation centers, or university training program clinics. Clinical research may also be carried out by practitioners in all these settings where the clients exhibit a particular disorder, participate in a specific treatment regimen, or benefit from innovative services.

Independent Settings

In independent settings for treatment of communication disorders, clinicians may offer part-time services through informal home visitation to selected clients in whom they are interested and at a cost below the community average. Full-time and part-time private practices accounted for 30% of employment among ASHA members in 1988 (Shewan, 1989), and the number continues to increase (Feldman, 1988). Private practices of speech-language pathologists or audiologists are businesses, which may be organized as sole proprietorships, partnerships, or professional associations (PAs, corporations) (Battin & Fox, 1978) and whose sellable product is service. Each service unit must stand on its own merits. Success of the practice depends on client satisfaction with the professional services and the maintenance of proficient relationships within the highly competitive business community.

An independent practice may be limited to one clinician who sees clients on one or more days per week, working either part-time or full-time; or it may consist of a large group practice offering speech, language, and hearing services in conjunction with psychology, physical therapy, occupational therapy or other related health care professionals. Still another collaborative relationship of the private practitioner can exist in a community network of specialists who utilize patient referrals and share information and opinions. In independent practice, the individual is both employer and employee, and stratified management is usually absent. The need for continual communication between the practitioner and resources in the community is critical. The independence and challenge of the private practice setting are not suited for every clinician. The freedom to set policies and service practices follows only after the application of astute business sense and continual public relations in addition to excellent work. A degree of financial independence from the business itself offers an added measure of security.

Conaway (1989) indicated that problems for succeeding in private practice, like reasons for the slow increase in numbers of private practitioners, lie in the lack of basic professional training. Although university training programs continue to graduate nurturing, helping clinicians, those same programs leave graduates unprepared to deal with today's institutional and economic environment. Guthrie (1988) pointed out that 80% of ASHA's members are women, and Crane and Cooper (1983) described a sample of women graduate students as passive, compliant, stereotypically feminine, sensitive, anxious, highly imaginative, creative, and energetic. Like other studies, the Crane and Cooper report implies that those are characteristics of therapists, but points to the continuing and growing need for professionals who are also astute in organizational structure and competent in management of service programs. Figure 5.2 displays some of the many directions in which the energies and attentions of the private practitioner are drawn. It is no wonder that multidimensional demands and stress levels of the private practitioner scare off even those individuals whose professional abilities can certainly stand on their own merit.

❧ ❧ ❧

TREATMENT SETTING INFLUENCES COUNSELOR ROLE

In each treatment setting, whether institutional or independent, counseling relationships between clinicians and their clients and caregivers are ideally dictated by the needs and abilities of each individual involved in treatment. In some settings, however, according to the policies or practices

Figure 5.2
Multidimensional involvement of the private practitioner

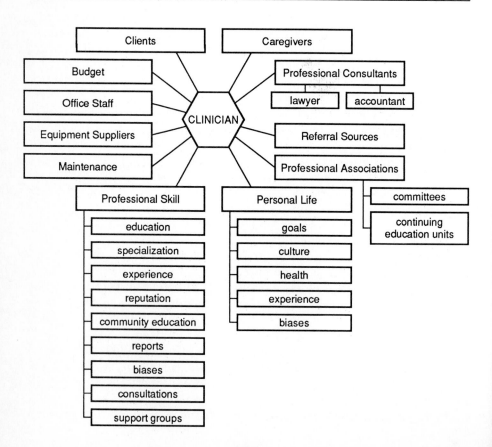

in place at any given time, counseling may be considered the domain of another discipline. Fischer (1978) reported that professional affiliation has no influence on a counselor's ability to help clients. However, some administrators and professional colleagues hold that counseling of any sort is simply not to be done by the communication disorders personnel.

Effect of Policy and Tradition on the Counseling Role

Time limits, heavy caseloads, extensive paperwork demands, administrative duties, and other factors imposed by the clinician's job description in some work settings preclude opportunities for counseling clients with communication disorders or their caregivers. In some of these situations, clinicians have been known to provide the help they believe is needed outside their normal work hours, without compensation or with minimal reimbursement. In other settings, activities that are called *counseling* and carried out by speech-language pathologists and audiologists are essentially informational or instructional relative to the particular communication disorder being treated. In such cases, adjustment aspects of the therapeutic experience may depend on referral to available resources of psychological and support services, or they may be left for clients to resolve on their own.

Many communication disorders professionals continue to believe that *counseling* is an activity defined only in the traditional manner of psychotherapy. In a setting where this belief is held by administrative personnel, the communicologist should be cautious in pursuing the need to include counseling by that name in the clinical management of clients. To do so may be perceived as contrary to the policies and practices espoused by the employing institution. Further, to act contrary to the institutional policies is to risk loss of employment there. It is comforting to remember that Rogers (1951) adopted the term *helping* to circumvent essentially those same criticisms. Through his long-term demonstration of the success of his ideas, he introduced the whole new way of thinking about the tasks of human services professionals. Nonetheless, in each service delivery setting, there must be the entity of the establishment or business that offers the service, and there must be loyal clinicians who represent the interests of the establishment by providing that service to clients.

Areas of potential conflict with colleagues, supervisors, or employers may result from differences in traditions, philosophies, or office management procedures and are possible in any communication disorders service setting. Resolving such differences and preventing conflict introduce another opportunity for the clinician to use the same interpersonal communication skills that apply in counseling. Experts who help clients change behavior can selectively apply those same helping techniques to modify their own reactions, their interpersonal interactions, and the behaviors of others observed in the work setting.

Effect of Counseling Skills on the Work Environment

Use of counseling or helping skills among personnel in the work setting can be a means of achieving a better professional product for the client. Helping skills can influence worker morale as well as practices and policies in the client treatment setting. Practices are the activities or customs carried out in the daily routine. Policies are the stated intentions of the parent organization, that is, the institution or independent practice. To gain a better understanding of the use of helping skills in the work setting, we need to continue exploring the clinician's many dimensions of personal investment, interaction, and influence in speech, language, and hearing treatment environments.

First, we must recognize that there are two basic entities continually interacting: the *establishment* within which the clinician works and the *clinician.* Each is capable of influencing the other in overt and subtle ways. The size of the establishment may range from a large megacorporation with a national base of operation to a sole proprietorship serving clients from a local district. Regardless of the size of the facility or the number of professional colleagues in the setting, the clinician's interaction with the setting's physical and human environment must have a beginning and a continuity.

To participate equitably in a program within an institution, clinicians must understand and appreciate the goals and philosophy of the establishment. That appreciation arises from knowing their own goals and expectations and recognizing how they fit into the establishment's milieu. Thus, we can consider the clinician's participatory experience in the work setting in two phases: selection of a work setting and work relationships in daily practice.

Selection of a Work Setting

Selection of a speech, language, or hearing employment setting may be approached in many ways. University placement services, professors' personal contacts within the community, educational internships, or clinical externships may introduce the beginning clinician to a potential employer. Some clinicians know and like the exact career parameters that suit them best. Clinicians who are generalists in professional skills as well as in interest may involve a number of considerations in the selection of work setting, although each clinician may have different priorities. Important considerations of job selection include availability, location, Clinician Fellowship Year opportunity, age of clientele, communication disorders treated, job description, rewards/benefits, and acceptability of the institution's philosophy. Based on information and impressions about the work setting, clinicians decide whether the proffered employment meets their current needs as a viable work setting.

A viable work setting invites clinicians to do what they do best and to enjoy doing it. A viable work setting offers a means to achieve current goals. Employment at a particular setting may be seen as achieving the next step on the way to realization of career plans and toward personal fulfillment or self-actualization. According to Maslow's (1943) theory of human motivation, the new position enables the clinicians to satisfy some of the needs within their developmental sequence (Figure 5.3). Selection of a new work setting concurs with placement in the hierarchy that differs for each clinician at the start and throughout the duration of a lifetime career.

Beginning clinicians, especially those with school loans to pay back, may start on the first step of Maslow's hierarchy of needs. That is, the dominant need is to achieve food, shelter, and solvency independently from parents or other former providers. A first position may assure the satisfaction of physiological needs only. Beginning clinicians may complete their Clinical Fellowship Years, an ASHA requirement for the CCC, in one setting and then seek other employment to satisfy needs for professional and personal stimulation. With experience, a clinician may decide to change jobs and accept new responsibilities because such a change is perceived as more prestigious. Thus, following Maslow's progression toward self-actualization, this individual has satisfied physiological needs of nutrition and safety, attained a stimulating and secure environment, elevated personal and professional social status, and now seeks to enhance self-esteem.

Figure 5.3
Developmental sequence following Maslow's theory of human motivation

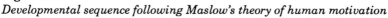

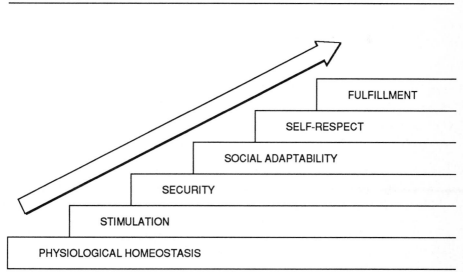

Further pursuit of self-esteem and self-discovery may involve clinicians looking for an opportunity to exercise creative talents and demonstrate an advanced level of expertise in diagnosis or standardization of application of a treatment protocol, which they have developed and proven over a period of concentrated work. Such a change or development may also apply to the clinician who decides to accept a supervisory or administrative post. Ideally, the supervisor or administrator takes to the new position all the skills of interpersonal interaction that served so well in clinical expertise. The reader should not assume that every clinical expert is also a promising administrative expert. These occupations demand different strengths and skills; neither career position is suitable for everyone.

Interpersonal Relationships in Daily Practice

The experiences of clinicians moving toward fulfillment denote dual motivation, both internal and external. The intrapersonal needs of the clinician comprise one source of motivation and the stimuli from the work environment comprise the other. By combining Maslow's hierarchy of needs with the two-factor theory suggested by Herzberg (1966), the administrator and total work environment act as the external motivator as the employee moves toward self-actualization. The external factors discussed by Herzberg are the ability of the establishment to maintain an environment conducive to doing the needed tasks and the ability of administrators to motivate employees to do the tasks. Figure 5.4 shows the relationship between internal and external motivational forces. This is the ideal coordination of the individual's needs satisfaction with the motivational powers of the employer, supervisor, or manager, which is espoused in human relations theory (Likert, 1961). It is this compatible match between the work setting and the clinician that allows and encourages progress along the continuum toward personal goals of the clinician and product or service enhancement for the employer.

Personal Needs In the Workplace

Various degrees of involvement in helping relationships occur in daily interactions within the environment where we work, study, and relax. The communicative exchange between co-workers is often casual and soon forgotten. Just as often, verbal and nonverbal messages shift the direction of thinking and feeling for the sender as well as for the receiver for a considerable period of time.

The need for the application of helping skills among colleagues, peers, and superiors holds some similarities to the need in the clinician's relationship with clients and caregivers. Although clinicians have no caregiving obligations to their peers, as mentally healthy people they view and react to all people in similar ways. In a mentally healthy environment,

Figure 5.4
Interaction of internal and external motivation

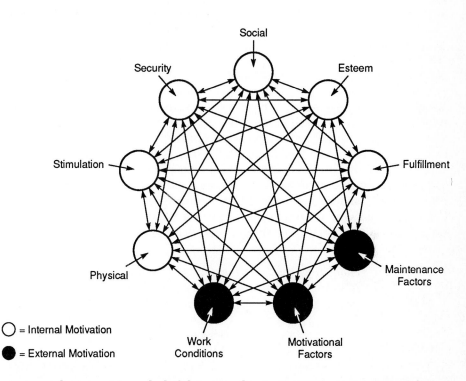

reciprocal support is as helpful in mundane situations as in stressful, creative, or experimental endeavors.

Job descriptions define and limit professional interaction among personnel in a work setting. That professional interaction is often extended and transposed into personal communication and friendship. We expect competency among fellow clinicians and share with them mutual respect because of that competency as well as individual differences that extend the expertise of the discipline. The same attitude is held for and displayed toward support staff whose jobs enable clinical services to be offered in smoothly coordinated ways day after day. Competent management provides opportunity for all staff members to utilize their strengths and develop new skills.

An essential task of administration or management is decision-making. Arbitrary decisions that are made as a part of daily routine can distract clinicians from their clinical work and call attention to inequities and injustices among personnel. Tensions that arise from real and imagined issues must be resolved immediately to prevent harmful morale problems from developing. Tensions often arise in response to the announcement of a decision that has been made. Sometimes tension noted in a group originates in misperceptions and misunderstandings. The proven way to prevent or dissipate debilitating tensions in a work group is through a competent network of communication that is found to be reliable over time. Through that medium, concerned individuals can gain insight into the rationale and justification of the decision, even when they don't like or agree with its results.

Stein (1985) indicated that decision-making in the clinical setting is very complex. Decision-making includes both conscious and unconscious issues. Among these are inner conflicts, assumptions, fantasies, expectations, beliefs, vulnerabilities, problem-solving abilities, values, and attitudes. Add to those elements trained observation, data collection, and assessment skills, and decision-making begins to take on aspects of the actual complexity involved. Decision-making in nonclinical matters is not limited to administrators. Instead, every interaction or communication involves decisions by both participants, that is, action and reaction. The following situations represent decisions that were made and require additional decisions to prevent or resolve disruptive outcomes.

1. Use of the school copy machine for personal business is strictly prohibited. A newly employed clinician at the school requests and receives permission to use the copy machine to make five copies of an 87-page thesis.
2. Ms. Mucherson put the audiometer's earphones in her desk again last night and locked the drawer for safety.
3. Mr. Haiotka, the senior clinician, wears a cologne to which Mrs. Washington, his assistant, is allergic.
4. When Dr. Brown-Pryor, the founding audiologist of the group, retired, her office space was assigned to the clinic director's administrative assistant because of its proximity to his office.

Such seemingly petty conflicts can undermine work relationships in any setting. The reader is invited to consider ways to resolve these disruptive situations with the use of helping characteristics and behaviors. First, list the individuals involved in the outcomes of the decision. Identify the investment of each of those participants. Then imagine inviting those people to interact in a constructive way to reduce the impact of differences they see and the negative feelings caused by those perceived differences.

Situations that arise at work are not essentially unlike those likely to occur in the everyday life of ordinary people, families, and student groups. In such situations, workers are invited to participate in conflict-resolution by applying helping skills.

❦ ❦ ❦

THERAPEUTIC POWER AND THE COUNSELOR

These highly regarded management theories of internal and external motivation can be applied to people in any job or position, any profession or career, or any geographical or cultural region. The combined hierarchy of needs and motivation-maintenance model is not unlike the ideal relationship between the client/caregiver and communication disorders therapist. Achievement of self-actualization in communicative abilities is believed by the clinician to be the goal of each client. Clients participate in interpersonal interactions with the clinician, whose astutely applied treatment techniques and counseling skills have a large part in motivating the client to move steadily toward that goal. Figure 5.5 presents an adaptation of the motivation-maintenance progression to suggest the harmony

Figure 5.5
Adaptation of hierarchy of needs and motivation-maintenance theory to motivational value of client-clinician relationship

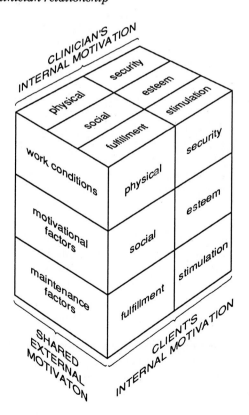

between counselor behavior and client progress. It indicates that client progress and client-clinician interaction are ongoing. In this sense, one can see how therapeutic power, which was introduced in chapter 2, is developed and maintained in conjunction with but separate from techniques for speech, language, or hearing therapy.

Therapeutic power is defined as selection of activity plus timing plus application. That is, the counselor selects the appropriate action for or reaction to the presence or activity of the client/caregiver; the counselor's selected activity is correctly matched to the client's or caregiver's expressed or intended message; the form and manner of the counselor's performance of the selected behavior is appropriate for the perceived client/caregiver need. Figure 5.6 displays an adaptation of this equation, listing the elements of each segment of the equation. Exchanges between parties are often so brief and rapid that many are missed in behavior counts made during direct observations. As suggested earlier, videotaping is a useful tool for analyzing the application of therapeutic power. A sequence might go like this:

- Clinician enters room and looks at the client.
- Client smiles, reaching out to touch the clinician's chair.
- Clinician smiles.
- Client makes eye contact.

The therapeutic power in the therapist-client relationship is based on the counselor's perception of the client, the client's performance and attitude, and the client's ability to elicit clinician behavior through the use of cues, which the counselor can and does interpret. That is, when the therapist's behavior—technical or counseling, action or reaction—is correctly matched to the client's need and the therapist's manner of response is acceptable to the client, the client's interest and reaction or response is elicited. Matched behavior by the therapist reassures and encourages the client. The client is then ready to participate in the next communicative exchange. This, in turn, confirms for the clinician the correspondence of the treatment paradigm to the client's communicative status and motivates the clinician to pursue yet another step in the protocol of client behavior change.

We can also rewrite the therapeutic power equation in terms of client/caregiver's perception of *achievement,* one aspect of client/caregiver motivation:

Communicative ability + Use of learned technique + Controlled activity → Therapeutic progress.

For the client/caregiver, therapeutic progress represents positive steps in satisfaction of the hierarchy of needs toward actualization of better com-

Figure 5.6
Therapeutic power: elements found in equation segments

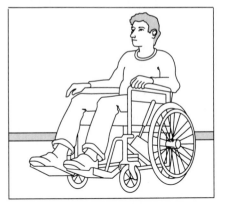

a) Nonverbal client sits waiting.

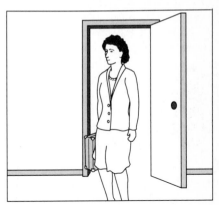

b) Clinician enters the room.

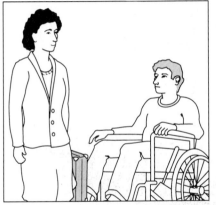

c) Client makes eye contact with clinician.

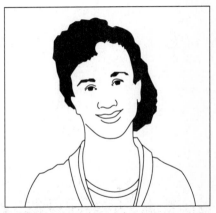

d) Clinician smiles.

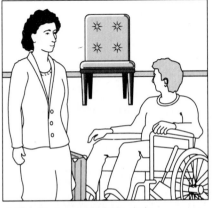

e) Client looks at clinician's chair.

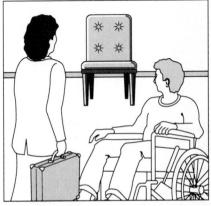

f) Clinician moves toward the chair.

municative ability. Progress acts as a motivational factor in achieving success and avoiding failure.

Although communicative activities by either the client or clinician may be verbal or nonverbal, as discussed in chapter 2, here we are limited to use of a verbal dialogue to demonstrate some elements of therapeutic power. Table 5.1 presents a series of statements made by a client. Each is followed by several choices of ways the helper may have responded. As you read the statements, select the counselor response in each group that seems most likely to provide the appropriate attending message to elicit the subsequent client statement.

❦ ❦ ❦

PERSONAL VALUES RELATED TO COUNSELING

Counselors As Self-Actualizing Persons

Human relations concepts can be applied by all the personnel of an establishment to all the people who work there. That is, self-actualizing employees, clinicians, and other staff as well as clients experience similar sequences of needs satisfaction. They react to internal and external stimuli, although at any given time each person may be in a different phase of achieving self-actualization. McConnell (1974, p. 631) restated Maslow's characteristics of self-actualizing people. They are summarized in the following statements:

- They are realistic and comfortable with reality.
- They understand and accept themselves.
- They behave simply and naturally and lack artificiality.
- They are interested in problems, issues, and philosophical questions.
- They like privacy and tend to be detached.
- They are relatively independent and rely on themselves.
- They appreciate blessings and enjoy the pleasures of life.
- They experience limitless horizons of the mind.
- They have a deep feeling of kinship with others.
- They develop deep ties with a few other individuals.
- They are democratic but not indiscriminate, although they tend to be unaware of differences.
- They are goal-oriented and ethical, with moral standards and conventional attitudes.
- Their humor is philosophical, not hostile; they are more serious and thoughtful than spontaneous.
- They are original, inventive, and creative.
- While they exist well within the rules of their cultures, they live by their own laws.
- They make mistakes that they recognize and to which they respond with ordinary feelings.

Table 5.1
Client statements and clinician responses. Select the response that best fits the preceding client statement and elicits the subsequent client statement.

Client: Well, as I told you, I stopped going out. I found that I couldn't talk to strangers without losing my voice.

Response: a. Did your husband complain?
　　　　b. It must have been difficult for others in your family to make excuses for you all the time.
　　　　c. And then . . .

Client: For a while, I couldn't visit my in-laws unless I had a few drinks.

Response: a. Are you an alcoholic?
　　　　b. Tell me more about that.
　　　　c. How much did you drink?

Client: (Looking down at the floor) Well, I started out having just a little.

Response: a. And then it got to be more and more.
　　　　b. Well, let's talk about something else.
　　　　c. It's difficult to talk about this.

Client: (Silence — 30 seconds)

Response: a. Can you tell me what's the matter?
　　　　b. How many drinks do you have during an average day?
　　　　c. (Attentive silence)

Client: I haven't told this to anyone before. I drink from the time I get up until my family comes home.

Response: a. Do members of your family drink?
　　　　b. I guess it's not easy to talk about.
　　　　c. Alcohol is quite expensive.

Note. Responses that the clinician actually made are identified in the Exercises section at the end of this chapter.

Fulmer (1974) combined the self-actualization characteristics named by Maslow (1943) and Rogers' goals of normal, human behavior (1951) and reduced them to six easy-to-remember statements, which describe mentally healthy and emotionally mature people:

1. They can accept the way things really are.
2. They are not afraid to get close to others.
3. They are efficient judges of situations.
4. They are creative and appreciative.
5. They are self-reliant.
6. They are willing to learn from anyone.

It has long been the contention of psychiatry and psychology that only mentally healthy and emotionally mature individuals should carry out psychotherapy. The role of counselor does not replicate treatment processes of psychoanalytic psychotherapy (Rousey, 1974, 1982), which is appropriate in special settings and requires extensive study in psychology. It does, however, draw the clinician into ongoing participation with the client in a close interpersonal relationship that affects the life of the clinician as well as the client (Klevans, 1982). It follows that professionals with such profound influence on the lives of their clients must likewise be knowledgeable about human behavior, especially their own.

Knowing Ourselves—Our Values

Characteristics of proficient, enduring speech-language pathologists and audiologists (Stone & Olswang, 1989; Rollin, 1987) reflect those that comprise the psychologically healthy individual, whose traits disclose a whole, fully functioning person and an effective counselor (Carkhuff and Berenson, 1967). Cole (1982) repeated the long-held principle that the effectiveness of helping depends not so much on what the clinician knows as the kind of person the clinician is. He discussed the helper's intrinsic personal values as less tangible qualities that influence the therapist's behavior and influence on others. He defined values as beliefs, attitudes, standards, or philosophy of an individual (p. 25). Strupp (1980) formulated specific statements of essential values held by mentally healthy self-actualizing people. These values comprise helpers' perspectives on humankind inclusive of themselves and others and hold that:

1. Every individual has the right to personal freedom and independence.
2. Members of society have rights and privileges as well as responsibilities to others.
3. Individuals are responsible for independently conducting their own lives.
4. Individuals are responsible for their own actions, but not for their feelings or fantasies.
5. Individuals deserve respect and should not be controlled, manipulated, or indoctrinated.
6. Individuals must make their own mistakes and learn from daily living.

These statements of values express ideals common in society. Rarely does the reader find someone who disagrees with the philosophy they express regardless of ethno-cultural origins. However, translation of these abstract statements of ideals into the practical daily experience finds a less universal agreement.

As a general rule, the way in which each person internalizes and acts upon a set of values begins in his/her relationships with adults during early, formative years. From that time onward, ordinary daily living has called on the maturing, adult individual to make decisions within and outside of the home environment, among circumstances and influences that are continually changing. A single incident has dramatically different influences on each involved individual, even though all participants may come from the same socio-cultural background. That is, each person formulates a unique perspective on experience relative to an internalized value system. This personal value system is truly unique, different from all others. The difference is much like the difference between the reports of several eyewitnesses of an incident. They may be similar, but different. Generally, personal valuing is not a conscious action but automatic experiential phenomena that occur as if by reflex, to delineate the unfamiliar (i.e., new or different), the unexpected (i.e., distracting or shocking), and the unacceptable (i.e., disregarded or destroyed).

The same stimuli can diversely affect clinicians, clients, and caregivers, depending on their backgrounds and perceptions of the stimuli. They likewise affect individuals who are supervisors, professors, employers, professional colleagues, politicians, neighbors, and members of the same family in different ways. It is often a puzzle how such differing people can set aside their own unique perspectives and work in harmony with one another. The initial step toward appreciation of all the variability among people, like appreciation of the people themselves, requires that we gain insight into our own perceptions, valuing system, and reactions to the world around us. In that way, we can reduce the chances that our impressions and expectations of ourselves and others are contaminated by personal biases.

Socrates, the ancient Greek philosopher, knew and taught the wisdom of self-knowledge: *Know thyself, know your strengths and your weaknesses, your potentials and limitations; take stock of yourself.* In doing so, mentally healthy people can accurately assess their needs, their value systems, and their goals in life and realize that these change over time. In other words, normally developing people have accurate self-images and feel content with those self-images. The contentment or satisfaction is positive self-esteem. Thus, self-knowledge, self-image, and self-esteem are intimately linked together and act concertedly to create self-directing individuals. Under self-direction, each person selectively interacts with influential stimuli and proceeds toward self-actualization, for each marches to a different drummer.

Learning, maturing, and growing are all part of self-valuing, and self-actualizing. The initial goal is to learn about oneself. This cannot be done only by reading about and studying the self as a separate abstract entity. Instead, understanding of self comes from action in and interaction with a multivariate society. Comparisons and contrasts between actions and reactions can be seen and discussed, and differences of values, opinion, and experience explored. In that way, each participant begins to recognize and understand that basic personal values on which behavior is predicated differ in significant, glaring, subtle, and intricate ways. Divergence of values systems becomes apparent among close acquaintances as well as among members of different social groups and different ethnic groups. One way we discover differences in personal values systems and valuing processes is through exploration of differences among the people with whom we interact to discover their needs, values, and personal philosophies.

Among present and future clients and caregivers, clinicians can expect to find exciting, inspiring, and trying challenges. While each interpersonal interaction is unique, the underlying goal for all human services is the betterment of the quality of life for the client. Achievement of that goal does not follow a single or simple pattern, nor is it always possible. In some instances, conflicts introduce and give priority to other goals; in other instances, help is rejected.

Case Studies: The Client, Clinician, and Others Who Matter

Below are three traditional, realistic case studies, followed by commentaries on the participants and discussions of points of interest. These tales invite the reader to consider each situation and the values evidently held by each participant and determine the effects of those values on outcomes for the client. Participants in each story react in unique ways to the described set of circumstances. Some professionals are more involved than others with helping, as various constituents of the clients' environments are seen to serve different functions in the clients' rehabilitation.

I. The Case of Adrian Wienowski. Adrian is a 24-year-old man who has cerebral palsy. His Full-Scale IQ Score as measured by the Stanford Binet is 130. During his waking hours, he is confined to a motorized wheelchair which he propels by means of a manual lever. Dysarthria interferes with his oral expression of language. He has learned to use a computerized voice generator to facilitate his communication. Although his speech is slow, when he is required to rely on speech alone, he is judged by Ms. Smythe, his current speech-language pathologist at the University Speech and Hearing Center, to be approximately 60% intelligible. Adrian has been in communication therapy most of his life. He can now manage to express himself clearly in public places and social gatherings when listeners are accepting of his communicative differences. During his college career, his communicative abilities have been sufficient to meet the demands of the academic program in which he was enrolled.

In three weeks, he will have completed all the requirements for a Bachelor of Science degree with a dual major in mathematics and computer engineering. His university records confirm a 4-year grade point ratio (GPA) of 3.87. He will graduate with honors in a class of 5,478 students. Adrian has been an out-of-state university student. His parents live almost 1,500 miles away, where both have responsible jobs that they do not plan to leave. Adrian has demonstrated that he can live alone and care for himself. He now lives in an apartment that was modified for his use.

Adrian was informed by Dr. Montgomery, his major professor, of a local job available at Enis Computer-Engineering Company. Mr. Enis is a long-time acquaintance of Dr. Montgomery. The professor assured Adrian that he was qualified for the position and encouraged him to apply for it. With excitement and confidence, the student filled out the application forms and asked Dr. Montgomery to review his answers to several of the questions on the form.

After completing and mailing the forms and his resume to the company, Adrian was scheduled for an appointment with Ms. Hodge, director of personnel. When Adrian arrived for the initial interview, Ms. Hodge was polite and friendly in a formal, businesslike way. She opened a folder on her desk, glanced at the papers inside, and assured Adrian that he was overqualified for the open position. She did not indicate any need or interest for continuing their conversation beyond congratulating him on his resume and the work represented on it. She also discouraged Adrian from making an appointment to meet with Mr. Enis to discuss the position. Adrian was stunned and found no adequate response except to thank Ms. Hodge for seeing him.

Upon leaving the Enis Company, Adrian returned home where he first telephoned Dr. Montgomery, and then Ms. Smythe, his speech-language clinician, as he had promised to tell them about the interview. He spoke as clearly as usual, but his voice quality revealed that he was distressed. In each phone call, he told the listener that he was upset and angry that he had to go to the interview in a wheelchair. He indicated that the reaction to his disability had occurred prior to his initiating speech. He was able to tell them just the bare minimum about the conversational exchange during his visit to the Enis Company.

Commentary. There is limited information about Adrian and his experience with which we may explore the personal values and reactions of the involved parties. Acknowledging that limitation, we can still recognize some patterns in behavior, and we can venture an educated guess as to what each participant wanted or valued from the work-related situation.

Adrian's reactions show he is disappointed in the progress and outcome of the interview; angry that he was not given an appointment with Mr. Enis; suspicious that the personnel manager judged him on the basis of his wheelchair; dissatisfied with himself because he was not able to change the personnel manager's mind; and embarrassed because he thinks that he disappointed his professor and feels bad that he couldn't talk readily and rapidly during the interview.

What Adrian wants is to get the job; prove that he can get a job; show that he can do what Dr. Montgomery believes him to be capable of; and have Mr. Enis hire him to do what he does well. He also wants to please Dr. Montgomery and assure Ms. Smythe that he can communicate satisfactorily for a responsible position in the world of work.

The reactions of Ms. Hodge, the personnel manager, reveal that she is relieved that the interview is finished; certain that she made the right decision; satisfied with the outcome of the interview with Adrian; convinced that she did the right thing in discouraging the young, disabled man. She thought his university performance was outstanding and indicated that he could contribute greatly to a computer-engineering program in all areas important to the Enis company, and it would look good to have a statement about hiring the handicapped in the company's annual report. However, hiring Adrian would necessitate the purchase of expensive modified equipment and furniture that only he could use; if his ambition matches his academic record, job-satisfaction needs would change faster than the plans and budget of Enis would satisfy; and with that limitation on his growth and development, Adrian would leave the company for another, more challenging position. Ultimately, company expenses for modification of facilities would be wasted.

What Ms. Hodge wants is to get on to the next candidate so she can fill the position described in the job advertisement.

Mr. Enis does not know that Adrian has been interviewed.

What Mr. Enis wants is a conscientious employee who can do the job needed.

Dr. Montgomery's reactions show that he is disappointed because he believes that Adrian would work out well in the described position. He suspects the personnel manager's concerns about company expenses and the duration of Adrian's employment and questions the accuracy of the announcement of the open position. He also has some concerns that Adrian's experience will discourage other students from following his suggestions to apply for positions that he recommends.

What Dr. Montgomery wants is to confirm his judgment in placement of the best candidate for a job; to talk to Mr. Enis to clarify the difficulty in hiring a graduate identified for a specific position; to try to influence Mr. Enis concerning Adrian's potential positive contribution to the company; and to confirm his ability to bring his influence to bear in achieving this goal.

Ms. Smythe's reactions indicate she is disappointed; certain that Adrian's oral-aural communication is more than sufficient within his specialization; suspects that the personnel manager reacted to Adrian's competent but slow speech production; saddened because she considers this interview experience an unfortunate one for Adrian; angered that the business world appears to continue to react negatively to individuals who are different; and defensive about her professional role and responsibilities.

What Ms. Smythe wants is to assert to Dr. Montgomery and Ms. Hodge that Adrian is communicating efficiently; reassure Adrian that his communication is adequate for his specialization and he is functioning at an acceptable level; and establish the right and adequacy of her specialization to make these judgments.

Discussion. Except for Mr. Enis, the participants have different experiences, reactions, and views of Adrian's potential. Each participant has a different investment in Adrian's experience, and each investment is endowed with internalized valuing elements of the individual. While all the participants may feel and express empathy, genuineness, and warmth for the student, their reactions include their own needs, expectations, and desires as well as Adrian's. They all see a cost to themselves in Adrian's experience. Their behaviors and wants suggest that those personal elements precluded any counseling behaviors on their parts. No two people reacted in exactly the same way, yet their behaviors could be construed as acting in Adrian's interest. They are recognized as caring, concerned people; concerned for Adrian and their own influences in his life; their responsibilities to their own reputations, careers, jobs, and establishments. These concerns take precedence over helping Adrian deal with his immediate concerns. If any one of them had responded as a counselor, interaction with Adrian would have been quite different.

A counselor's reactions would involve perceiving and accepting Adrian's anger, hurt, and disappointment; his concern for the way in which his professor and clinician might receive his news; his fear of their potential disappointment in him; his distress over his need to use the wheelchair; and his realization and fear that his disability may be more of an employment handicap than he had come to believe.

What a counselor would want is for Adrian to recognize his current thoughts and feelings; reaffirm his own worth; address and get a grasp of the situation in a realistic way, inclusive of positive and negative aspects of the experience; figure out what alternatives are available to him; make decisions as to which alternatives are worth following and what next step to take; review his goals and perhaps adapt those goals; devise realistic strategies to achieve goals; and begin to apply the strategies.

II. The Case of Jahara and Her Great Grandmother. Mrs. Maebelle Spencer Brown is an 87-year-old widow, a proud great grandmother. She is recovering from a stroke, which left her a little weak on the right side of her body with a minor degree of upper limb apraxia and with poor auditory comprehension of spoken language and transitional mild speech apraxia. She has lived for 9 years with her granddaughter, Pearl Crosley, who is a single parent, and her 9-year-old great granddaughter, Jahara.

While Pearl advanced through responsible positions in her work at an insurance company office, Mrs. Brown helped take care of their home, meals, and the family laundry. She was there each day when Jahara got home from school and when the child had a holiday or was ill and needed to stay home from school. Mrs. Brown accompanied Jahara to the Community Speech and Hearing Center for several assessments during pre-school. She was also in the practice of meeting Jahara after school so they could walk home together. Three days each week, Miss Watson, the school speech-language pathologist, saw Jahara individually for 20 minutes of fluency therapy. On those days, Mrs. Brown met her great granddaughter at the front door of the school because it was close to the speech therapy room. Mrs. Brown has felt quite comfortable at the school's speech and hearing center. Mr. Allen, the school's audiologist one day a week, seemed like a nice man. He had tested Mrs. Brown's hearing several years ago at the Community Health Center when she discovered that sometimes people said one thing and she heard another. She remembers that Mr. Allen told her that her hearing loss was related to her age. Since then she has taken the hearing problem for granted, even though she has noticed at times that her hearing seems to be getting worse.

The shared living arrangement has met the family's needs for 9 years, and Jahara loves and respects her "gramma," who is her best friend and confidant. In fact, talking to her great grandmother has been the only communication experience for Jahara in which she is consistently and completely fluent. Similarly, Mrs. Brown has believed that her hearing problem is less noticeable, certainly less bother, when she is alone with Jahara. She has never had trouble understanding what Jahara was saying to her. Of course, Mrs. Brown knows that she could not hear anyone over the noise of the sweeper or the electric mixer. The two of them did a lot of things together, work and play, at the kitchen table. They would sit across the table from each other and talk, play, laugh, and sometimes sing. They would share stories of their day's adventures, read books, and plan activities for the time they would have available on Saturdays and Sunday afternoons.

One Saturday morning, Mrs. Brown got up to make breakfast, as was her custom. Twenty minutes later, Jahara went to the kitchen and found her great grandmother lying on the floor, unable to get up. Mrs. Brown seemed dazed and confused, unable to recognize Jahara. Jahara ran to wake her mother, who then called the emergency medical services. While they waited for help to arrive, Pearl telephoned a neighbor and asked if Jahara could stay there while she went to the emergency room with her grandmother. After the ambulance arrived, Mrs. Brown was taken to the hospital, where a medical team used computerized brain mapping to diagnose an ischemic CVA or occlusion in a secondary branch of the left middle cerebral artery. Mrs. Brown was admitted to the hospital for observation and stabilization. The attending physician, an internal medicine specialist, told Pearl that the patient would be in the hospital for at least a week, but would eventually be expected to regain about 80% of her prior body function. The specialist said Mrs. Brown might need extended care in a nursing home following dismissal from the hospital, and that several weeks would pass before her speech would clear up. Her condition was called *minor Broca's aphasia*. The report further suggested that Mrs. Brown was experiencing considerable confusion in understanding what was said to her. The physician explained that this might be a worsening of her known hearing loss, but had found no damage to the ear or eighth nerve during examination. The receptive problem appeared to be centrally located and nonreversible.

About 5 hours after Pearl had left home, Mrs. Brown was resting comfortably at the hospital. Weary and tired, Pearl then returned to collect Jahara from the neighbor's house where she had stayed. She found Jahara frightened and agitated, with the child's dysfluencies so frequent and profound that she became alarmed. The mother and daughter went home and huddled together on the sofa for mutual comfort.

The following day, Sunday, Jahara and her mother visited "gramma" at the hospital. The patient seemed alert and pleased to see Jahara, whom she immediately recognized. She tired quickly, however, so the mother and daughter left her to sleep and promised to return after Jahara's speech-language therapy Monday afternoon. Pearl planned to take time off from work to make sure Jahara would get to therapy on time.

At school the next day, Jahara was very quiet, even more so than usual. When her teacher asked if she was feeling all right, Jahara responded that she was okay, just tired. She did most of her school assignments and took only a little bit of written work to complete at home. When it was time for speech class, Jahara grabbed her books and papers and hurried to Miss Watson's room.

Miss Watson was startled to observe the severe increase in Jahara's dysfluency. To avoid calling attention to the dramatic breakdown in communication skills, Miss Watson re-introduced materials that would assure Jahara success in performing the tasks. By not allowing Jahara the opportunity to be more dysfluent, she increased the child's success with fluency. These experiences also served to stabilize fluency at a lower level than Jahara was capable of producing at the end of the previous week (Carlson, 1990).

As the session was ending and Jahara was gathering her papers, she told Miss Watson that she and her mother were going to visit "gramma." Miss Watson expressed interest in the pending visit and discovered the story of the illness and hospitalization that had occurred over the weekend. While Jahara relayed this story, Miss Watson accompanied her to the front of the school where her mother was waiting. She expressed her concern for Mrs. Brown and extended empathic best wishes to Jahara's mother. She then told Jahara good-bye and congratulated her on "good working," and promised to be ready for her on Wednesday. Miss Watson was relieved to learn what lay behind Jahara's severe relapse. It eased her concerns about the child. It was disappointing to see such a large step backward, but at least Mrs. Brown was on the mend.

Commentary: The reactions of people involved during Mrs. Brown's illness reveal differences in their perceptions and their inner valuing of those perceptions. While age may explain some of those differences, others relate to the degree and duration of attachments and dependency. The suddenness, unexpectedness, and severity of the illness focused their attention on the startling realization of the advanced age of the key-stone of a household. Jahara and her family react to fundamental problems far more threatening than those acknowledged by any character in the case of Adrian Wienowski.

What all characters want in the story of Jahara and her great grandmother is for the illness and its effects to go away. Fear and anxiety permeate the household and interpersonal relationships. However, confronted with the realities of daily survival, the needs of each character are met in simple compensatory ways which signify the socio-cultural and personal values of Jahara's family and therapist. The following descriptions indicate some of the characteristics of their environment which erupted into their awareness and overshadow all else.

Mrs. Brown's reaction involved her feeling physiologically threatened and dependent, representing the first of Maslow's (1943) steps. Her conscious awareness came and went during the critical hours of onset of the illness, and her awareness was directed toward survival, the will to live. As she recovered and acknowledged the changes in her body, she felt grief for the loss of physical stamina. She could not talk or swallow. She began to fear the possible outcome of this illness, of either not recovering or recovering with diminished capacity. However, Mrs. Brown's courage and determination to continue her loving relationship with Jahara added to her will to survive and become independent again, or to achieve physiological need-satisfaction.

As the crisis passed, Mrs. Brown regained the ability to swallow and to move her tongue. Six weeks later, after recovering in a nursing home, she returned home. She was required to rest several times during the day and take her medicine regularly. She walked steadily, but slower than before. She used a crab cane, and because of her illness and residual right side weakness she was restricted in the chores she could do to her own satisfaction. This limitation annoyed her, but Jahara was a big help. Working together after Jahara came home from school provided an opportunity for each of them to practice her communication skills. Each agreed that the late afternoon and early evening are the best parts of the day.

This determined, aging patient was able to manage most things for herself. Her work load was reduced, with her family participating more in the management of the home, but Mrs. Brown remained a proud woman and gladly let everyone know who really "runs the place." Her increased appreciation of her own mortality intensified her attention to the people around her. She learned quickly to delegate small jobs and to spend some precious energies in starting to teach Jahara how to become an independent survivor, too.

Jahara's reaction initially was being terrified to find "gramma" on the kitchen floor. She could only run to her mother for help. After that, her part in caring for Mrs. Brown largely involved staying out of the grown-ups' way and going ahead with routine in spite of the terrors of anxiety, fear, and anger that boiled inside her. Her relationship with her mother may have become closer, but her need for "gramma" continued to be evident in her distractibility and eagerness to visit the hospital, and later the nursing home. Each subsequent visit to see her great grandmother was anticipated with great energy. Each visit was all too short, and saying good-bye was very sad. In this anxious fashion, Jahara slowly shut out the terror that almost suffocated her when gramma got sick and was taken away in the ambulance.

When Mrs. Brown returned home again, Jahara saw for the first time how old her great grandmother appeared. She and gramma developed a modified routine that incorporated her gentle but clumsy care of "gramma" and help with household chores. As the days passed and her great grandmother's speech cleared up, Jahara's ability to speak more fluently with her slowly increased. She was very careful to be sure that she faced her gramma when talking to her, because that helped to get ideas across. She learned that her gramma could hear sound if Jahara was beside or behind her, but she understood best when she could see Jahara's face. Jahara felt that the more she did to help her gramma, the better the chance of keeping her well and strong. Jahara felt responsible and learned to adapt her own behavior to accommodate others.

Jahara didn't think much about being dysfluent at school. Except for class participation, her grades were good. She tended to be even quieter while other children eagerly wanted to respond in class. When a teacher called on her, she often said she didn't know the answer, although she really did. In speech therapy, Jahara could work quietly with Miss Watson. She liked Miss Watson, who was very nice and proved during every session that Jahara really could speak fluently by following the exercises they had worked on. Although the child was compliant at school, she was easily distracted. Jahara was preoccupied with getting things back to normal at home and keeping them that way. It was really hard to make everything seem okay everywhere she went, because so much had changed. Jahara was unsure what might happen next, especially while she was away from home.

Pearl's reaction initially was shock at her grandmother's illness. The shock was followed by great anxiety and fear of the unknown. She had always loved and depended on Mrs. Brown as a mother instead of a grandmother. She feared that perhaps she had taken the changes of aging too much for granted. She felt guilty for having not been able to prevent the

CVA by more and better caring. Pearl struggled to control her feelings of anger at the destruction brought on by old age, fear of her grandmother's dying, and being threatened with losing the security of having "gramma" as a constant source of strength at home with Jahara and a resource of mature wisdom for herself, a young career woman. She believed that her own dependency was almost as strong as Jahara's, and she realized that she must assume a larger part in maintaining continuity of the household and stability for herself and Jahara. She knew that she must also persist in her high level of performance at work. Pearl believed that these things were matters of survival for herself as well as her daughter.

Miss Watson's reaction, as a competent, conscientious speech-language pathologist, involved her immediately observing the need to provide Jahara with fluency success in her therapy sessions. During the early weeks following Mrs. Brown's illness, she inquired about the patient at the beginning of each visit and rejoiced with Jahara at evidence of her improvement. She sent "get-well" cards to Mrs. Brown at the address Jahara had provided. Under Miss Watson's guidance, Jahara earnestly pursued the fluency skills which she had gained and lost, but the work was slow and required great patience and continual monitoring on the part of the clinician. After a week's work, re-evaluation of Jahara's speech was necessary to adjust the program of therapy to meet the new development. Miss Watson initiated the process of reviewing and redesigning Jahara's Individual Education Plan for speech therapy. Records of the procedure were updated in compliance with the student's status. They reflected the sudden deterioration of fluency as well as a plan to treat the dysfluency. She had to arrange a parent conference, too, but with the family upset, anticipated a delay.

Miss Watson generated many new techniques and materials to catch Jahara's imagination and keep her attention and interest. When completed, many of the materials were available for Jahara to take with her on visits to "gramma." This evidence of Jahara's good work became delightful rewards for earnest efforts during therapy and treasures for Jahara as well as for gramma. Miss Watson and Jahara talked about "some day soon" when the child and her great grandmother could again walk home together from school after therapy.

The medical team consisted of the ambulance emergency crew, hospital staff, attending physicians, and rehabilitation specialists, including the audiologist, occupational therapist, physical therapist, and speech-language pathologist. The hospital setting utilized the problem-oriented system of care management. The efficiency with which Mrs. Brown's diagnosis and appropriate medication were established attested to the merit and quality of their work. The primary contribution of each of the rehabilitation unit's specialists was assessment with recommendations for services, once Mrs. Brown was placed in a nursing care facility and after she was again at home.

At the time of discharge from the hospital, the attending physician instructed Pearl in the management of Mrs. Brown's health care. He told her that the physical and occupational therapists would begin their work with Mrs. Brown at the nursing home by assessing her spontaneously recovered abilities. He reported that Mrs. Brown's vision and balance were not impaired by the ischemic attack. He also provided test results and recommendations from the audiologist and the speech-language pathologist who had seen Mrs. Brown as a service of the hospital's rehabilitation unit.

Audiometric records revealed a hearing threshold that is typically expected in the geriatric female patient. The measure of sensori-neural loss was not unusual for a woman of Mrs. Brown's age. No vertigo was found, but mild tinnitus was present. With the results of assessment, the audiologist did not recommend amplification for this patient. In discrimination testing, there was greater difficulty understanding speech than could be accounted for by the hearing loss alone. There was no evidence of cognitive incompetence. After careful explanation of the hearing loss, Mrs. Brown appeared to understand the difference between her hearing and her understanding of speech. She insisted that she could understand her great granddaughter. Close questioning revealed information suggesting that Mrs. Brown was quite astute in speech-reading the child's expressive verbal language.

The audiologist recommended that Mrs. Brown see Mr. Allen for audiological services at the Community Health Center, since her previous records were there. The audiologist suggested that would be the appropriate site for re-testing in one month and for acquiring needed therapeutic intervention. Suggested therapies included speech-reading and auditory training to increase Mrs. Brown's comprehension of spoken language. The speech-language pathologist at the hospital concurred with the audiologist's recommendations, adding that he expected Mrs. Brown's distorted speech to clear up on its own in a few weeks. Participation in speech-reading and auditory training would be excellent intervention and also provide an opportunity for the family to maintain access to clinicians who could monitor the speech and apprise the family of Mrs. Brown's progress.

Discussion: The case of Jahara and her great grandmother involves three generations of women faced with the realities of the life span. The child perceives restraint and calm as normal behavior of her significant adults. In her distress over her great grandmother's illness, Jahara does not cry or act out in an unpleasant way. She suppresses such behavior as well as her feelings and tries to carry on. The child has exacerbated her dysfluency, but to the holistic therapist that is the lesser problem and only a symptom of her current turmoil. In her short life, Jahara has come to depend on feedback from her great grandmother to confirm her worth and sustain her courage. Jahara has not begun to establish a realistic perspective of herself as a separate, intact, unique, or acceptable person. Although she is still a child, she is immature for her age. She remains dependent on a person whose willingness to sustain the dependency has perpetuated Jahara's immaturity and protected her from experiences of conflict with other children and adults. Jahara has not been toughened to face and resolve inner conflicts.

Mrs. Brown has known for a long time that she cannot understand everyone. She has learned to speech-read Jahara's communications and knows that her understanding is accurate. Jahara uses slow, careful, rhythmic speech and maintains a moderate loudness when talking to "gramma." In their daily conversations, each complements the other, bypassing their separate disabilities. Gramma has feared that Jahara was not and could not be normal.

Pearl has been distant from the close personal relationships that blossomed in the household. She has accepted and sanctioned the secure closeness of Jahara and "gramma." No stranger to conflict in her earlier social life or at work, she has been pleased to witness its absence at home. However, like Jahara and gramma, she can no longer ignore the fragile nature of life. One CVA indicates that another can happen at any time. Destabilization of Mrs. Brown's homeostatic condition must be guarded against, but the responsibilities of work, school, therapy, and the household cannot be set aside. Pearl will need help in meeting these newly realized responsibilities to her family, her employer, and herself.

If Miss Watson had counseling skills and experience and if the school had a resident child psychologist or psychiatric social worker, a natural reaction to Jahara's dramatic and sudden dysfluency and the story of Mrs. Brown's illness would have been to refer the child for psychological consultation. The clinician recognized some inner distress in Jahara's dysfluency. This appeared to be associated with Mrs. Brown's illness, and Mrs. Brown was getting better. The clinician proceeded to meet her commitment to provide exceptional student services for Jahara as defined. Thus, the work setting was exerting an influence on the work of the clinician.

Jahara has needed and continues to need help in identifying and diminishing the terrors that can bring her to silence or near silence and that perpetuate her stifling dysfluencies. Her mother and great grandmother cannot help her beyond offering assurance of their love and protection. They, themselves, are distressed; they need their shared closeness and evidence that Jahara is okay to sustain them. Family counseling is eminently appropriate for all three members of the household; however, Jahara is in critical need of individual help. She seems to be trapped between the stimulation and security levels of needs satisfaction. Her stimulation has been largely perceptual and intellectual with protection from a range of emotional stimulation. Her security has been based in "gramma," with little independence or give-and-take with her own mother.

She cannot get on with her life or her fluency without resolution of the inner turmoil she is experiencing.

The clinician as counselor strives to understand the stutterer's inner feelings (Van Riper & Emerick, 1990, p. 336). In treating Jahara, the counseling role of the clinician begins with discernment of her emotional status as she manages the dysfluencies, her interactions with people, and her responses to a variety of situations, including the crisis in her home and internalized distortions of reality that were contributed by her home communication environment.

Early in working with Jahara, the clinician would have utilized instances of dysfluency to introduce open discussions of feelings at the moment of dysfluency. That would have provided an opportunity to use the language of emotion when the feelings were of a manageable strength. Jahara could learn that feelings can be accepted as a part of all of us, and that it's all right to acknowledge and talk about them. With that security firmly in place in the therapy background, the clinician could have created an opening to assist the client in identifying underlying feelings when the dysfluency crisis occurred. Desensitization is an accepted procedure in the treatment of communication disorders. In Jahara's case as described, however, the sensitive inner world remained dark and secretive.

Communication disorders literature on stuttering provides clearly described procedures and techniques that facilitate client exploration of inner feelings, perspectives, and values. Rollin (1987, chap. 4) is an excellent resource. Therapy experiences are designed for both individuals and groups and can be used in treatment of families. Thus, even if Jahara's treating clinician had no access to psychotherapy or a family therapist for Jahara and her family, there would remain proven alternatives such as client-centered therapy postulated in treatment of the communicative disorder itself.

The treatment proposed for Mrs. Brown recognizes her long-standing hearing loss due to aging and the accompanying language comprehension problem. She has sustained brain damage through the aging process, but the recent CVA apparently did not add to the auditory comprehension problem. Audiologically, she is within the limits of expected competency for her age. Her experience in communicating verbally with Jahara appears to have given her highly useful speech-reading skills. Even though she may not have recognized this latter fact, the ability to comprehend the child's spoken language suggests that by monitoring their interaction, the clinician can easily build a program from successful comprehension of vocabulary, appropriate rate for the speaker, and articulatory effort expected to be appropriate for Mrs. Brown to read. Note must be taken of the current dysfluencies being experienced by Jahara and whether or not they interfere with Mrs. Brown's normal level of comprehension.

In the best of situations, the clinicians who are treating Jahara and Mrs. Brown would confer and collaborate on the therapy plans. The therapy plans could facilitate family counseling. Appropriate techniques could be included to help educate the great grandmother about Jahara's speech problem and her innate normal abilities. The grandmother could be of help in Jahara's recovery; they both must identify and admit the reality of their separate existences and reduce their mutual dependency. By structuring their work together, the clinicians could extend therapy beyond the clinic and into the home. To satisfy the need for additional exposure to a broad range of speech-reading and auditory training, other speakers would be introduced. Adding new acquaintances to the formerly two-way communication process would expand the communicative experiences of Jahara and "gramma."

III. The Case of Jennifer Longrun.   Jennifer, a much-wanted first child, was born with a bilateral complete cleft of the lip and palate and hypertelorism. As the granddaughter of a prominent physician in the community, she had the best of care available from St. Luke's Hospital's interdisciplinary team and its consultants. The baby progressed beautifully through her staged surgeries, middle-ear management, and oral-motor adaptation. Her mother had been an elementary school teacher; with the help of team specialists, she learned quickly how to apply her knowledge and love of children to give Jennifer the best of good early stimulation and monitor her behavior for signs of conductive hearing loss. Jennifer's father, also a teacher, remained the constant, supporting husband and patient, gentle father throughout the seemingly endless hours of her early life in and out of the hospital. The mother and father became local and state activists in the Cleft Palate Parent Association. They were aggressive in making contacts among influential citizens and nurse educators in the several local hospitals.

By the age of 3, Jennifer had blossomed into a "little lady" with obvious intelligence, extensive vocabulary, and communication skills that would be enviable in a 5-year-old child. She was beautiful in appearance and behavior, a delight to be around at any time. Because of expert care and development, there had been no need for formal auditory discrimination training or speech-language therapy, and the tubes in her ears needed only routine periodic monitoring by Mrs. Perry, the pediatric audiologist. The family had achieved success-status in dealing with the birth defect and its sequelae. They were proud of the child as well as themselves.

The day after her third birthday party, Jennifer became very ill. She was hospitalized, and a few hours later her diagnosis was confirmed as bacterial meningitis. Ototoxic drugs were administered to control the disease and save Jennifer's life. The episode resulted in immediate profound bilateral central deafness.

During the months of Jennifer's recovery as she regained strength, parents and grandparents searched and explored every known way to regain auditory access to information for Jennifer. The child's advanced oral language abilities may have misled the parents and grandparents at that time that there was no risk to her continued use of that mode of communication without drastic change. Mrs. Perry and her colleagues on the cleft palate team, professional contacts in the community and at respected otological and aural rehabilitation research institutions were interviewed. The family's struggle to have a normal child led them to discuss her future, their future, and the maximum load of effort the family could and would support.

The family realized the controversy among the choices of oral, manual, and total communication for Jennifer. They could never seriously consider the use of gesture language in any form. No expense was spared, no examination or trip for medical and educational advice was bypassed. The final decision by the mother, father, and maternal grandparents was that Jennifer was to be placed in preschool at a local oral school for the hearing-impaired and continue to learn and be taught through the use of spoken language only. They believed that decision would offer Jennifer the greatest opportunity to realize her full potential and be a normal child and adult. With this decision made, the family moved their residence to be near the selected preschool and immersed themselves in Jennifer's training as they had previously dedicated their energies to the cleft palate group. Their newly busy lives essentially cut them off from former communicological and cleft palate parent support groups. They no longer utilized the cleft palate team, but relied on the grandfather's long-time colleagues for Jennifer's medical treatments. No additional surgeries were performed. News notes from the oral school often carried items about Jennifer. During the next 5 years, the family occasionally sent holiday greeting cards to Dr. Bothwell, a community private practitioner in speech-language pathology, and Mrs. Perry, both of whom had served on the cleft palate team.

Five years after the onset of deafness, when Jennifer was 8 years old, Ms. Longrun telephoned Dr. Bothwell. In spite of many hours of daily work, Jennifer's formerly beautiful speech had deteriorated to unintelligible gibberish. The mother was interested in locating a speech pathologist who would be able to clear up Jennifer's speech. During the friendly telephone conversation, the mother reported that Jennifer has excelled in vocabulary acquisition, and her teacher has indicated that her written syntax has reached adult standards. She has achieved proficient speechreading among her acquaintances, both children and adults. According to the mother, the only communication problem with which they continued to struggle was her lack of speech intelligibility. Only the mother could comprehend what Jennifer was saying, and she knew that she depended on context cues. Ms. Longrun was very insistent that she was looking for an experienced speech pathologist who would provide Jennifer experience with a moto-kinesthetic feedback method of speech articulation. She appeared knowledgeable of difficulties and probable prognosis of the undertaking, but her determination did not waiver.

Dr. Bothwell reviewed the community roster of therapists, and identified two possible resource clinicians with whom Ms. Longrun might pursue the desired articulation therapy for Jennifer. He gave names and phone numbers to Ms. Longrun. He made follow-up telephone calls to the Longrun home, but only reached an answering machine, and the calls were not returned. In casual conversations at subsequent professional meetings, Dr. Bothwell learned that the two suggested clinicians had not been contacted by the Longrun family. About 6 months later, he learned through medical colleagues that Jennifer had been provided a cochlear implant device at an out-of-state medical center. Following the surgery, the child's original school placement continued. Eighteen months later, a visiting audiologist happened to mention that she had been on Jennifer's cochlear implant team and wondered how the child was progressing. A response from another audiologist indicated that the electronic stimulator had not achieved what the family had believed to be its potential.

Commentary. The reactions of Jennifer's family reveal convictions and determination based on their values and expectations and driven by their individual hopes, ideals, and goals. What the family members wanted was Jennifer's normalization.

The ability of the grandfather to command the critically needed aid during the early days of caring reinforced his place of authority in the family structure. In fact, this tremendous contribution seemed to have fixed or perpetuated a notion that remediation of any of Jennifer's problems could be possible if only those responsible for her care looked for it in the right places. It is important to note that the family resided in a community where American Sign Language was still not considered a language. In fact, the local public school system had not succeeded in graduating a deaf child with a regular academic diploma, although two of the upper-level vocational schools had employed interpreters to serve deaf students enrolled there.

Jennifer was very intelligent, willing to work, and undiminished by her craniofacial birth defect. She became secure in her family, her school, and her work. As she matured, she was often lonely for peer company, and her participation in neighborhood activities was curtailed by the demands on her time for vocabulary and English exercises. Her learning situation has resulted in a tightly structured daily routine and limited experience in socialization with other children.

Ms. Longrun has dedicated her life to her family. She devotes her entire energies to her husband and Jennifer. She believes that Jennifer can achieve her potential and function normally, like other girls her age. Ms.

Longrun seems convinced that she can make things all right for her deaf daughter by continuing to find new scientific developments.

Ms. Longrun's life has been influenced by her parents, who have long been powerful and respected individuals in local society. She works diligently at each stage of Jennifer's development and continues to search for an answer to each new problem that arises. She expects to discover a way to give her daughter an advantage. This apparent sense of desperate hope seems to permeate this mother's behavior and is fueled by her perception of the expectations of those around her. One must question her understanding of Jennifer's handicap and need to communicate with people whose speech she has been reading for years. The influence of exclusive oralism has selectively restricted Jennifer's friends and associates, much as the parents said they feared that introduction of gesture communication would do.

Mr. Longrun has remained the steady and firm backbone of the family. He continues to teach school and support his wife and daughter with moral strength and belief in them and whatever they undertake. He cooperates with the programs in which they are involved daily and spends special time with Jennifer. They go places and do things together. They especially like a quick tennis match on Saturday mornings.

Mrs. Perry has not been seen by Jennifer since the onset of her deafness. Because of the family's choices, ongoing follow-up for middle-ear monitoring purposes was discontinued. However, according to Mrs. Perry's best information, audiological theory and techniques have been part of the medical considerations concerning Jennifer.

Dr. Bothwell has remained accessible to the family, and the mother has used that accessibility. As a community resource and a source of information or direction whom the mother had known in the local Cleft Palate Parent Group, the speech-language pathologist has responded when asked, provided services when requested, and made suggestions that were politely heard. As a helper, however, Dr. Bothwell assessed the receptivity of his skills and recognized the family's determination to pursue their own decisions unaided by nonmedical opinion and consultation. Although he did not agree with decisions and plans made by the parents and grandparents, he decided not to argue with them and risk their alienation. Instead, he accepted the family members as they are, and kept communication channels open with the mother and father. He chose to remain readily accessible and to suggest current alternatives available for Jennifer so that the family could stay abreast of their realistic choices.

Discussion. When a family that is used to exercising authority makes a choice, they assume responsibility for the decision as well as its outcome. Where there is honest difference of opinion between family and counselor, the counselor does not strive to change the family decisions. Acceptance of Jennifer's family as they insist on normal oral-aural communication for

Jennifer supports their perception of themselves and their belief that they are doing what is best for their child. Their invitation to the counselor to stay available but distant and not to expect them to participate in an interaction signals that their daily effort is at times overwhelming, but they are functioning in their community. When that functioning is threatened, the counselor will be available if needed.

Dr. Bothwell realizes there are legitimate differences of opinion about methods of teaching and communicating with children who are deaf. He has clearly stated his opinions and preferences to the Longrun family. They have said that they understand the ramifications of various methods of communication for the deaf. Continuing to repeat his professional opinion would be futile, since the family is not accustomed to changing decisions. On the other hand, for the counselor to refuse any contact with this noncompliant family would be to negate potential future opportunities to help them. In the event that the family decides to seek closer contact or professional services some day, Dr. Bothwell chooses to retain an open mind and reserve a place in his professional life for the Longrun family and others like them.

Unmet Client/Caregiver Needs

These three case studies point out individual differences of communication disorders specialists in carrying out their professional duties. The work settings involved in these stories include a public school, hospital rehabilitation unit, university, community health center, hospital interdisciplinary team, and private practice. The clinicians cannot be faulted for their work on the communication disorders or their commitment to that work. In each case, there was apparent need among the clients/caregivers for counseling and support. In the first two cases, that need was as yet unattended; gaps in available services are apparent. In the third story, although the clinicians maintained helping attitudes and availability, their efforts were acknowledged but rejected.

Upon reflection, each of the case studies could involve members of any one or more of the ethno-cultural communities in America. With only minor changes, they could include people from any socio-economic group. Across the many potential differences among participants, the types of communication disorders might remain the same; however, the concomitant need for help would be expected to vary among people from different environmental backgrounds.

Ethno-cultural Diversity and Professional Flexibility

While the majority of ASHA's certified clinicians are white and female, the American Speech-Language-Hearing Association is interested in increasing the numbers of professionals from other cultural backgrounds

(American Speech, Language, and Hearing Association, 1985). There is interest, too, in recruiting more males into the profession. Also, the majority of clients typically served have been members of the white middle class population. ASHA has identified underserved populations: linguistic minorities, economically disadvantaged, institutionalized, remote/rural, Native Americans, and populations in developing regions (Flower, 1985). Current and anticipated cultural diversity across the United States, as well as around the world, presents clinicians with unique characteristics of colleagues, clients, and caregivers among whom to test their helping skills of acceptance and understanding. As experts in human communication, speech-language pathologists and audiologists must be open to the rich diversity of modern American culture.

Boorstin (1987) described the encounter of cultural differences due to the composition and distribution of American citizenry as *verges*. The successful speech-language pathologist and audiologist will recognize, respect, and rejoice in those verges (Herer, 1989). By learning about human differences in all cultures, we no longer fear people because they differ from us. With tolerance and understanding, we can help ameliorate trust among others.

Cole (1989) presented the cultural diversity of America as becoming less European and more an integrated collection of distinct cultural heritages. As populations become more homogeneous, there is a tendency to emphasize and reclaim former differences, if only in a symbolic way. Such emphasis on tradition and heritage represents and maintains the melody of languages and the harmony of customs, manners, and values. These ingredients are truly the recipe for the blend of socio-cultural citizenry that the United States was founded to accommodate (Boorstin, 1987).

Cole (1989) suggested that, within the next few decades, one third of all clients will be members of minorities. Some of the characteristics that signal cultural separateness are known. These known factors form a basis to create appropriate assessment and therapeutic materials. However, the helper's interaction with individuals of another cultural background is less dependent on that background than on the helper's ability to accept, appreciate, and respect the personal philosophy, value system, and goals of the communication partner.

Constraints on clinicians who work with current underserved populations may have more to do with the professional's acquisition of the minority language than with insight into the customs of the minority culture. The situation resembles earlier difficulties in finding clinicians who were sufficiently proficient in American Sign Language to work with the deaf population. Some communication limits of clinicians can be traced to the origins of the profession of communication disorders. Expansion of the required skills or eventual specializations within the field are signs of the maturation and growth of the discipline. Likewise, satisfactory means of providing services to rural, remote, and developing regions has not been resolved. Much like the problems raised in continuing services to those who were de-institutionalized, complexities in service delivery create more of a problem than performing the treatment. Changes in service management are slow to come, but they must evolve if the claims of providing services to those who need and want them are to be legally satisfied.

Service to prisoners has been restricted by the institutions that house them and control their lives. There has been resistance within the criminal justice system to admit or utilize communication disorders personnel to provide rehabilitative services for prisoners. Provision of speech, language, and hearing services to institutionalized psychiatric patients has likewise been limited. Rousey (1974) and Prizant (1989) have demonstrated the types of work needed by those patients in appropriate diagnoses and therapies for communication disorders complicated by concomitant mental and emotional problems.

This brief reference to future opportunities for expansion of services to individuals with communication disorders indicates pending change in the discipline, training programs, treatment sites, and client management methodologies. Flexibility and staying current are the watchwords for astute career personnel in speech-language pathology and audiology. As the field grows and matures, situations described in this chapter, whether interactions between clinicians and clients/caregivers or among co-workers, will demand keen interpersonal communication abilities. Situations that can be expected are not unlike those that occur in the everyday life of ordinary people, families, and student groups. In the following exercises, the reader is invited to undertake conflict-resolution by applying helping skills.

EXERCISES

RESPONSES TO ITEMS FOUND IN TABLE 5.1:
C, B, C, C, B.

The items listed below suggest realistic situations in which there is conflict between individuals in a clinical setting. The reader is invited to join in role-playing the characters introduced here. If videotaping is possible, players can review their performances to look for points at which conversations were directed in specific ways. The tape can be stopped to discuss intentions and feelings at interesting or confusing moments in the experience.

Take the information given here as the starting point for developing interaction that prevents or resolves the indicated conflict. Suggestions made in this and previous chapters can assist the characters in compromising and drawing rational conclusions that are emotionally acceptable and appealing.

As the items are acted out and discussed, each participant will be able to see differences between inner reactions and those communicated by other members of the group. These differences comprise behaviors, both verbal and nonverbal, based on the conscious and unconscious responses of the communicator.

1. You are completing your third year of employment as the assistant clinical audiologist in a rehabilitation center. Since coming to this center, you have received positive reinforcement for your work as well as encouragement to try new things. During the past month, you have become aware of a difference in the director's manner when she talks with you. Today is your appointment for your annual evaluation and discussion of next year's contract with the organization.
2. You are an aphasiologist who has accepted a contract with a national firm to provide language therapy to three patients in the Meadows' Nursing Home. A geriatric patient, Melissa Green, has observed you as you come and go to do the therapy in a room that is down the hall from hers. Ms. Green has reported to the director that you have taken a valuable piece of jewelry from one of your patients. Indeed, the jewelry is missing. The director of the nursing home undertakes an inquiry, during which you are quizzed concerning the affair. While you are in the room with the director, you open the language master and there is the missing lapel pin.
3. Mr. Hiram Wertz is a patient in the Coriss Memorial Hospital. He has been admitted with a diagnosis of laryngeal cancer. The attending physician has invited a surgeon to discuss partial removal of the larynx within the next few days. As the new coordinator of allied health services, you go to visit Mr. Wertz and his wife in his hospital room to discuss the pending surgical visit and any questions they may have concerning Mr. Wertz's illness. The surgeon has not yet indicated the extent of the laryngectomy.
4. You are one of the communication disorders clinicians who serve on an interdisciplinary pediatric diagnostic team. A young couple with a 4-year-old son who is mentally retarded found out last week that the wife is pregnant again. The father is anxious about the potential condition of the new baby, and he insists that his wife have an amniocentesis. She is frightened. They have arrived early for their son's team visit so that they can talk to you about their situation. They believe you will hear what they are trying to say and help them do the right thing.

REFERENCES

American Speech, Language, & Hearing Association. (1985). Racial/ethnic demography of ASHA membership. *ASHA, 27*(6), 27.

Battin, R. R., & Fox, D. R. (1978). *Private practice in audiology and speech pathology*. New York: Grune and Stratton.

Boorstin, P. J. (1987). *Hidden history*. New York: Harper and Row.

Carkhuff, R., & Berenson, B. (1967). *Beyond counseling and therapy*. Toronto: Holt, Rinehart, and Winston.

Carlson, R. (1990). *Personal communication*. Tampa, FL: University of South Florida.

Cole, D. R. (1982). *Helping*. Toronto: Butterworths.

Cole, L. (1985). Racial/ethnic demography of ASHA membership. *ASHA, 27*(6), 77.

Cole, L. (1989). E pluribus, pluribus: Multicultural imperatives for the 1990s and beyond. *ASHA, 30*(11), 65–70.

Conaway, J. (1989). Legal counsel's column. In *The American Academy of Private Practice in Speech Pathology and Audiology Newsletter*. July, 8–9.

Crane, S. L., & Cooper, E. B. (1983). Speech-language clinician personality variables and clinical effectiveness. *JSHD, 48,* 140–145.

Dale, E. (1969). *Management theory and practice* (2nd ed.). New York: McGraw-Hill.

Feldman, A. S. (1988). Some observations about us and private practice. *ASHA, 30*(1), 29–30.

Fischer, J. (1978). *Effective casework practice: An eclectic approach*. New York: McGraw-Hill.

Flower, R. (1985). 1985 national colloquium on underserved populations report. *ASHA, 27*(11), 31–35.

Fulmer, R. M. (1974). *The new management*. New York: Macmillan.

Guthrie, T. J. (1988). Adaptation and progress in times of change. *ASHA, 30*(8), 27–30.

Herer, G. R. (1989). Inventing our future. *ASHA, 31*(12), 35–37.

Herzberg, F. (1966). *Work and the nature of man*. New York: World Publishing.

Klevans, D. R. (1982). Techniques of therapy based on principles of counseling and self-management. In W. H. Perkins (Ed.), *Current therapy in communication disorders*. New York: Thieme-Stratton.

Likert, R. (1961). *New patterns of organization*. New York: McGraw-Hill.

Maslow, A. H. (1943). The theory of human motivation. *Psychology Review*, 370–396.

McConnell, J. M. (1974). *Understanding human behavior*. New York: Holt, Rinehart, and Winston.

McLuhan, M. (1964). *Understanding media: The extensions of man*. New York: McGraw-Hill.

Oyer, H. J. (Ed.). (1987). *Administration of programs in speech-language pathology and audiology*. Englewood Cliffs, NJ: Prentice-Hall.

Prizant, B. (1989). Speech-language pathology in a psychiatric setting. *ASHA, 30*(6–7), 91–96.

Rogers, C. (1951). *Client-centered therapy*. Boston: Houghton Mifflin.

Rollin, W. J. (1987). *The psychology of communication disorders in individuals and their families*. Englewood Cliffs, NJ: Prentice-Hall.

Rousey, C. L. (1974). *Psychiatric assessment by speech and hearing behavior*. Springfield, IL: Charles C. Thomas.

Rousey, C. L. (1982). Techniques of therapy based on principles of psychotherapy. In W. H. Perkins (Ed.), *Current therapy in communication disorders*. New York: Thieme-Stratton.

Shewan, C. M. (1989). Adaptation and progress in times of change. *ASHA, 30*(8), 27–30.

Stein, H. F. (1985). What ever happened to countertransference? The subjective in medicine. In H. F. Stein & M. Apprey, *Context and dynamics in clinical knowledge*. Charlottesville, VA: University Press of Virginia.

Stone, J. R., & Olswang, L. B. (1989). The hidden challenge in counseling. *ASHA, 31*(6–7), 27–31.

Strupp, H. H. (1980). Humanism and psychotherapy: A personal statement of the therapist's essential values. *Psychotherapy: Theory, Research, and Practice, 17*, 396–400.

Van Riper, C., & Emerick, L. (1990). *Speech Correction* (8th ed.). Englewood Cliffs, NJ: Prentice-Hall.

CHAPTER SIX

❦ ❦ ❦

Helping—Throughout a Career

Issues

❦ *The personal and professional experiences of each clinician have an impact on the role as counselor or helper in the daily practice of treating clients with communication disorders.*

❦ *An individual's cumulative experience both influences and is influenced by personal philosophy and agents of change in the world.*

❦ *Current and future social and technological trends demand creative abilities as essential ingredients for realizing a satisfying and rewarding career as clinician or counselor in the field of communication disorders.*

❦ ❦ ❦

THE INFLUENCES OF PERSONAL AND PROFESSIONAL EXPERIENCES

In the preceding chapter, we discussed some of the internal and external influences that lead to the selection of a work setting for the practitioner in audiology and speech-language pathology. We also discussed external influences in the work setting itself that shape the counseling involvement of the individual clinician. In this chapter, we take a look at the self-actualizing clinician progressing through a career, adding the complex influence of time.

Aristotle defined *time* as the measure of motion according to before and after. In the context of the clinician, the activities that comprise daily living and the clinical practice of treating clients and their families represent the *motion* in Aristotle's definition. We tend to remember events rather than dates as we scan the past progression of our careers and those of others. Sometimes the pressure of meeting a deadline, taking an examination, or beginning a new project marks a particular day, month, or year as significant. We are even more likely to recall acquiring a much-needed and valued piece of equipment, the experience of working with a significant other, or a city where we attended a conference. This tendency of memory often causes us to fail to account for our subtle responses to internal and external influences that are incidental to progression toward self-actualization.

With the passage of time, advancing of skill, and accumulation of knowledge, the clinician will experience changes in professional maturity in as many ways as one can imagine. However, barring a devastating personal experience, an individual's personal philosophy remains essentially the same. The internal system of values by which a person lives will sustain the individual's rationale for maintaining existence, drive selected modes of behavior, and support the continual striving for self-fulfillment. Personal experiences contour and mold the personality, but among survivors of the world of clinical practice, the nuclear regard for the quality of life remains constant.

Some clinicians may remain in a single setting for an entire career, content and highly productive. In doing so, they demonstrate that the setting suits them personally and meets their defined needs for professional activity. They also confirm through their colleagues that their clinical skills are maintained at a level that is proficient and up-to-date with current trends in the discipline. By preference, those skilled practitioners perfect their service in a selected domain of client treatment to ensure that their clients have access to the best that is currently available in the profession. This is often found to be the case among clinicians in public school settings. The thousands of children whose communication abilities are screened or treated by a single public school clinician attest to the professional's personal philosophy and continual commitment. Another example of a single-setting career can be found in the clinician who works in a health-related setting with one or more interdisciplinary teams. Interactions among colleagues and patients in these settings often have profound and dramatic effects on clients and their families. The clinician may screen or treat less than 1% of the number of potential clients seen in a school setting within a comparable time frame. However, the challenge to the clinician in a medical setting tends to be both extensive and stimulating. In either of these two settings, the opportunities of educating and interacting with men and women in other professional disciplines provide continuing challenges and frequent rewards to audiologists and speech-language pathologists.

At the opposite extreme are clinicians who need or prefer to change positions every 2 to 5 years. These changes often become necessary because of personal obligations or nonprofessional commitments. Family obligations often shape careers, in part because of the predominance of women employed in the communication disorders profession. A change of residence because of a spouse's work situation, the arrival of a new baby, or a change in school placement of an older child are typical reasons for the interruption of a career or a change of work setting.

❦ ❦ ❦

THE INFLUENCE OF PERSONAL PHILOSOPHY AND EXPERIENCE

Other alterations in a professional career may result from a desire for additional education, the opening of a new facility with a tempting and open position, or the acceptance of an administrative position. As in other aspects of the discipline, the personal factors that converge to result in the sequential moves within a career are unique to each clinician. Table 6.1 suggests some features of communication disorders clinicians that affect early position selection and shape careers.

The Beginning Clinician

At the beginning of a career, graduate students who enroll in programs of audiology and speech-language pathology find curricula that draw on most known fields of knowledge. Programs that are currently available in the United States generally assure their graduates of meeting the minimum standards for practicing these specializations in treatment of the communicatively disordered. This guarantee is a strong foundation on which the beginning clinician can depend. Consequently, the initial step into the responsible world of professional clinical practice is eased and may be expected to proceed without major adjustments in knowledge base or therapeutic interactive skills.

The first work setting for the clinician who wants to achieve the Certificate of Clinical Competency (CCC) from the American Speech-Language-Hearing Association (ASHA) is one that offers the Clinical Fellowship Year (CFY). This period of supervised employment is a modi-

Table 6.1
Personal, professional, and societal influences on early career choices

The Beginning Clinician		
Resources	**Challenges**	**Rewards**
Personal philosophy	New responsibilities	Salary
Education	Decision making	New information
Family support	Flexibility	Work satisfaction
Clinical training	Critical thinking	Encouragement
Self-confidence	Professional	Self-esteem
Professional association	responsibilities	Recognition
	Family responsibilities	Improvements in field
	New technology	Broadened interests

fied professional internship for audiologists and speech-language pathologists. For various reasons, not every clinical setting offers the supervised CFY experience. A common obstacle is the demand on the time of a certified clinician to supervise the intern. The time needed for supervision is time that the clinician may prefer to spend in direct treatment of clients.

The Clinical Fellowship Year (CFY). In clinical settings where a CFY is available, that position may offer a half- or full-time position with a partial or full caseload and a minimum salary. Proprietors of these settings typically construct those positions to meet their own specifications as well as to accommodate the entry level needs of the beginning clinician. These matters are not yet regulated by ASHA, as is the requirement for supervision of clinical services during that time. Lack of resolution of questions about the CFY may relate to its short duration and the need of beginning clinicians to move on to other situations and resolve other more immediately pressing considerations. That is, the CFY clinicians themselves are not in place long enough to address existing or potential problems of the overall situation.

Schools have been popular settings for CFY placement since almost half of ASHA members are employed there (American Speech-Language-Hearing Association, 1990). As a scarcity of clinicians continues, school systems are generally pleased to offer CFY placement along with the probability of continued employment following satisfactory completion of the supervised internship. However, not all school districts or state departments of education require that communication disorders clinicians hold a graduate degree or the CCC. In these areas, a beginning clinician may find the CFY is not available or needed. However, a later move into another geographical area controlled by a different education system with CCC requirements may restrict career advancement of the noncertified communication disorders clinician.

As the size and influence of ASHA continue to increase, requirements for professional practice will become more broadly recognized among policy-makers and funding agencies. The beginning professional who enters the field with academic and clinical credentials in compliance with ASHA requirements has achieved a significant step toward assuring professional security and self-esteem.

During interviews for the CFY, the applicant may be told of possible continuation of the position as a permanent placement. Upon completion of the CFY, a clinician may be invited to remain in the same clinical setting and take a staff position with additional responsibilities, less regularly scheduled supervision, and increased financial remuneration. Quite frequently, this proposal is a welcome invitation to the beginning clinician, and the arrangement is satisfactory to all parties. In other cases, post-CFY clinicians may feel the need to find another employment opportunity.

Reasons for this decision may be as diverse as dissatisfaction with the experience of the CFY, a need to get away from problems at home, or discovery that clinical practice at this level of training is not sufficient and more education is essential.

Differences in the potential for arranging ongoing employment after completion of the CFY often influence the graduate student's initial selection of CFY placement. On the other hand, it is not unheard-of for a beginning clinician to want a change in work setting after the CFY to undertake treatment of a different type of client in a different type of setting. At the extreme, some beginning clinicians who have completed the requirements for the CCC will choose to alter their life course by entering an allied profession, such as law, medicine, clinical psychology, education, business management, gerontology, or other newly identified disciplines.

Personal Attributes of the Beginning Clinician. Before we leave these thoughts about the beginning of a career, there is an additional consideration of personal attributes that needs to be mentioned. With changes occurring rapidly in the profession and even more so in the diversity of the American population, the demand for bilingual clinicians continues to grow. Spanish is the most common foreign language in the states, although many Oriental languages such as Vietnamese are spoken in school districts and business communities throughout the country. The clinician who has mastered English and another spoken or gestured language will have an advantage in any CFY or permanent employment setting in which the dual language ability is in demand.

Other abilities that can help a beginning clinician seeking a position include a background in emergency medical services, nursing, musical performance, counseling, or creative art. While their specific skills have not been measured, women who return to school after staying at home and become communication disorders clinicians often demonstrate managerial skills and insights into their own behavior and that of others that are significant assets in their new profession. Because of the broad spectrum of human behavior encompassed by the field of audiology and speech-language pathology, graduate students and beginning clinicians are well advised to examine carefully their own experiences and abilities to be sure that none are tucked away and forgotten because they are considered no longer useful. By applying abilities that were useful in other endeavors, a clinician will often introduce a new technique or operating procedure that enhances clinical work and clinic management.

All the internal and external influences involved in seeking and accepting employment are agents that shape and change careers in the field of communication disorders. The reward for the clinician who is aware of those influences and uses them in career planning and goal-setting will be an efficient process with a successful outcome.

The Experienced Clinician

Many features of the experienced clinician that are shown in Table 6.2 are dependent on the passage of time. The shape of a career is significantly modified by the opportunities, challenges, disappointments, and rewards that are part of each interaction with clients or caregivers, colleagues, and members of the community. In addition, careers are molded by new developments and emphases in the discipline, as well as by increases or decreases in funding for services, equipment, space expansion, travel, continuing education, and research.

Time alone does not account for the acquisition of essential insight and skill that are observable in the work of the most successful clinicians. Each clinician must build a career one day at a time and find or make a niche in the overall scheme of the discipline. To do so successfully demands that the individual establish goals and plan steps to achieve those goals, following an old axiom that says, "Failure to plan is planning to fail." While plans may change, having direction from the outset gives a clinician a standard against which to measure progress, success, and the need for change. The idea of planning a career in the complex and changing field of communication disorders demands that the clinician be highly competent in critical thinking and highly skilled in flexibility. These abilities are essential for the continued renewal of clinical performance and the prevention of *burnout* from the fundamental routine that is essential to managing the communicative needs of every client or caregiver.

Table 6.2
Personal, professional, and societal influences on ongoing career choices

The Experienced Clinician

Resources	Challenges	Rewards
Personal philosophy	Routine, boredom	Security
Experience/skill	Professional association	Reputation
Colleague rapport	New colleagues	Work satisfaction
Continuing education	Research change of	Recognition
Professional contacts	position	Privilege
Community support	Problem-solving	Self-esteem
Community change	Community	Contentment
Realistic goals	involvement	Collaboration
Family support	Conflict resolution	Creativity
Financial security	Family responsibilities	acknowledged
Professional association	Fund-raising	Support for projects
Self-knowledge	Public relations	Awards
Creative insight	Profession's evolution	Promotion
Faith and hope	Technological advances	
Inner toughness		

❦ ❦ ❦

THE EFFECT OF SOCIAL TRENDS

As we noted in chapter 1, the evolution of society led to the development of audiology and speech-language pathology as it exists today. Similarly, social, political, environmental, and cultural mixes affect the role and scope of the profession throughout a single clinician's career. This is especially true as we approach the 21st century with the rapid world-wide changes in the identification of societal problems and the political and economic strategies to resolve them, as well as the technology explosion and increases in ideological conflicts. The accumulation of new scientific and technical information is vast, as are the desires and demands of entire populations that are changing global boundaries. All these influences are reflected not only in the working world but also in aspects of leisure such as the performing, graphic, and structural arts.

Some ramifications of one example can illustrate concerns of the discipline of communication disorders on such broad-reaching societal changes. In 1990 the national census bureau reported that the number of men in their 20s exceeded the number of women in their 20s by almost 2 to 1. One result of this shift might be an increase in the number of men who enter the communication disorders profession. Should this happen, job placement for women would be challenged in ways not currently experienced. Inclusion of these men in other segments of the nation's work force might also produce a change in the apparent societal trend toward a proportional increase of working women in all wage-earning positions. Such work-force modifications would affect child care and early childhood education.

An increase in the number of men who survive into middle age can also be expected to modify future statistics of the aging population, which has been traditionally dominated by women. Hearty young men not lost to or damaged by physical trauma may live to demonstrate characteristics of aging not previously observed in the elderly population. On the one hand, fewer aging parents may have to face the tragic memories of having lost a child or cared for a disabled one. On the other hand, those parents potentially will have an extended support network through the longevity of their children.

The world-peace initiative that began in 1989 suggested the possibility of a reduction in the number of men and women injured in military service. Such a trend could decrease the need for veterans' hospitals and associated facilities for long-term care and rehabilitation of patients with disorders related to military service.

Current and anticipated complex technical and social changes will affect individual clinical careers (Herer, 1989). To fully explore all the possibilities of this idea, we would have to be fortune-tellers. It may be useful, however, to consider expected and planned developments in the world as we know it. In view of the great number of writings on the future of the

United States and world societies that appeared in print in 1989 and 1990 alone, we may discern some circumstances that will affect audiology and speech-language pathology.

Jarratt (1989) listed seven social trends that appear to be continuing long-term directions and the primary consequences of each. Those trends included change in demography of the work force, women's increased commitment to work and education, new generations' values and attitudes, sedentary occupations, global consciousness, expanding public ignorance, and technological change. Even a cursory examination of trends and predictions for the next 2 decades could be overwhelmingly complicated. Societal changes will certainly affect both the individual clinician and the entire profession of communication disorders. A manageable plan for our discussion becomes imminently important. At the risk of oversimplifying this challenging task, we can initiate a discussion of *helping* across a clinical career by considering some of the developments that are anticipated and how they may shape the individual, the tool of counseling, and modify the direction of the profession.

In chapter 2, we discussed ways in which four determiners of communication abilities could be seen to affect clients and caregivers across the life span. In this chapter, we will discuss anticipated changes in the realm of each of those determiners of communication abilities. Then we can venture an educated guess as to how careers in speech-language pathology and audiology will be influenced, because the changes will affect the profession as a whole and the clinician as an individual.

❦ ❦ ❦

THE EFFECT OF SOCIAL AND TECHNOLOGICAL TRENDS ON FUTURE CAREERS

Anticipated advances in information, technology, and skill can be found in every field of knowledge. Many of these topics have been introduced in earlier chapters. This chapter contains a selection of specific developments that are expected to have an impact on the profession of communication disorders during the next decades. Hope as well as superstition may influence thinking and planning in human services as we begin a new century. Hypothesizing about the future, however, offers an opportunity to lay a foundation of knowledge that will sustain helping careers for years.

A discussion of anticipated changes that can dramatically change the effect of the four determiners of communication abilities and disorders can provide a glimpse of some ways in which careers of clinicians may differ in the future. Changes can be expected to augment or challenge different aspects of the discipline of communication disorders and the individual clinical practitioner. By doing so, societal changes shape the behavior of clinicians and influence their perceptions of themselves and the world in which they live.

Remembering that the personal characteristics of the clinician are key elements in establishing and maintaining helping relationships, it is easy to understand how societal trends and changes may challenge the field of communication disorders and individual clinicians. The selection of the four topics listed in Table 6.3 is arbitrary and does not imply that these are the most significant or dramatic societal influences to be encountered. Instead, the topics are presented with the intention of stimulating the reader to think about current events, either personally observed or reported in the media, and reflect on the fact that even isolated experiences generate twists and turns through the history of a career. The discussion that follows considers some aspects of each topic in relation to an individual clinician's career as well as in terms of the profession as a whole.

The "Decade of the Brain"

Long held in awe, the human brain has been raised to the pinnacle of public valuation by becoming the focus of national research efforts for all disciplines interested in neuroscience. These include speech, language, hearing, psychology, neurology, neurogenic disorders, neurological diseases, neuropsychology, gerontology, embryology, and computerized brain imaging and cortical mapping technologies. Advances in neurological and neurochemical sciences touch many lives across the age span, including people who are well, healthy, deformed, or diseased. Major scientific discoveries and technical developments can prevent biological conditions that underlie large numbers of communication disorders. Research in neuron replication may become the alchemy of the 21st century. Targeted groups include neurologically impaired neonates who are damaged in utero, the aging population who face loss of normal neurological function, and traumatically brain-injured patients of all ages.

The President of the United States declared the 1990s to be the "Decade of the Brain." That federal attention has potentially wide-reaching outcomes for the many aspects of brain function and dysfunction.

Table 6.3
Selected topics that affect the determiners of
communication abilities / disorders

Determiner	Topic
Biology	"Decade of the Brain"*
Cognition	Applications of technology
Psycho-social adaptation	Substance abuse
Environment	Pollution

* On July 25, 1989, the President of the U. S. signed
legislation declaring the 1990s the "Decade of the Brain."

Federal agencies such as the National Institutes of Health (NIH) can use that designation to support requests for increased congressional funding of their programs. Medical ethics related to sustaining life through dramatic efforts of specialists and machines may receive more scrutiny from social and legal perspectives. In education, continued research into learning and social behavior may discover that students who become school dropouts do not fit the system because it was not flexible enough to have met their needs. To acquire the desired factual knowledge and critical thinking skills, such students require learning settings, methods, and interaction with teachers beyond the scope of those typically furnished.

The American Speech-Language-Hearing Association may increase emphasis on neurogenic communication disorders and invite closer alliance with medicine and psychology for diagnostic and treatment protocols; encourage a broader definition of communication disorders to which speech-language pathology and audiology apply; vigorously pursue interdisciplinary measures to increase the prevention of communication disorders; and intensify research efforts in brain function and dysfunction in receptive and expressive communication.

Federal and professional emphasis in neurobiology and neurogenic disorders can be expected to find an increase in curricular demands of university training programs. Academic courses and clinical experience in the science of nerve structure, function, and dysfunction will need to be enhanced to accommodate newly emerging information and treatment techniques. Practitioners already in the field will need continuing education courses to update their information and skills. Public information must be made available to inform colleagues in other professions and future clients of the services that become available. Certainly not least of the implications for the field of communication disorders in expanding emphasis on the brain and its function is the inclusion of modern technology in diagnosis and treatment methodologies.

Neurology and Communication Disorders.   With increased attention to behavioral differences based on neurological dysfunctions, it can be expected that patients with diagnosed neurological and behavioral problems will be referred for communication services more frequently and earlier in the development of the disorder. Clinicians will see more of these patients and see them earlier in the course of their development of dysfunction or behaviors that demonstrate the presence of the dysfunction. Expertise of audiologists and speech-language pathologists may be called upon for close consultation and intervention earlier in the health-care or educational planning for these patients.

Three types of communication disorders that may be represented in current and new research derived from the Decade of the Brain include dysfunctional perception, central processing, and psycho-motor function. All three of these areas involve both audiology and speech-language pathology. Current clients may exhibit hearing or vision loss, depressed acuity of hearing or seeing, auditory-visual comprehension, intersensory synthesis of meaning, memory or retrieval disorders, encoding, or neuro-motor coordination of the speech mechanism.

Other Influences on Speech-Language Pathology and Audiology. Decreases in normal function cause depression and withdrawal in many clients. In its simplest form, the role of the communication disorders expert will necessitate a thorough knowledge of the anatomy and physiology of the nervous system, its effect throughout the normal cognitive, emotive, and physiological function, and its distortion of human intra- and interaction when tissue-specific dysfunction is present. Additionally, the clinician must be acquainted with the importance of timely use of drugs to increase or reduce neural firing, as well as the side effects of those drugs. Comfortable use of the skills required to meet the needs of family members who work with these clients will become a prominent aspect of daily clinical practice.

Anticipated increases in the incidence of neurologically impaired neonates, the occurrence of traumatic brain injury, and the diversity in the gerontological population are sure to modify the role of the communication specialist. Patients who require temporary or prolonged life-sustaining measures with implications of brain damage will affect the demographic characteristics of clients and even of ASHA members. Specialists in pediatric audiology and developmental behavior may be overwhelmed with demands for their services.

Delivery of services to residential and homebound clients of all ages will offer new practice sites. Current training programs fall short in offering instruction in parenting of young children. Child care specialists in nurseries and preschool programs will need additional information and skill in managing children while parents work. Through organized collaborative efforts, their assistance in early stimulation may reduce the severity of language-learning disabilities. Caregiving for affected elderly clients is another weak area in training and service programs. For example, very few communication disorders programs require graduates to be proficient in cardio-pulmonary resuscitation. Also, informed providers of respite care desperately need programs that offer training for helping complex-care clients of all ages. They must be trained in ways appropriate for the clients whom they serve.

Also, the clinician who meets the demands of the 21st century may deal more often with dying clients and their families who need support through their grief. Neurological dysfunctions involved in cases of progressive diseases, malignant brain tumors, repeated strokes, or autoimmune deficiency syndrome (AIDS) can affect anyone at any age. The incidence of these conditions is expected to increase. There is special concern for expected increases in the number of AIDS patients, and this issue is addressed later as an aspect of psycho-social adaptation. Certainly as the awareness increases, communicological services will be sought for more patients with progressive diseases and their families.

Even with continued deinstitutionalization, urbanization may cluster many neurologically impaired clients in a small geographical area, but rural or remote areas can also have high incidences of neurologically involved clients. To intervene with these underserved populations, clinicians of the future must provide a means of access to the services besides the expert services themselves. The means of access must include funding, transportation, acceptable methodologies for the culture indicated, and clinicians who are dedicated to a mode of clinical practice that is less traditional and institutional.

These thoughts touch on emerging developments in the biological determiner of communication abilities and their implications for change in the profession. Their relation to the individual specialist in communication disorders emphasizes the need for skill in the use and creative design of sophisticated equipment to facilitate diagnoses and therapies. To explore some of the emerging trends in the field, we will consider how telephones, television, and computers form the beginnings of an explosion in treatment technology.

Explosion in Treatment Technology

In the modern space age, real-time hours, minutes, and seconds no longer mask the tiny movements, pauses, or sounds that have come to be the working material of the speech-language pathologist and audiologist. To examine cognition and resulting language behavior that we claim to resolve or modify, it is now possible to probe infinitely small particles of oral language generation and sound perception. Modern technology has come to the assistance of the informed clinician who must maintain accountability to clients and caregivers, professional standards, and third-party reimbursement resources.

Reports from among those speech-language pathology professionals have typically contained a good deal of subjective information reflecting the nature of traditional services, much more so than the reports of audiologists. However, this situation has changed with the advent of computers and software to drive programs of speech and language assessment. It is no longer necessary to struggle for substantiation of one's "good clinical ear" alone. Common understandings of phenomena can be facilitated by shared respect for objective evidence of behavioral outcomes. Electronic instruments are available to analyze speech, voice, respiration, and resonance. Other instruments selectively amplify frequencies within the speech sound spectrum through frequency-modulated radio waves and infrared light rays. Still other instruments can record the electronic transmission of energy waves across the cortex upon stimulation by impulses initiated by response to acoustic or light energy. Brain function can be mapped in colors that indicate vascular activity. These instruments are too expensive to be available in every treatment setting. Instead, local or regional diagnostic facilities may be the wave of the future.

To function fully in the modern competitive world of allied health professions, the clinician must be knowledgeable about modern instruments, the capacities in which they serve, and the degree of reliability they offer. We must recognize the limits of current technological reality and be able to read reports intelligently based on high-tech findings. Dreams for better client management that exceed the limits of known instrumentation and techniques can only materialize if clinicians become involved in making those dreams come true (Holley, 1988; Thornton, Krishnaiyer, Young, Moore, & Johnsrud, 1989). Practitioners must be continually alert to recognize major breakthroughs, which often occur accidentally and may go unnoticed. Many times a minor adaptation to a tool used elsewhere can provide a much-needed device for the communicatively handicapped. Consider the significance of the development of the tracheo-esophageal puncture and valving instruments and techniques in voice management of post-laryngectomy patients.

Development of technological advances can be found in several levels of complexity. Engineers are developing new, more sensitive, tougher, and more resilient materials that can perform functions only imagined in the past. Some of these materials can be used inside the human body without fear of infection or rejection. Surgical steel, which sometimes rusts and necessitates removal or replacement, no longer need be depended upon for mending bone breakage or restoring bone loss. Plates, screws, pins, and wires made of rare metals such as titanium and their alloys have been used successfully for years without negative effects. More recently, biomaterials of ceramic admixtures have been introduced into bone grafting to strengthen the graft sight and to increase the substance of the bone itself (Habal, 1989a). Some of these bone grafts are widely used in habilitation of congenital or acquired craniofacial anomalies, and are examples of the process of combining two well-known materials to produce a material with unique characteristics of its own. Combinations of materials are being developed, and devices composed of them are being tested for compatibility with and within the human body.

One thrust in the creation of new materials involves miniaturization. One ideal product that many researchers dream of developing must be small enough to drive cellular units of the living body and microcomputer components. To meet these needs, there is interest in developing molecular-sized particles or mini-microchips, with properties that can act as real-time stimulators for other body parts or cells. They would be electronic time-release capsules. For example, a subcellular-sized stimulator could assist neurons in producing and secreting the components of neurotransmitters into synapses. Such a device could have a major effect on the outcomes of brain damage and the severity of dementia, aphasia, or emotional disturbance due to trauma, disease, or developmental dysfunction. Another proposed development in miniaturization relates to the use of the artificial molecule as a catalyst or other activator, such as one that would change the pigment in rods or cones to stimulate the optic nerve, or substitute for the lost hair-cell function in the organ of Corti and thereby stimulate the eighth nerve. Such bio-molecular devices are no longer merely dreams or components of futuristic fantasies. Their design and use are well within the realm of possibility.

In some craniofacial centers, clinicians now utilize three-dimensional computer-reformatted-imaging to visualize the internal and external features of the skull as a routine part of complete diagnosis for certain clinical cases. The result of this technique is a three-dimensional pictorial replica or "picture" of the inner and outer configuration of the deformed, damaged bones or missing fragments of the cranium and face. The picture is produced by digitized points of light fed into a computer from a CATscan and then reassembled to replicate the contour of the bone and present it on a full color film (Habal, 1989b; March & Veneer, 1985).

Devices like those described above would dramatically modify the day-to-day work of speech-language pathologists and audiologists and their availability would greatly affect the lives of clients who need them. Readers may want to explore the contents of recent journals on biomaterials research to learn more about the application of biomedical technology to potential devices for use with rehabilitation of oral-aural communication. Increased sophistication in every field of knowledge and greater availability of new services to the average person significantly improves the chance for prevention of communication disorders. Unfortunately, the availability of these tools and the expertise to handle them also elevates the cost of allied health services, as we align the profession of communication disorders even more closely with biomechanics technology and neurobiological-materials sciences. It follows that the results of these technological advances, while welcome and even ideal, would impose dramatic changes on all aspects of the communication disorders profession and on individual clinical responsibilities. Not the least of these is the urgency for clinicians to become comfortable with use of the emerging equipment and conversant with the language of the technological developments (Paul, 1990).

Substance Abuse

Rampant among all social classes during the close of the 20th century is access to and abusive consumption of chemical substances, which change human tissues in structure, modify their function, diminish total physiological and mental performance, and addict the consumer to the use of more and more potent substances. (See Appendix F.) This social phenomenon is not new. Historically, the use of herbal toxins to stimulate or suppress unusual physical, mental, and emotional experiences has been a part of religion and medicine. The addition of synthetic stimulants has gained in popularity more recently. Because of the addictive properties of these substances, they have a devastating result for the consumer and a dramatic impact on the economy of the society in which they flourish. Because of the illegal status of their production, distribution, and use, they have a negative impact on the social perception of producers, merchants, and consumers.

In the last two centuries, the Opium Wars of the Far East exemplify the international political control which can be imposed through domination by drug addiction. Drug-related armed conflict within and between countries of both hemispheres has more recently focused attention of democratic governments on the horrors of the supply-and-demand cycle of addictive substance abuse. Within the profession of communication disorders, psycho-social implications of substance abuse require close attention to the competency of the mature or developing client who is exposed to drugs.

Substance abuse involves people of all ages and all socio-economic classes. The substances include forms of alcohol, tobacco, inhalants, marijuana, cocaine, hashish, and heroin. Of these, the first three are available on the open market; and access to the first two is restricted by law only in terms of the age of the purchaser. The remainder of substances named here are sold by "dealers" who may be as diverse as an elementary school student, a junior high school or high school dropout, an inner city resident, a teacher, a physician, a lawyer, or a corporate executive.

The appeal of drugs, whether legal or illegal, to the individual consumer today is similar to that of the past. Many people use drugs in pursuit of wellness, freedom from pain, psychological escape from bad or undesired feelings and situations, or making good feelings better. These attitudes toward improving one's experience are probably related to the pursuit of wellness and the public widespread misconception that there is a cure or answer for everything. Evidence of this idea is found in the consumer's support of thousands of nonprescription medicines found on shelves in pharmacies and supermarkets. Further proof is the high visibility of pills, capsules, and elixirs shown and praised in television advertisements and color inserts in daily and weekly newspapers that feature price-reducing coupons. The result of the situation is that people of all ages can develop physiological and psychological conditions from substance abuse that may result in communication disorders. A brief review of some of the related problems will be helpful.

Alcohol.   The direct effects of alcohol on the body of an aging person or a newborn baby illustrate the permanent damage that can be caused by this cheap and readily available drug. Alcoholism occurs in 10% to 15% of the aging population (Oppeneer & Vervoren, 1983; Price & Andrews, 1982; Trapp & Spatz, 1988). In the aging individual, the use of alcohol to reduce the awareness of loneliness or assuage depression not only introduces the drug into the neurological system for interference with normal nerve firing, but most frequently reduces the normal intake of nutrients. This combined damage to metabolic homeostasis increases the rate of mental or cognitive dysfunction, and may do irreparable organic damage to the brain. Additionally, the combined intake of alcohol with prescribed drugs can produce further adverse reactions. Clinicians who work with the aging population must be alert to the interference of drugs and/or alcohol to testing or treatment being administered.

In the neonate born to an alcoholic mother (1/2500 births), the condition of fetal alcohol syndrome (FAS) is well known (Jung, 1989). While the severity of FAS varies with period of pregnancy and amount of alcohol ingested, its symptoms include: short palpebral fissures, hypoplastic philtrum, thinned upper lip, ptosis, low nasal bridge, epicanthic folds, midface hypoplasia, and posterior rotation of the ears with poorly formed concha (Jones & Smith, 1973). These children may also be found to have microcephaly with accompanying central nervous system dysfunction, mental retardation, and deficits in all aspects of language. They may have heart defects, cervical vertebral defects, cleft palate, small teeth with faulty enamel, and renal anomalies. Their growth rate is typically 1/3 to 1/2 that of normal children. General impairment of mental function and hyperactivity include impulsivity, cognitive and perceptual deficits, and multiple social and academic problems (Lippman, 1980; Sparks, 1984).

An indirect effect of alcohol is the high incidence of automobile accidents related to driving while intoxicated. According to the 1988 Bureau of Statistics reports, 40% to 60% of all automobile accidents involve driving while intoxicated. One fifth of the deaths caused by these accidents involved adolescents, and 130,000 additional injuries occurred in these accidents. The dead and injured may have been either the driver or a passenger. Survivors of these accidents frequently have traumatic brain injury (TBI) or closed head injury (CHI) to the brain. Such damage to the brain results in a range of cognitive and behavioral disorders, which may or may not respond to remediation techniques currently known. These patients often experience intense emotionality. Treatment of these communicatively involved patients requires interdisciplinary rehabilitation services (Committee on Interprofessional Relationships with Neuropsychology, 1989; Committee on Quality Assurance, 1989).

Speech-language pathologists and audiologists will find that clients whose lives are so drastically affected by alcohol demonstrate needs for all areas of communication services. Knowledge of the effects of alcohol and its interaction with other consumed drugs is critical to the adequacy of care that a clinician can provide these clients. A clinician who discovers that therapy is complicated or impeded by the client's abuse of alcohol should seek help through social and psychiatric services available in most communities. An inquiry at the local library or a local medical clinic can usually steer the clinician in the right direction to acquire the needed help for the client. In some instances, it is desirable or necessary to postpone treatment of the communication disorder until the client begins to get help with the alcohol problem. Modification of scheduling for treatment requires collaboration among the counselors dealing with the client.

Drug Addiction.   Using *drug addiction* as an inclusive term is misleading. The actual relationship of the consumer to legal and illegal drugs may be described as one of the following several categories (Cole, 1990; Marlow & Redding, 1988; Smith & Deitch, 1987; Trapp & Spatz, 1988).

Chemical *dependence*: repeated use of a drug that results in an altered psychic state and/or behavioral responses
Drug *abuse*: persistent or sporadic use of drugs that is inconsistent with or unrelated to medical practice or social customs
Drug *addiction*: overwhelming involvement with the use of a drug, obtaining a supply, and a high tendency to use drugs again after withdrawal
Drug *tolerance*: the need to increase dosage to maintain the same effect
Recreational or social *use* of drugs: experimental or incidental use of drugs

Some drugs are known to cause more extensive and severe neurobiological problems than others. The use of drugs and their effects on the structure and function of the body involve all socio-economic classes from the very young to the very old. Reaction to any drug depends to some extent on the drug, its purity, the amount used, the frequency of use, and the condition of the user. Appendix F at the end of this chapter summarizes drug types and their effects biologically and psychologically.

In addition to the internal physical and psychological disruption caused by chemical toxins, there are social implications for the ease of obtaining illegal goods, the temptations that professionals must confront in their personal lives, the enormous amounts of money to be made by furnishing drug supplies, and the extreme poverty sustained by masses of dependent drug users. Crimes from petty theft to professional malpractice to murder are ascribed to the sale and use of drugs. Clinicians should be cautioned about the potential effects of such marketing and legal involvements for themselves, their clients, and their colleagues.

Individuals who are dependent on the use of drugs certainly have intrapersonal communication problems according to current societal standards. However, the clinician is more likely to encounter a client whose communication disorder came first and who began to use the licit or illicit drug as a means to assuage the disorder. When such a person becomes a communication disorders client, the clinician must decide the relative importance of the contributing components through review of records and conversational interaction with the client and others, professionals and nonprofessionals, in the client's life. For some of these clients, team-coordinated treatment is excellent. For others, postponement of therapies is necessary until the substance abuse can be brought under control. For the casual drug user, it is necessary to investigate effects of the drug on the speech, language, or hearing problem and advise the client of that finding. In all these cases, keeping careful records is critical. For example, if a client is on a medically prescribed drug, the clinician must know its value for normalizing or impeding communication abilities. The clinician's consultation with client, caregiver, and physician will help the client gain a better appreciation of how the body and mind interact in acquiring and stabilizing better communication.

Clinicians should be aware of problems that occur in babies born addicted to drugs. The addicted mother's use of drugs during pregnancy often leads to premature birth of the baby, low birth weight, tremor, and poor muscle tone and reflexes. Experienced early childhood educators indicate that preschool children who were born addicted to cocaine exhibit disorders that include:

- Emotional disturbance, anti-social behavior
- Short attention span
- Poor coordination of gross and fine motor movement
- Developmental delays

The continuing of drug use by the mother or the primary caregiver for the child may be even more detrimental to the child's development than fetal drug exposure (Cole, 1990).

However, further consideration of problems that affect drug-addicted babies include the sequelae of low birth weight. They are at risk for developmental disabilities including disturbances of the central nervous system. The range of possible disorders has not been fully traced among addicted infants.

It seems probable that cocaine addiction does not have the massive destructive effects on the central nervous system that are identified with narcotics addiction (Marlow & Redding, 1988; Smith & Deitch, 1987). Within 24 to 72 hours of birth, the effects of narcotic addiction (i.e., heroin, morphine) are discernible (Merker, Higgins, & Kinnard, 1985). Besides increased activity in utero at times when the mother needs drugs, the narcotic effect includes:

- Bilateral coarse or fine tremor
- Hyperirritability, abrasion of skin from rubbing the bedding
- Rigid limbs, hyperreflexia responses

- Fever, rapid respiration, high-pitched cry
- Sucking fist, poor feeding, poor sleeping, decreased moro reflex
- Regurgitation of food, vomiting, diarrhea, dehydration
- Yawning, sneezing, frequent convulsions, myoclonic jerking
- Respiratory depression, apneic attacks

An additional problem interlaced with the use of illicit drugs by injection is the transmission of AIDS. Prior to the 1980s there was no screening process to differentiate contaminated blood from among blood donors. Sale of blood to blood banks was a ready way for the drug-dependent individual to access money to purchase drugs. Contracting AIDS was formerly associated with homosexual transmission of the virus. However, the well-publicized cases of Aliena Martinez and Ryan White have increased awareness that the disease may be transmitted through transfusions of infected blood. In the early 1980s when the virus was identified, blood banks and hospitals created multiple blood-screening techniques to prevent this from happening. As the search for prevention and cure of AIDS continues, many elective surgery patients today donate their own blood prior to surgery to be safe from accidental contraction of HIV virus.

Another connection between drug use and the spread of AIDS is the practice of sharing contaminated needles to inject drugs intravenously. Drug users may not tell their sexual partners about sharing needles and the possibility of their own infection. The results not only affect the drug user but the sexual partner and any fetus which is conceived by them and carried by the infected mother. Neonates with prenatal or perinatal infection with AIDS are born dying.

The role of the speech-language pathologist and audiologist in treatment of these patients often comes in the latter stages of the disease (Committee on Quality Assurance, 1989; Flower & Sooy, 1987). Risk of transmission of the disease to these professionals is extremely low. However, appropriate precautions must be known and maintained. Institutions that provide care for AIDS patients have established precautionary practices concerning handling of materials, equipment, and waste products. Specific precautions for speech-language pathologists and audiologists were spelled out in the ASHA Committee on Quality Assurance report (1989). Of particular note is concern for "interactions that involve an inherent potential for mucous membrane skin contact with blood, body fluids, or tissues, or a potential for spills or splashes of them" (p. 35). Also, caution must be exercised in handling of instruments that are placed in the mouth or probes that are used in the external ear canals. These must be cleaned or disposed of according to the decontamination procedures of the care facility. Clinicians wash their hands before and after each single routine daily activity.

Until a vaccine is developed to prevent the spread of the HIV infection, clinicians must take responsibility for containing contaminants through routine measures. Information about new discoveries, developments, and data in the work with AIDS patients is available from the Centers for Disease Control, National Institutes of Health, and the Food and Drug Administration. Readers who are interested in the latest information on the precautions needed in the treatment of AIDS patients are encouraged to inquire from these resources, check with the government documents section of a library, or telephone the local department of public health. Appendix E offers some basic information associated with AIDS.

Pollution.   Pollution is a fact of life throughout the world. It is a modern problem related to physical matter and energy forms. Air, water, and land are damaged by the dumping of waste from industrial and personal waste. Chemical, electrical, and radiation energy overflow into the environment from the use of materials and equipment that support the economics of the life style demanded by today's urbanized culture. Smog, dust, smoke, sulfur, hydrocarbons, and ozone are common words in the vocabulary of school children. All of these can and do affect the respiratory systems of thousands of people, especially those who have respiratory distress ailments. While this population has not been a major target for communication disorders research, the involvement of respiratory efficiency relates to the satisfactory performance of daily communication needs. This may prove to be an additional area of exploration for future communication disorders personnel. Certainly, individuals who have irreparable damage to the linings and structures of the respiratory and vocal tracts will need the intervention of the speech-language pathologist when the damage reaches levels of dysfunction.

Because of their prolific use, chemical pesticides and fertilizers have saturated the soil and entered households in the plants and food we use every day. Inhaled and ingested chemicals are known to contribute to allergic reactions such as sinus, middle-ear and pharyngeal irritation, and laryngitis. Ingestion of other chemicals commonly used in foods causes physiological disorders and discomfort. A common example is the "hotdog headache" produced by ingestion of nitrite preservatives in some foods (Lockey & Bukantz, 1986). Mercury, frequently found in water contaminated by industrial waste, is toxic to the central nervous system. Its ingestion produces reactions of:

- Parasthesias, weaknesses, apathy, poor concentration, memory loss
- Ataxia, tremors, chorea
- Hearing loss, conductive and sensori-neural, coma, seizures

Lead poisoning, another chemical threat to the central nervous system, is more common in children than in adults (Ehrnman, 1982; Needleman, 1990). A transplacental poison, lead is frequently ingested by individuals who suffer from *pica,* compulsive consumption of nonfood substances. Pica is associated with environmental stress and with children born to affected mothers. Lead poisoning, like that of other chemicals, affects the normal function of the central nervous system. Resulting damage to the brain of a surviving patient requires long-term rehabilitation. Communication training in speech, language, and hearing is included in the needs of these patients.

An enduring threat to the welfare of modern society is the presence of radiation contamination in the environment. At risk are the genetic material of future generations as well as the normal function of the neurophysiology of men, women, and children living today. Since the beginning of the atomic age, nuclear fission and fusion have haunted the average citizen as material of doomsday. In reality, except for isolated incidents, quality controls have restricted the realm of danger from nuclear radiation contamination at energy-generating sites. Of course, there are very real yet unknown factors of human survival and damage to present and future generations following tragedies like the explosion at the Chernobyl nuclear site. Radioactivity that was carried immediately through the atmosphere and later in contaminated products may have reached millions of unsuspecting people throughout many countries. Effects of that and other accidents may contribute to the caseloads and research questions in communication disorders in years to come. Safe disposal of waste from these facilities is a growing problem and remains to be resolved. Because of the invasive nature of radiation energy, the potential disruption of human physiology is presently unpredictable and has been the core of much science fiction in all the entertainment media. Of course, that application has bypassed inferences of communication disorders, perhaps because of the media format and imaginary characters. Certainly, the imaginary characters produced in these stories often represent fearful intruders treated by authors and screenwriters as barbarians, monsters, and outlaws. There are exceptions to this, however, in the heroes found in the popular television, film, and print series called *Star Trek* and cartoon characters such as the *Mutant Ninja Turtles.* Readers who are not interested in science fiction should remember that many realities of modern technology appeared first as prototypes of the future in the imaginings of earlier creative minds.

As an environmental contaminant, light energy must be considered here as contributing to the concerns of specialists in communication abilities and disorders because of its relation to epilepsy. An epileptic seizure may be caused by a reflexive reaction to a strobe light, a shimmering fluorescent light, a flickering television picture tube, the repeated rhythmic beat of a sound or musical tone. Epilepsy is considered a hidden disorder that may arise at any age and is found in 3 to 10 per 1000 (Ferry, Banner, & Wolf, 1985). The clinician is wise to be alert to symptoms of seizure activity, whether *partial* (e.g., beginning in thumb or mouth, exhibiting symptoms from somatosensory variations or clonic jerking to anxiety, sensory hallucinations, sudden change in motor activity of face and limb followed by confusion, sleepiness, or headache) or *general* (e.g., bilateral motor tonic, clonic involvement, and unconsciousness). Seizures, central nervous system activity, and communication disorders are discussed in language courses and upper-level specialization courses that deal with neurogenic communication disorders.

Mechanical energy within the sound spectrum, called *acoustic energy*, likewise contributes pollution to the environment. Industrial, military, and entertainment noise often exceeds the limits of acceptable volume. Consideration of the duration of noise exposure varies from incident to incident. Audiologists know well the importance of hearing conservation in industrial and military occupations, and they have more recently become interested in effects of sustained loud sounds at rock concerts. Loud sound invades many aspects of the environment, in work and social settings, in automobile radios and tape decks with stereophonic speakers, or in isolation where listeners use earphones. Regardless of the setting or the method of input, the presentation of very loud sounds to the human ear eventually results in hearing damage. As yet, the number of people affected and the degree to which they have sustained auditory impairment from modern acoustic technology is not fully known. Specialists in all phases of communication disorders must be prepared to meet the needs of clients with such hearing losses.

As evidence of the effects of pollution on physiology and behavior becomes more available, clinicians will continue to identify differences in their daily work. This is further reason for conscientious record keeping. Documentation of minute differences often signals the identification of unexpected combinations of structures and functions. By carefully observing those differences, the clinician can make modifications in treatment and avoid errors of clinical judgment. These interests support the concept of counseling every client or caregiver to assure a mutual understanding of the experiences and impressions of the individual who has lived with the condition being presented.

Comment. These topics represent social problems that remain unresolved. Each problem is complex in nature and far-reaching in effect. These problems require complicated, long-term solutions involving many people all over the world. The solutions themselves will inevitably alter many aspects of our diversified culture. Within a limited community, local conditions present similarly confounding problems. The identification of problems sets the stage for resolving them. These ongoing steps of adaptive maturation are a large part of the external and internal influences that shape a professional career over time.

EXERCISES

1. Select an article about local news from a newspaper. Gather information about the reported item from local politicians, merchants, community service people, and homemakers.

   a. How do the people you interviewed believe the newsworthy item affects them?
   b. How does the topic of information affect you?
   c. How can this topic potentially affect your future career?
2. Interview someone who is two or three times your age. Conduct an interview to identify two or three specific personal and professional factors that influenced or shaped the interviewee's career over time. Be sure to reserve extra time as you prepare for this exercise. Apply helping skills during the interview to understand responses from the perspective of the person you select as an information source.
3. Carefully review the last 6 months of your life. List external influences, internal responses, and decisions you have made. How did these affect your life during that time? How will they influence your anticipated career?

REFERENCES

American Speech-Language-Hearing Association. (1990). A report to the members. *ASHA, 32* (3), 9–11.

AMA Division on Drugs. (1984). *Drug Evaluations,* (5th ed.). Chicago, IL: American Medical Association.

Cole, C. (1990, April). Unpublished remarks at a workshop for the Juvenile Welfare Board of Pinellas County. St. Petersburg, FL.

Committee on Interprofessional Relationships with Neuropsychology. (1989). *ASHA, 31* (4), 328–329.

Committee on Quality Assurance. (1989). AIDS/HIV: Implications for speech-language pathologists and audiologists. *ASHA, 31* (6–7), 33–38.

Ehrnman, K. (1982). Community involvement in the prevention of childhood lead poisoning. *Health Education, 13* (1), 38.

Ferry, P. C., Banner, W., Jr., & Wolf, R. A. (1985). *Seizure disorders in children.* Philadelphia: Lippincott.

Flower, W. M., & Sooy, C. D. (1987). AIDS: An introduction for speech-language pathologists and audiologists. *ASHA, 29* (11), 25–30.

Habal, M. B. (1989a). Ceramic-bone composite implant: A new method of augmentation for bone regeneration. *Biomedical Materials and Devices, 110,* 245–310.

Habal, M. B. (1989b). New concepts in pediatric plastic surgery. *Journal of the Florida Medical Association, 76,* 617–621.

Herer, G. R. (1989). Inventing the future. *ASHA, 31* (12), 35–37.

Holley, S. C. (1988). The new ASHA: Preparing for the future. *ASHA, 30* (12), 19–22.

Jarratt, J. (1989). Trends shaping U.S. society: 1990–2005. *ASHA, 31* (12), 33–35.

Jones, K. L., & Smith, D. W. (1973). Recognition of the fetal alcohol syndrome in early infancy. *Lancet, 2,* 999–1001.

Jung, J. H. (1989). *Genetic syndromes in communication disorders.* Boston: Little, Brown.

Lippman, S. (1980). Prenatal alcohol and minimum brain dysfunction. *Southern Medical Journal, 73,* 1173–1174.

Lockey, R. F., & Bukantz, S. C. (1986). *Principles of immunology and allergy.* Philadelphia: W. B. Saunders.

March, J., & Veneer, M. W. (1985). *Clinics in plastic surgery, 12* (2), 279–291.

Marlow, D. R., & Redding, B. A. (1988). *Pediatric nursing.* Philadelphia: W. B. Saunders.

Merker, L., Higgins, P., & Kinnard, E. (1985). Assessing narcotic addiction in neonates. *Pediatric Nursing, 11* (4), 177.

Needleman, H. L. (1990). Low-level lead exposure: A continuing problem. *Pediatric Annals, 19* (6), 208–214.

Oppeneer, J. E., & Vervoren, T. M. (1983). *Gerontological Pharmacology.* St. Louis: Mosby.

Paul, R. (1990). Increasing computer literacy in speech-language pathology students. *ASHA, 32* (4), 63–64.

Price, J. H., & Andrews, P. (1982). Alcohol abuse in the elderly. *Journal of Gerontological Nursing, 8* (3), 16.

Smith, J. E., & Deitch, K. V. (1987). Cocaine: A maternal, fetal, and neonatal risk. *Journal of Pediatric Health Care, 1* (1), 120.

Sparks, S. M. (1984). Speech and language in fetal alcohol syndrome. *ASHA, 26* (4), 27–31.

Thornton, J. R., Krishnaiyer, R., Young, M., Moore, R., & Johnsrud, C. S. (1989). Technology transfer. *ASHA, 31* (12), 38–40.

Trapp, E. P., & Spatz, T. (1988). Considerations for the practitioner with older clients. In B. Shadden (Ed.), *Communication behavior and aging.* Baltimore, MD: Williams and Wilkins.

CHAPTER SEVEN

❦ ❦ ❦

Evaluating Counseling Skills of Clinicians

Issues

❦ *Evaluation of counseling skills in training and practice may be carried out in various ways by many individuals.*

❦ *Objective self-study necessitates feedback from communication partners through meta-communication and / or the use of audio- and videotape recording equipment.*

❦ *Performance Evaluation Training (PET) prescribes self-observation and mutual review of recorded interactions with a client, either real or role-played, in the presence of a skilled instructor to assist and protect the participants.*

❦ *Self-study of clinical and counseling skills is applicable throughout a career in the field of communication disorders.*

❦ ❦ ❦

VARIETY OF TECHNIQUES TO EVALUATE COUNSELING SKILLS

Evaluation is an essential part of professional accountability in the field of human services. Evaluation of the counseling aspects of communication disorders treatment also enters into accountability to clients. In fact, whether or not the interactive behaviors described as counseling skills are assessed by a third party, they are evaluated as a part of the interpersonal interaction. The search for ways to evaluate helping in the treatment of speech, language, or hearing disorders can be approached from four perspectives: tradition within the profession, academic and clinical teaching programs, expectations of clients and caregivers, and self-perceptions of the clinician.

Evaluation of Counseling in the Treatment Process

Traditionally, the approach to evaluation of counseling skills in speech-language pathology and audiology has been one of caution. The caution reflects concerns that counseling is really psychotherapy and that the practitioners are ill-prepared to undertake responsibilities that could harm clients and caregivers or even generate incidents of professional malpractice. Greater emphasis traditionally has been placed on protecting clients from what counseling is not than on analyzing or evaluating what it is. This nearly universal caution may relate to the origins of the communication disorders discipline and its continued alignment with health care services. Attitudes and perceptions of the clinician's role may represent a carryover of exaggerated reverence for medical and psychological precepts of territorial domains. However, the ASHA Code of Ethics (American Speech-Language-Hearing Association, 1989) supports the concept and application of counseling skills in the treatment of clients.

Because of the recurrent use of the term *counseling* in the literature of communication disorders, one must believe that the concept of interpersonal interactions (Luterman, 1984) of many sorts is not abhorrent to the governing body of the professional association. As a discipline, members seem to have held an underlying belief or trust in the nurturing goodness of fellow clinicians and a respect for outcomes of individual practices much like the popular attitude toward classroom teachers. There has been little effort to arrive at a consensus of what counseling is and how it is to be included in the repertoire of clinicians.

The diversity of traditional opinions about counseling in speech-language pathology and audiology requires a level of caution, but not to the extent that clinicians restrict their roles to the transmission of information. In fact, limiting the role of counseling to transmitting information relates to one of the leading criticisms of clients about the practitioner's interactive communication skills with clients and caregivers, especially during crisis situations (Martin, George, O'Neal, & Daly, 1987). The austerity of the clinician's role suggested by informational counseling alone belies the use of the term counseling except in the legalistic sense, that is, instruction and advice giving.

The rigid parameters of counseling as information sharing may be illustrated by considering a stereotypical surgeon who visits a hospitalized patient to gain the information necessary to perform the anticipated dissection. Having learned what the operative procedure will require, the surgeon then goes to a dictaphone, records findings and orders to be typed by a remote secretarial service, and leaves the room. In that controlled contact, the patient and family visually and auditorily identify the surgeon with whom they communicate through carefully correct responses to succinctly posed questions, but there is a void of personal involvement or association for either the surgeon or the patient and family. The interaction is imbedded in an external phenomenon, that of the family's trust in and dependence on the reputed ability of the surgeon. Neither the surgeon nor the family exceeds the minimum level of communication required to enable the anticipated procedure. As in an efficient assembly line process, when the operation is completed, follow-up care of the wound is left to the nursing support personnel and follow-up care of the patient and family is left to a family doctor or no one at all.

The place of counseling in the communication disorders profession may have developed as a result of attitudes common in other fields and an attempt to emulate colleagues who practice in those specialties. On the other hand, either in ignorance or in awe of psychological and emotional reactions or illnesses of some clients or caregivers, we may have neglected to become as broadly educated as need be (Klevans, 1982; Rousey, 1982). Emerging cultural diversity across the nation and within the profession of communication disorders demands a flexibility in each clinician that has not been required in an earlier, more limited view of communication disorders. Increasing demands for services in diagnosis and treatment for newly described communication disorders require that each professional be equipped to meet the needs of clients and their families in settings not yet described.

The attitudes of professors and supervisors toward teaching and evaluating counseling skills have not been surveyed. Student evaluations of classroom teaching and clinical supervision have only hinted at the effective use of counseling abilities among training program faculties. This is to be expected, since the discipline itself has not yet determined what it means by counseling. Thoughts about counseling among current instructional personnel in the field may be as varied as the individuals. Historically, teachers of new generations of clinicians may have taught aspects of counseling through experiential interactions in classrooms and practicum settings. If so, "naturalistic" pedagogic good fortune has sustained an appreciation of the abilities of isolated clinicians in limited communities from one generation of clinicians to the next. Backus (1960) and Rollin (1987) addressed concerns about the psychological distance and detachment between clinician and client that overprofessionalism can cause.

The number of professionals employed in the communication disorders profession is expected to exceed 83,000 by the year 2000 (Holley, 1988). Such a large number of practitioners increases the risks associated with independently identified counseling roles and undefined personal limits for counseling, making those risks professionally unacceptable. As a discipline, communication disorders still needs to establish a consensus of the meaning and boundaries of the various aspects of counseling.

Counseling Instruction for Clinicians

The ideal opportunity to instruct clinicians in therapeutic values of interpersonal communication and assistive "counseling/helping" experiences exists as part of their regular speech, language, and hearing training programs and should not be left to chance. The mystery and confusion surrounding the concept of *counseling* must be recognized for what it is. Professional curricula must recognize the commitment of the clinician in the counseling or helping role, thereby reducing the fear of either harming the client or caregiver or overstepping imaginary boundaries between disciplines. Routinely accepted oral examinations differentiate clients who need immediate medical intervention from those who need articulation therapy. Similarly, clinicians must have the breadth of knowledge, experience, and ability to discern and differentiate which clients have psychological or emotional conditions that interfere with therapeutic progress and call for counseling and which warrant referral to psychotherapeutic specialists.

Counseling or helping is not only an academic concept to be gained from lectures and discussions, nor is it just casual conversation that is perfected in social contexts. Rather, it is the timely and judicious application of an intricate bank of behaviors that enable accurate "idea transplant" back and forth between people of all ages, races, and cultures, in any setting, with any disorder, and in spite of all the internal and external personal impedimenta to dyadic communication. Concepts, language, and observable behaviors of counseling may be introduced and described in classroom discussions. Becoming proficient in the use of counseling demands involvement of the student-clinician in monitored, direct, one-on-one counselor-client interactions to identify, reinforce, critique, and perfect helping skills.

One approach to training and evaluation of counseling skills was described in chapter 2. Through introductory courses to clinical work and through mentorship by clinical faculty or supervisors, student-clinicians can test the limits of their abilities to recognize and address details of client characteristics. Under clinical supervision, they participate in planning and analyzing interpersonal interaction with peers and supervisors. Through effective working relationships, they also learn about therapeutic implications of the psychological and emotional status and needs of clients and their families (American Speech-Language-Hearing Association, 1985; Pickering, 1989).

The ideal clinical supervisor teaches helping skills by offering insight into the student's interpersonal strengths and weaknesses and guiding the student-therapist's interaction with clients and caregivers. Thus, the ideal clinical supervisor is a proficient counselor who applies counseling skills to instructive interactions with student-clinicians. However, the practical restrictions on personnel and time allotted for supervision for each session often emphasize the administration of specific tests or the use of certain treatment techniques and prohibit enhancement of the student's interpersonal skills. In some training programs, extension of the clinical supervisory role to incorporate enhancement of specific counseling or helping skills may not be very different from current policy and practice. In other programs, incorporating interpersonal communication as a component of the practicum experience would pose a different sort of problem. With some degree of consensus on the definition of *counseling,* modern clinical supervisors may want or need training and experience in mentoring and teaching those behaviors as a category of treatment skills.

If therapy is both art and science, it may be that the *art* of therapy, if fully described, would closely match counseling or helping. Traditional practicum experience supervised by *artists* in the field may have provided a forum for teaching undefined, unnamed, and even unrecognized applications of counseling techniques. If so, like a spectrographic analysis of speech sounds, the discipline needs a minute dissection of the interactive communication behavior, nonverbal and verbal, among supervisors, clinicians, and clients and caregivers. Such work has been accomplished in other fields, but it has not been fully applied to the treatment of clients with speech, language, or hearing problems and their families. A word of caution must be repeated here. As discussed in this book, to create rigid norms for counseling skills would defeat the whole purpose of the effort. Instructors and students must remember that the application of helping skills varies with personality, setting, disorder, and the unique attributes of each participant.

To follow the clinical psychology training model would require special practica devoted to experience in counseling the communicatively handicapped. However, as an intricate part of treatment, helping is not an exclusive technique but a pervasive one; as such, it must be deliberately recognized and incorporated into each client-clinician encounter. Training for mentorship should be made available to potential teachers and clinical supervisors, as not all successful professionals in the academic setting are expected to be natural helpers or skilled mentors of helping skills.

Clients and caregivers demonstrate their approval and appreciation of clinicians' services by returning to subsequent treatment sessions, complying with requests for practice, using equipment, and referring relatives and neighbors who seem to need similar services. Reports of formal evaluations of counseling by clients and caregivers are relatively scarce. Martin, George, O'Neal, and Daly (1987) found divergence of opinion between parents and audiologists relative to parents' feelings and needs for counseling services offered at the time of diagnosis of their child's hearing loss. Coulter, Scheuerle, Laude, & Habal (1991) surveyed parental stress levels in relation to services at a craniofacial center. They found that stress increased relative to family characteristics and decreased with the time, support, and counseling received from center staff members.

Client/caregiver evaluation of counseling services may be a prime target for the development of a bank of research. To do this, services at any treatment setting should be divided into subcategories. Those recognized as counseling services can be coded in any questionnaire designed to elicit consumer responses. If marketing strategies apply at all to speech-language pathology and audiology, they would seem to apply here. Ongoing satisfaction of the consumer is essential to maintenance and growth of the service (Battin & Fox, 1978). If services can be enhanced by increased emphasis and incorporation of counseling skills, practitioners will be wise to explore and strengthen their own abilities in this area.

Self-evaluation of counseling or helping abilities is yet another perspective of evaluating the effectiveness of therapeutic techniques (Casey, Smith, & Ulrich, 1988). Most intervention in communication disorders is carried out by a single practitioner or a sequence of single practitioners. Clinicians should evaluate their own areas of proficiency in interactive communication and maintain awareness of their professional uses of and responses to the verbal and nonverbal communication behaviors described as counseling skills (Anderson, 1988). The ways of doing this during training generally depend on curriculum management within the academic department of communication sciences and disorders. In addition to classroom faculty and clinical supervisors' assessment of students' abilities, student-clinicians may be asked to give subjective assessments of their own work and their individual comfort levels in each of several practicum settings. Also, videotaping may be provided to assist student and supervisor in recalling and reviewing therapy or diagnostic techniques and procedures. These self-monitoring experiences have been found most helpful when they emphasize the positive strengths of the student-clinicians. The same procedures can be adapted for the monitoring of helping behaviors, as suggested in Tables 2.6 and 2.7.

Following the design for identifying individual behaviors, as discussed in chapter 2, objective behavior counts can be made and used for discussion of the behaviors, their performance, and their desired increase or decrease. For observation purposes, the clinician's helping behaviors can be clustered in four naturalistic categories (Kagan, 1976): exploratory responses, listening responses, affective identification, and honest labeling.

Exploratory responses are those that encourage the client to pursue a line of thought. These verbal or nonverbal behaviors may be open or closed questions, minimal encourages, or silence. Appropriately applied, these counselor responses elicit continued exploration by the client. The result may be a clarification, the addition of detail, or an indication of tangent actions, thoughts, and feelings. Exploratory responses are posed in such a way as to maintain equality in status between the clinician and the client or caregiver. In this way, the relationship is free from the clinician's authoritarian control of the client. Exploratory responses ensure that the whole problem is presented and considered in as many aspects as possible. Exploration should never be used solely for the accumulation of information by the clinician, but rather for clarification of the client's thinking.

Listening responses of the clinician or counselor are those identified as paraphrasing and restatements. The ability to reverbalize the intended message of the client confirms the counselor's role as a partner in the therapeutic effort. These types of responses also provide the client an instantaneous opportunity to review the message as it has been received by the communication partner. Listening responses keep the communicative exchange on topic, clarify the client's intended message for both partners, and demonstrate the acceptability of whatever aspect of the self the client has presented. In this way, the clients are encouraged to be honest with themselves, even when dealing with a difficult topic.

Affective identification refers to the counseling strategy of recognizing and naming client feelings, asking the client about affective dimensions of discourse, and sharing emotional reactions to client behaviors. These helping techniques often show the client an aspect of self that was previously hidden even to the client. Hidden feelings of clients, caregivers, and clinicians sometimes result from cultural influences. In some cultures, people have learned to emphasize the cognitive domain and teach successive generations of children that it is unacceptable to express or discuss feelings publicly, especially negative ones. Affective identification focuses on the feelings of the client.

Honest labeling is closely associated with the identification of affect. It calls for the clinician to be forthright as well as aware of the client's cognitive and affective states. In this way the clinician assures that recognized responses of the client are seen and named for what they are in the client's life. With this behavior, the clinician can avoid the risk of seeming cruel while being accurately reflective. The clinician must always be careful to stay on target when applying this behavior and avoid misrepresenting or misperceiving a client condition. The clinician must also be cautious not to allow deliberate distortion to enter into the labeling process. Remembering that humor is often a simple distortion of reality, the clever clinician may see the humorous side of a client's dilemma, but must not use it as a therapeutic moment unless the client has indicated readiness for that type of response.

The potential for supervisors to interact with student-clinicians has been greatly enhanced by the capacity to videotape practicum sessions for later review. However, there is often an incorrect assumption that the use of this tool will be properly handled by all who choose to use it. Little attention has been paid to teaching supervisors the advantages as well as the risks inherent in capturing the student's best efforts on tape. Certainly this concrete evidence of a student-clinician's performance suggests areas for caution in the interaction between supervisor and student. The clinical supervisor has the responsibility for coaching the best in the student, while the student is commanded to face the self. When used carefully and effectively by a clinical supervisor astute in the application of helping skills, early videotaped samples of therapeutic technique in a practicum experience can be compared with later ones to estimate the advancement of skills and improvement of client communication.

Supervisors generally find that students who watch themselves perform a skill, administer a test, or make a silly mistake learn quickly to appreciate their own efforts. Just as Allen Funt's *Candid Camera,* the humorous television program of the 1980s that looked at ordinary life, helped audiences to see themselves as others see them, videotape recording prohibits denial of the reality of behavior and invites recognition of strengths and weaknesses for what they are. If handled improperly, these confrontations with self can impose stressful experiences with negative outcomes on the student.

These four descriptive categories of helping behaviors, like those found in other texts, are easily understood and may not seem new or different. However, learning the language to describe counseling behaviors and identifying them in actual treatment sessions are quite different undertakings. The clinician may obtain additional evaluative feedback by inviting selected, experienced clients and caregivers to participate. In such an exercise, the focus of review or critique expands to include the relationship between the clinician and client as well as the personal capacity of the clinician.

Evaluation of Clinician and Client/Caregiver Interaction

In clinics where clients gain skills for coping as well as communication or the handicaps of their communication disorders are reduced, clients and caregivers are often invited to complete evaluation questionnaires. As an in-house component of accountability procedures, these questionnaires can be effective in reinforcing practices, supporting procedural changes, or instituting new programs. In some instances, positive comments from clients and caregivers may also enhance a clinician's standing on the professional staff at times of annual performance review. In university teaching clinics, parents and adult clients may be asked to assess the services of students of speech-language pathology and audiology as a component of the semester's grading process. Little information is available about the types of questions typically asked. The questions we have reviewed emphasized satisfaction with the client's progress in gaining clearer communication abilities. However, consumer feedback is valuable for whatever purposes the questions are designed to fulfill.

Another type of evaluative feedback contributes directly to perfecting counseling or helping skills. *Meta-communication,* or communication about communication, opens an opportunity to recall and influence the interactive behaviors of both parties in a dyad. Most adults have probably experienced conversational exchanges that recall and modify previous communications or miscommunications, such as the following examples:

"Oh, no. That's not what I mean. It's . . ."

or

"I didn't mean to say that. I'm sorry if I gave you the wrong impression. What I meant was . . ."

or

"Do you really feel that . . . I'm so relieved."

or

"Remember what we were talking about earlier? I'm really anxious that nobody else knows about that."

or

"Last week I thought you approved. How do you really feel . . .?"

or

"Yeah! That's it. Exactly . . ."

Clarification of meaning through exploratory communication can be applied to learning and improving counseling skills. Because of time constraints, many professional schools adopt classroom techniques of showing films, one of *good counseling,* where excellent communication is evident, and one of *poor counseling,* where inadequate communication is rife. The class is instructed to discuss the effectiveness of the two portrayed counselors. Discussions may include critiques of verbal and nonverbal communication abilities, apparent attitude and concern of the counselor, or underlying social causes of such behavior. Sometimes the class discussion focuses on the physical actions of the communicator. Observed behaviors may give clues to simultaneous covert processes of thoughts and feelings. The client's need for more or different interaction with the counselor may become apparent.

In communication disorders, materials for studying good and poor counseling skills may be readily available through the use of clinical teaching tapes. However, one must be very careful to protect the people displayed on videotapes that are to be critiqued. Legal and ethical considerations require that individuals whose images and voices appear in the recorded session give permission for use of the tapes. Viewers must respect the people in the tapes, even when disagreeing with techniques and methods used.

A basic need exists to observe and understand the differences between good and poor counseling, and good and poor interpersonal communication, during a treatment session. Recognizing that difference is an essential step toward becoming an effective counselor or helper. Using the appropriate behavior at the appropriate time and producing the reactions that are labeled as good counseling are even more demanding than recognition. The doing requires the helper continually to set aside the self. This is a high-energy and demanding task. Remember that the speech-language pathologist and audiologist does not expect the communicatively disordered client to achieve rehabilitation in one or two visits. In much the same way, gaining proficiency in the use of good counseling skills requires carefully staged involvement in performing the measures that are known to be effective.

It is important to have a ready vocabulary to label the expressed or apparent underlying emotion of the speaker. Not all observers are competent in this, and some may need to be taught how to label various looks, acts, and sounds that signal changes in feelings. Additionally, not all people express similar feelings in the same way. Regional, cultural, and ethnic diversity have been mentioned earlier. A demonstration and class discussion often brings this out, and it needs to be reemphasized in this context.

The ability to recognize and label affective dimensions of behavior accurately is based on observation of verbal and nonverbal behavior. Learning to label the affective state or intent of another person accurately often requires a dialogue in which the counselor indicates the perceived affective message and seeks confirmation of that perception. Because of a client's differences in custom or habit, a counselor may incorrectly label an affective state. Assigning a verbal label to what the counselor observes offers the client the opportunity to confirm, reject, or correct any such perception. That is, the verbal exchange concerning feelings negotiates the mutual understanding of the actual affective state and assigns acceptable language to it, as in the following examples.

Caregiver: (swinging foot rapidly and speaking loudly) When Michael comes home late and smells of beer, I know he's not telling me everything.

Counselor: It's upsetting not to know what's going on.

Caregiver: Oh! I know what's going on, or at least I think I do. But I've not dared to ask.

Counselor: You're afraid of what you may learn.

Caregiver: Yeah. I'm sure I'll not be pleased even if it's only a beer with the guys in the carpool.

Counselor: You're feeling angry about what you suspect.

or

Child: (slowly and quietly) My dog died last night.

Counselor: Oh, I'm sorry. You must feel very sad.

Child: Yes. A big truck hit him on the street. He wasn't supposed to chase cars and things. He just couldn't help it.

Counselor: You tried to teach him how to be safe.

Child: I yelled for him to come back, but he was barking and running out of the yard when the truck came down the street fast and kept on going.

Counselor: It makes you angry that the truck driver didn't even stop.

Child: Yeah. My daddy said that truck driver wasn't a good citizen to kill my dog and run away.

The progression toward perfecting mutual understanding must include practice that consists of exploratory and confirming dialogue. Through meta-communication, two people can study their communicative strengths and weaknesses. Review of interpersonal communication may be carried out casually from memory or in a more structured way with stimulation by audiotape and/or videotape. Guided review of recorded sessions in conjunction with the client, real or role-played, allows the communicating partners to cross-match their impressions, intentions, relations, and feelings.

❦ ❦ ❦

GUIDED SELF-STUDY THROUGH META-COMMUNICATION

The progression of self-discovery and self-evaluation for counselors or helpers can be undertaken with careful guidance by an experienced counselor-instructor who is trained in helping skills. Such guidance is necessary because of the nature of the interpersonal communication that inevitably occurs under these circumstances and the fact that it is being taped for review. Regardless of how self-assured the partner, whether the client or the actor who is role-playing the client, or how experienced the clinician, there are instances in honest, open communication wherein inner personal traits are divulged and no longer remain covert (Kagan, 1975, 1976). In these instances, performers are vulnerable to the critical awareness of any viewer, especially to themselves as observers. Part of the risk lies in the seeming permanence of the recording, a factor that may be disturbing to participants who have not yet developed a secure self-image. Once a behavior is captured on tape, it remains there with the possibility of being repeated, unchanged and unchangeable until the tape is erased. Another aspect of the risk is that the initial reaction to one's own image on videotape is sometimes startling. Desensitization normally occurs with repeated exposure, practice, and positive guidance.

Although it is easy to erase a videotape, the ultimate purpose of the procedure being proposed is for the clinician and client to view the tape together to stimulate their memories of what happened, the sequence of happenings, how the participants felt from moment to moment, and what they thought while the recorded action was taking place. To do this, the participants must move beyond their immediate reactions to the review process and concentrate on the actions that occurred during the taping of the session.

When participants are initiated into this procedure, rules for mutual respect and confidentiality must be explained. At the outset, they must be advised of methods to be used and cautioned about the rights of others who may participate in the interviews. The rationale is not only humane but also practical, considering modern civil rights law dealing with invasion of privacy. To assure protection, both legal and ethical, the presence of an informed, experienced instructor and consistent attention to simple rules are essential to the success of the review-recall guided self-study.

Simple rules form an important part of the introduction to the procedure. Immediately upon introducing this study-of-self type of evaluative process to clinicians, students, actors, and clients, it is necessary to specify their individual rights and the limits of the demands that can be placed upon them. A participant who feels the need at any time to withdraw from the procedure must be allowed to do so under the principles of mental health. The candidate for withdrawal may privately inform the instructor of the desire to cease participation in the activities. Participants who view the work of others on video monitors must be cautioned about their behavior and commentary during such viewings. Viewers must be aware of the vulnerability of clinicians, clients, or actors who role-play those characters. To this end, we have found it beneficial to allow only positive comments during the review of the tape. Participants who wish to analyze their own taped performances in more detail are invited to do so privately at an appointed time with the counselor-instructor. As a general rule, self-viewers tend to see more faults in their performances than items to praise. The requirement to identify praiseworthy behaviors enables clinicians to learn to assert their strengths. The instructor need never fear that weaknesses will be missed entirely.

Basic, common language is needed to prepare for full participation in this application of meta-communication. Each member of the group must be able to identify emotions by name and description. Most participants will have had some experience in recognizing behavioral signs of the more commonly experienced emotions. Some time should be spent discussing this to ensure a general consensus of the intent of the communicator when emotionality is a component of the expressed message. Another necessary discussion must address the counselor's reaction to the client's expressed emotion when the message is directed toward the counselor. It may be desirable to invite an actor from outside the participant group to portray several states of emotion. Common displays of anger, fear, joy, sensuality, anxiety, and frustration will usually suffice for participants to begin to recognize the initiation of response in their own bodies. Videotapes of counseling are also available. One set of communication/psychology videotapes from which to select is the Public Broadcasting System's (PBS) *Bradshaw on the Family* series. The 10 tapes can be used in sequence, or single tapes may be selected to study participant behaviors. Titles of the 1-hour tapes offered in the Bradshaw collection are:

The Family in Crisis (Symptoms)
The Healthy Family (A model)
The Unhealthy Family (Dysfunctional)
The Compulsive Family (Preaddictive)
The Persecuted (Abuse)
The "Bad" Child (Self-concept)
The Most Common Family Illness (Co-dependency)
Help for the Family (Forgiveness)
Health for the Family (Problem identification and intervention)
Hope for the Family (Self-esteem)

These and other appropriate videotapes are often available through an academic department of mass communication or a media library. Affective vignettes such as those by Kagan (1975) are excellent for this purpose. They are brief, and the actors utilize verbal and nonverbal behaviors to send specific affective messages. Motion pictures such as *On Golden Pond* invite affect identification, although full-length films may consume too much class time. Selected portions of such films have been useful and well-received by participants.

Once participants become conversant with the language of emotional reactions, they tend to identify more readily their own reactions and those of others. These initial practices of naming observed affective states and of identifying one's own physiological reaction to someone else's expression of feelings are the foundation for building a meta-communication evaluative process.

Performance Evaluation Training (PET) can begin when participants can readily identify frequent emotional reactions. Review of video-recorded sessions is best begun by borrowing a videotape from the clinic library of demonstration tapes. A seasoned clinical supervisor is an insightful resource for recommending a tape in which none of the current class of participants are shown. Viewers can identify and label the clinician's helping behaviors and the client's responses to them. They can stop the tape to label and discuss affective reactions that are apparent or implied by the behavior of both recorded participants.

❦ ❦ ❦

PERFORMANCE EVALUATION TRAINING (PET)

The next step in the guided study-of-self involves videotaping each participant performing the role of counselor. Having mastered the behaviors described in chapter 2, the counselor now integrates those skills into a therapeutic whole. During replay of the recorded session in the presence of the instructor, participants observe their own behaviors and stop the tape periodically to comment on performance and identify concurrent covert thoughts and affective processes. The recommended sequence of experiences for the playback portion of the project is (a) review of a prepared demonstration tape of a counselor, (b) review of the self performing as counselor in an interactive session, and (c) shared or mutual review of the interaction between counselor and client. Similar learning methods have been designed and used successfully in educational and training programs for professionals, paraprofessionals, and lay persons in both homogeneous and heterogeneous ethnic and cultural groups (Kagan, 1976; Scheuerle, 1985, 1990).

The first step in this procedure is instructional, and its primary focus is for the reviewer to learn to identify behaviors that denote nonverbal messages. This information, combined with verbalization by the counselor, provides the reviewer with a clear picture of the trend of the recorded session. The second step begins to involve the participant directly in the meta-communicative procedure. Replay of the videotaped stimulus allows the counselor-participant to monitor technique, stop the tape, and identify covert processes that accompanied and influenced recorded behavior. That process requires considerable objectivity in viewing the self while focusing on the recorded interaction. Guidance by an experienced counselor is important in this step. Achievement of these strategies may require several attempts. In a positive environment with consistent guidance, participants can master an enormous amount of self-assessment. Graduate students often learn to laugh at themselves while undertaking this exercise. On the other hand, instructors should remain very much aware during selection of candidates for the project that videotaping may uncover both positive and negative covert processes.

The third and final step of the PET offers a unique opportunity for the clinician and client to rehearse, revisit, and review communicative instances that would be transitory if not captured on tape. They explore their relationship, their mutual understanding and concerns, and especially their success in open, honest communication of ideas and feelings. This system of communication-about-communication holds a novel and appropriate attraction for the discipline of communication disorders because of the continually emerging diversity among clients, caregivers, and colleagues in the modern professional world. Video-stimulated review of communicative interaction has proven to be especially successful in working with people from different disciplines and cultures (Kagan, 1976; Scheuerle, 1985, 1990). The ease with which the method is adapted centers around successfully applying the principles of self-monitoring and self-exploration. A participant has no need to anticipate criticism from someone who neither understands nor appreciates cultural differences.

This method of self-study is useful not only for learning and improving counseling or helping abilities but also for evaluating them. In preceding chapters, we have seen that personal traits and internal and external influences wield great control in molding and shaping decisions, feelings, attitudes, and behaviors. Further, the relationship and trust between the clinician and the client are significant parts of the driving force, the power of therapeutic change. It is invaluable for clinicians to identify and recognize their own incidental or habituated actions and reactions. Some responses of each partner to multivariate stimuli may remain internal, hidden from the person producing the response as well as from an observer. Other actions may be overt and obvious to any observer. Shared review of a treatment session provides a format for clinician and client to explore and clarify their previous communicative attempts and recognize their influences upon each other. This meta-communication opportunity generates a context in which the counselor, the student-clinician, can feel secure as overt behavior as well as covert behavior are identified, labeled, and critiqued. More than that, the student-clinician has access to the communicative partner for direct feedback as to the minute-by-minute effectiveness of the counseling effort.

Through the review dialogue, under guidance of the experienced counselor-instructor, the participant progresses in self-discovery and self-evaluation. The participant also gains proficiency in establishing and maintaining a counseling or helping relationship.

❦ ❦ ❦

APPLICATIONS OF SELF-STUDY IN CLINICAL CAREERS

In our modern adult society, some people display emotional behavior, but few talk extensively about their feelings. In professional settings, one often finds a considerable degree of formality in discourse and a tendency to endow the professional with mythical traits of authority and even superiority. Clinicians who assume postures and manners that create psychological distance between themselves and their clients increase barriers to communication and consequent shallow understandings. Becoming a helper or counselor includes learning to reduce and relax communicative formalities and related barriers. Informal, friendly, caring approaches to clients, caregivers, and colleagues do not diminish the value or status of the professional clinician or reduce the authoritativeness of professional acumen. Whether a clinician knowingly utilizes distancing devices as a shield or a defense becomes an important question, if the therapist is striving to be a helper. Perceiving one's own behavior, overt and covert, realistically continues to be an important element in enjoying a successful career in communication disorders. Self-knowledge enables the clinician to make choices and effect changes.

McCormack (1984) emphasized that higher academic degrees cannot provide the graduate with more than a foundation of knowledge and an introduction to a discipline. Academic beginnings in communication disorders teach clinicians how to do their homework in preparation for client rehabilitation. Graduates may be less prepared to make tough decisions relative to employment settings or methods of initiating innovative changes in existing programs. Two additional areas of expertise that enable success in professional clinical practice are knowledge of people, or being able to *read people,* and knowledge of *the game,* or knowing how to create an impression (McCormack, 1984). This seems to suggest that clinicians must expand their self-knowledge to include understanding their interactions with people besides colleagues, clients, or their caregivers, that is, others who are not knowledgeable about the profession of communication disorders or clinical rehabilitation of communicatively disabled clients. This wide spectrum of others includes family members, friends, neighbors, employers, and potential funding sources. To face the infinite possibilities for encounters, the best preparation for a successful lifetime career is self-knowledge, self-understanding, and proficiency in the communication skills of exploration, confirmation, and negotiation.

As a family member interested in maintaining a career, family expectations must be considered. Parents, spouses, and children of clinicians have different perspectives of the person who is the clinician. They express those expectations daily, often in the form of demands (Ward, 1987). The clinician may find that conscientious responses to family demands tax the best of listening, reacting, and decision-making skills. Family members who work together find that the interactive behaviors that are appropriate in the business setting do not always fit the situation at home (Strickland & Thompson, 1989).

Differences in the needs and desires of the clinician and those of other people in the several environments challenge the clinician's ability to preserve integrity and self-hood. The clinician who has gained insight into the habits of reacting and inner processes will find interaction with others, including family members, much more manageable and less stressful.

In the progress of a career, clinicians may experience a *plateauing* effect. Bardwick (1986, p. 3) described plateauing of a career in saying that when "a major aspect of life has stabilized, as it ultimately must, we may find ourselves significantly dissatisfied." This feeling of stagnation may arise from the American philosophy of optimism and expansionism, that is, there is always room for growth, advancement, improvement. One often hears about climbing the ladder of success or moving up in the world. Clinicians may come to expect access to that upward mobility. However, societal changes include a broad diversity of jobs that combines with increasing numbers of employees, diminishing the possibility of advancement through promotion and salary increases.

In a more stabilized workforce of the future, new and different types of rewards are necessary. Goldman (1986) indicated that individuals must take the initiative in creating achievement awards and career rewards. This is exemplified by Kahler (1989), a successful, highly respected clinician who faced disenchantment with her professional role. She developed a method to reward herself by modifying her approach to her career. She changed from being a dialectician and grammarian to being involved in broader-based considerations for an entire school system in West Babylon,

New York, the American Speech-Language-Hearing Association, and clinical research.

In daily activities, the self-actualizing clinician gains trust in the self through a wealth of knowledge based on a lifetime of direct experience. Practical theories of human behavior grow out of that experience. Beliefs and theories are influential inner forces that affect behavior, attitude, and feelings. The inner strength to define and challenge the limits of a current situation, test the adequacy of the overall best function of a system, and grow creatively to fill gaps in service and research marks the joy and reward of a satisfying career in the profession of communication disorders.

EXERCISES

1. McCormack (1984) identified three statements that are hard to say, but necessary for professional success. They are:

   I don't know.
   I was wrong.
   I need help.

   a. Initiate a conversation with a classmate. Be sure to use each of these three statements during the dialogue.
   b. Initiate a conversation with a teacher. Be sure to use each of these three statements during the dialogue.
   c. Initiate a conversation with an adult client or caregiver. Be sure to use each of these three statements.
   d. How did you feel during each of the conversations when you introduced the three "hard-to-say" statements?
2. During the next 2 days, when natural situations arise that might be construed to be crises, pause and do not react. If asked what you think, respond, "No comment."
   a. Think about the crisis; give yourself time to be rational and consider all sides. Then present your response to the crisis.
   b. Compare your initial reaction to the rational reaction that you were able to compile, given a little time to think.
3. Stone & Olswang (1989) suggest that counseling boundaries must be considered in terms of focus or content and style or dynamics.

   Focus within boundaries refers to what you talk about, feelings in response to diagnosis, information about speech-language development, concerns about treatment results or prognosis, and treatment planning or decision-making (p. 28).
   Style within boundaries relates to how the clinician and client interact, share power, and assume responsibility (p. 29).

   Discuss this concept in terms of holistic treatment.

REFERENCES

American Speech-Language-Hearing Association. (1985). Committee on Supervision in Speech-Language Pathology and Audiology. A position statement. *ASHA, 27* (6), 57–60.

American Speech-Language-Hearing Association. (1989). ASHA Code of Ethics. *ASHA, 31* (3), 27–30.

Anderson, J. L. (1988). *The supervisory process in speech-language pathology and audiology.* Boston: Little, Brown, and College Hill Press.

Backus, O. (1960). The study of psychological processes in speech therapists. In D. A. Barbara (Ed.), *Psychological and psychiatric aspects of speech and hearing* (pp. 501–535). Springfield, IL: Charles C. Thomas.

Bardwick, J. M. (1986). *The plateauing trap.* New York: American Management Association.

Battin, R. R., & Fox, D. R. (1978). *Private practice in audiology and speech pathology.* New York: Grune and Stratton.

Casey, P. L., Smith, K. J., & Ulrich, S. R. (1988). *Self-supervision: A career tool for audiologists and speech-language pathologists* (Clinical Series No. 10). Rockville, MD: National Student Speech-Language-Hearing Association.

Coulter, M., Scheuerle, J., Laud, M., & Habal, M. B. (1991). Psychological aspects of parents of children with craniofacial anomalies. *Journal of Craniofacial Surgery, 2*(1), 9–17.

Goldman, R. (1986, January 6). Being there is not as satisfying as getting there. *The Wall Street Journal,* p. 20.

Holley, S. C. (1988). The new ASHA: Preparing for the future. *ASHA, 30* (12), 19–22.

Kagan, N. I. (1975). *Interpersonal process recall.* Office of Medical Education, Research, and Development, Michigan State University. East Lansing, MI: Education Publication Services.

Kagan, N. I. (1976). *Interpersonal process recall: A method of influencing human interaction.* Office of Medical Education, Research, and Development, Michigan State University. East Lansing, MI: Education Publication Services.

Kahler, L. B. (1989). Working in the public schools and loving it. *ASHA, 31* (1), 44, 60.

Klevans, D. R. (1982). Techniques of therapy based on principles of counseling and self-management. In W. H. Perkins (Ed.), *General principles of therapy: Current therapy of communication disorders.* New York: Thieme-Stratton.

Luterman, D. (1984). *Counseling the communicatively disordered and their families*. Boston: Little, Brown.

Martin, F. N., George, K. A., O'Neal, J., & Daly, J. A. (1987). Audiologists' and parents' attitudes regarding counseling of families of hearing-impaired children. *ASHA, 29* (2), 27–32.

McCormack, M. H. (1984). *What they don't teach you at Harvard Business School*. Toronto: Bantam Books.

Pickering, M. (1989, March). *Establishing and maintaining an effective working relationship: The first task of supervision*. Paper presented at Clinical supervision across settings: Collaboration and communication workshop, St. Petersburg, FL.

Rollin, W. J. (1987). *The psychology of communication disorders in individuals and their families*. Englewood Cliffs, NJ: Prentice-Hall.

Rousey, C. L. (1982). Techniques of therapy based on psychotherapy. In W. H. Perkins (Ed.), *General principles of therapy: Current therapy of communication disorders*. New York: Thieme-Stratton.

Scheuerle, J. (1985, May). How do I mean? Paper presented at a workshop of the Institute for State Libraries, Columbia, SC.

Scheuerle, J. (1990, March). *The complete communicator*. Paper presented at a meeting of the National Cleft Palate Association, St. Louis, MO.

Stone, J. R., & Olswang, L. B. (1989). The hidden challenge in counseling. *ASHA, 31* (6–7), 27–31.

Strickland, A. J., & Thompson, A. (1989). *Strategic management* (5th ed.). New York: Irwin.

Ward, J. (1987). *Keeping the family business healthy*. San Francisco: Jossey-Bass.

PART I

Annotated Bibliography: Perceptions of Outcomes of Counseling by Speech-Language Pathologists and Audiologists Reported Between 1975 and 1989

Drotar, D., Baskiewicz, B., Irvin, N., & Klaus, M. (1975). The adaptation of parents to the birth of an infant with a congenital malformation: A hypothetical model. *Pediatrics, 56,* 719–717.

> Twenty mothers and five fathers indicated that there are five stages of parental reactions to the birth of an infant with congenital malformation: shock, denial, sadness and anger, adaptation, and reorganization. Early crisis counseling in the first months of life may be particularly crucial in parental attachment to the infant and adjustment to having a baby with a birth defect.

Shipley, K., & McCroskey, R. (1978). Strengths and weaknesses in clinical procedures at university clinics. *Journal of National Student Speech and Hearing Association, 9,* 80–89.

> Responding to a questionnaire concerning their experiences at a university clinic, 82 parents most often cited their interactions with clinicians and other personnel as favorable. The most frequent negative comments were made about the use of communications, including explanations and discussions of the client and client's problems with parents.

Walesky-Rainbow, P., & Morris, H. (1978). An assessment of information-counseling procedure for children with cleft palate. *Cleft Palate Journal, 15,* 20–28.

> In a study of 32 cleft-palate children and their mothers who participated in programs at a particular clinic, the mothers indicated they had sufficient information, but the children did not. Findings suggest a need for more systematic procedures for providing information about treatment and treatment outcomes to the child with the cleft. Additional research about the general counseling process is recommended.

Madison, C., Meadors, D., & Miller, S. (1984). A survey study of a voice clinic program in a public school. *Language, Speech, and Hearing Services in Schools, 15,* 276–280.

> In a survey of 39 parents of clients, 91% of respondents said the clinic had been helpful to their children in some way.

Broder, H., & Trier, W. (1985). Effectiveness of genetic counseling for families with craniofacial anomalies. *Cleft Palate Journal, 22,* 157–162.

Pre- and post-counseling assessment of parent and patient feelings about the birth defect revealed that the majority of participants indicated more positive feelings following genetic counseling. However, 25% expressed negative feelings after genetic counseling.

Castellani, P., Downey, N., Tausig, M., & Bird, W. (1986). Availability and accessibility of family support services. *Mental Retardation, 24,* 71–79.

Several factors affect availability and accessibility of family support services. Employees among 133 agencies take into account the ability of the client to move from acknowledging a need for services to actually accessing those support services. Although families may share a common factor in the diagnosed condition of the client, particular services must be designed and implemented to fulfill the individual family's needs for support services.

Turnbull, J., & Olswang, L. (1989). A pragmatic analysis of speech and language IEP conferences. *Language, Speech, and Hearing Services in Schools, 18,* 275–286.

In analysis of tape-recorded samples of parent counseling sessions by four clinicians, the majority of communication units were found to be predominantly one-way. That is, most of the exchange consisted of clinician statements giving information to relatively passive parents.

Martin, F., George, K., O'Neal, J., & Daly, J. (1987). Audiologists' and parents' attitudes regarding counseling of families of hearing-impaired children. *ASHA, 29,* 27–33.

Parents of hearing-impaired children (N=268) responded that counseling was not meeting many of their needs for information and support concerning management of their children. Audiologists (N=85) were more positive in their perceptions of the outcomes of the counseling sessions with these parents.

Von Almen, P., & Blair, J. (1989). Informational counseling for school-aged hearing-impaired students. *Language, Speech, and Hearing Services in Schools, 20,* 31–40.

Audiologists who were subjects (N=255) in this survey indicated that they believe their role is to provide informational counseling. That is, they see themselves as responsible for sharing information relative to diagnosis, impairment, and its management. They did not perceive a role in support or behavioral management consultation for the parent of the child with a hearing disorder.

Andrews, J., Andrews, M., & Shearer, S. (1989). Parents' attitudes toward family involvement in speech-language services. *Speech and Hearing Services in the Schools, 20,* 391–399.

In a survey of opinions among 1,684 parents, 51% wanted family involvement in the school speech-language services to their children.

For 28%, their involvement should be more extensive than currently, and another 28% were satisfied with their current arrangements for services.

PART 2

Utilization of Counseling in Communication Disorders Literature

The term *counseling* is used in a variety of ways in the literature of the communication disorders discipline. Within the context of a given journal article or book, the term is defined, described, or identified as an activity. Some of the activities imply that counseling consists of multiple discrete, though undesignated, behaviors on the part of the clinician. Others suggest that the act of counseling is composed of a single behavior or a combination of activities such as giving or eliciting information. Without acknowledged consensus, however, there is an underlying suggestion that all practitioners of speech-language pathology or audiology should know what counseling is. Likewise, many of the suggested components of counseling are abstract statements with implied broad behavioral scope, while others identify a particular interpersonal communication technique.

The following list is offered of "counseling/counselor" characteristics of audiologists and speech-language pathologists that have been cited in the literature. The traits have been organized into categories that focus on their commonalities: definitions of counseling, provision of information, elicitation of information, communication skills, and abstract statements. Items were arbitrarily arranged in alphabetical order within respective groups to eliminate any impression of priority among the characteristics. A list of sources for these citations is also provided.

DEFINITIONS OF COUNSELING
- All the work done with families of clients with communication disorders
- Communication of cognitive and affective messages, allowing and engendering growth of the communicating partners
- Guidance
- Not eliminating psycho-emotional pain, but helping clients learn to detach feelings from self-defeating behavior, develop skills for more effective communication, and transfer and maintain those acquired effective skills in their natural environments
- Problem-centered mutual educational experience

PROVISION OF INFORMATION
- Communicating and interpreting clinical findings
- Communicating specific management recommendations
- Conveying information to family

- Discussing serious problems with the client and/or family that do not interfere with therapy
- Informing and instructing the prospective client for initial clinic visit
- Informing and instructing the client and family for cooperation with treatment plan
- Informing the client and family about the nature and impact of the communication disorder
- Outlining options for resolution of problems related to the immediate situation
- Providing appropriate referrals for problems that interfere with the progress of therapy
- Providing an empathic environment
- Providing information about the communication disorder, its consequences, and its management
- Providing relevant information as needed
- Sharing appropriate personal information
- Sharing client information with other professionals
- Sharing information with colleagues for the purpose of problem solving
- Speaking at an appropriate loudness level
- Speaking slowly enough to allow for questions and comments
- Suggesting appropriate resources for resolution of problems that interfere with the progress of treatment
- Suggesting to family members ways of changing their behaviors
- Summarizing discussions
- Verifying client and family understanding of information

ELICITATION OF INFORMATION
- Asking client and family to suggest solutions to problems
- Eliciting suggestions from the client to achieve independence
- Gathering as much information as possible
- Identifying appropriate time and type of referral needed for mental health consultation
- Identifying ways in which the communication problem is experienced by each member of the family
- Identifying what each member of the family has done to improve or reduce the effects of the problem
- Identifying what family communication strategies are effective in reducing the impact of the communication problem
- Identifying what family members perceive as needing change
- Obtaining information from parents

COMMUNICATION SKILLS
- Accepting and encouraging appropriate client participation in discussions
- Communicating effectively
- Encouraging appropriate client focus

- Encouraging client self-exploration
- Listening
- Providing client and family opportunity to talk
- Reading, comprehending, and responding to non-verbal messages
- Using attending behaviors
- Using open-ended questions

ABSTRACT STATEMENTS
- Ascertaining appropriateness of intervention strategies
- Avoiding inappropriate counseling
- Helping families clarify their attitudes, ideas, and understanding
- Improving the client's self-concept and social relationships
- Motivating clients to achieve their potential
- Perceiving the client as a whole person
- Providing a setting that will reduce anxiety
- Providing education and training for client and family
- Providing for client comfort during diagnosis and treatment
- Respecting the rights of client and family
- Setting a professional tone
- Supporting the family's beliefs in themselves
- Understanding classic stages of grieving
- Understanding the principle of behavior modification
- Understanding the role of nonverbal communication
- Using a variety of approaches to the client and family

SOURCES OF "COUNSELING" CITATIONS

American Speech Language Hearing Association. (1984). Professional Services Board: *Accreditation manual,* Rockville, MD: American Speech Language Hearing Association.

American Speech Language Hearing Association. (1989). Code of Ethics. *ASHA, 31,* 27–30.

Andrews, J., & Andrews, M. (1988). Counseling principles for family participation. In D. Yoder & R. Kent (Eds.), *Decision-making in speech-language pathology* (pp. 180–181). Philadelphia: B. C. Decker.

Andrews, J., Andrews, M., & Shearer, S. (1989). Parents' attitudes toward family involvement in speech-language services. *Language, speech, and hearing services in the schools, 20,* 391–399.

Chabon, S. (1982). Client preparation: A counseling imperative. *ASHA, 22,* 603–608.

Clark, J. (1982). Counseling in a pediatric audiologic practice. *ASHA, 22,* 521–526.

Cornett, S., & Chabon, S. (1988). *The clinical practice of speech-language pathology.* Columbus: Merrill.

Curlee, R., & Campbell, M. (1978). Disordered processes and clinical intervention. In P. Skinner & R. Shelton (Eds.), *Speech, language, and hearing. Normal processes and disorders* (pp. 147–172). Reading, MA: Addison-Wesley.

Douglas, L. (1988). Counseling parents of speech-language impaired children. *Seminars in Speech and Language, 9,* 223–236.

Emerick, L. (1988). *The parent interview: Guidelines for student and practicing speech clinicians.* Danville, IL: Interstate Printers and Publishers.

Emerick, L., & Haynes, W. (1986). *Diagnosis and evaluation in speech pathology.* Englewood Cliffs, NJ: Prentice-Hall.

Flower, R. (1984). *Delivery of speech-language pathology and audiology services.* Baltimore: Williams and Wilkins.

Kelvans, D. (1988). Counseling strategies for communication disorders. *Seminars in Speech and Language, 9,* 185–208.

Knepflar, K. (1976). *Report-writing in the field of communication disorders.* Danville, IL: Interstate Printers and Publishers.

Lavorato, A., & McFarlane, S. (1988). Counseling clients with voice disorders. *Seminars in Speech and Language, 9,* 237–256.

Luterman, D. (1984). *Counseling the communicatively disordered and their families.* Boston: Little, Brown.

Martin, F., George, K., O'Neil, J., & Daly, J. (1987). Audiologists' and parents' attitudes regarding counseling of families of hearing-impaired children. *ASHA, 29,* 27–33.

Matkin, N., Ringel, R., & Snope, T. (1983). Master report of surveys and discrepancies. *ASHA Report, 13,* 93–105.

McCarthy, P., Culpepper, N., & Lucks, L. (1986). Variability in counseling experiences and training among ESB-accredited programs. *ASHA, 28,* 49–52.

Meitus, I. J. (1983). Talking with patients and their families. *Diagnosis in speech-language pathology.* Baltimore: University Park Press, 311–338.

Monat-Haller, R. (1987). Speech-language pathologist as counselor and sexuality educations. *ASHA, 29,* 35–36.

Rollin, W. (1988). Counseling spouses of the communicatively impaired. *Seminars in Speech and Language, 9,* 269–282.

Sanders, D. (1982). *Aural rehabilitation.* Englewood Cliffs, NJ: Prentice-Hall.

Shelton, R., Hahn, E., & Morris, H. (1968). Diagnosis and therapy. In D. Spriestersbach & D. Sherman (Eds.), *Cleft palate and communication* (pp. 225–268). New York: Academic Press.

Stone, J., & Olswang, L. (1989). The hidden challenge in counseling. *ASHA, 31,* 27–31.

Webster, E. (1977). *Counseling with parents of handicapped children: Guidelines for improving communication.* New York: Grune and Stratton.

Webster, E., & Cole, B. (1979). Effective leadership of parent discussion groups. *Language-speech-hearing services in schools, 10,* 72–81.

APPENDIX B
Suggested interactive stimulus materials by age

BIRTH TO 3 YEARS OF AGE
    Bright colored objects
    Black and white objects
    Mobile, movable objects
    Noise-making toys, such as rattle,
        music box, ticking clock
    Soft, cuddly stuffed toys
    Mirror
    Small plastic boxes (pint or quart)
    Small toys, too large to swallow
    Variety of fabrics – different textures
    Pan – tub of water
    Blocks – 1" or larger
    Stacking toys
    Balls
    Baby doll and doll clothes
    Picture books
    Pull toys
    Small cars and trucks to push
    Rocking chair or rocking horse
    Scooter to push with feet
    Finger paints
    Crayons
    Clay
    Shovel for digging
    Mallet and block for pounding
    Puzzles and take-apart toys
    Beads for stringing
    Hollow blocks
    Interlocking toys

3 TO 6 YEARS OF AGE
    Tricycle or bicycle
    Climbing apparatus – play yard
    Hauling device – wagon, bucket
    Play telephone
    Play or real kitchen utensils
    Simple board games
    Cardboard cartons – large
    Empty spools
    Paper, scissors, markers
    Paste, transparent tape
    Simple card games
    Books, books, books

6 TO 10 YEARS OF AGE
    Bicycle
    Dollhouse
    Jump rope
    Balls
    Bats
    Puppets
    Musical instruments
    Phonograph records
    Tape player and tapes
    Videotapes
    Puzzles
    Computer games
    Books, books, books

10 TO 13 YEARS OF AGE
    Books about hobbies
    Library card
    Special interests
        Sports equipment
        Crafts books
        Game books
    Telephone
    Computer games

13 TO 16 YEARS OF AGE
    Sports equipment
    Musical instruments
    Crafts
    Collectibles
    Computer
    Computer supplies
    Books, books, books

16 YEARS OF AGE AND OLDER
    Workout equipment
    Motorized vehicle
    Electronics
    Specialty items
    Magazines and books
    Clothes, cosmetics
    Music
    Movies, films
    Books, books, books

APPENDIX C
Supplementary Reading

Supplementary light and very light reading is suggested to entertain and inform. These resources are suggested especially for the students of human nature who have already collected a substantial amount of information about their own cultural perspectives of the human life span and the personal values derived therefrom.

The following list of reading materials is a brief introduction to other ways of viewing the world and may be helpful in understanding and melding the many cultures and traditions that enter the clinical setting. For some of the items (Very Light Reading), the reader is encouraged to visit the children's section of the local public library or bookseller and browse. There you can sample brief volumes that are rich in different cultures, classes, real-life experiences, and myths and superstitions for insight into developmental concerns of the modern world. Other listed materials may be found in the adult section of most libraries or acquired through interlibrary loan if not locally available.

Light Reading (not light content)

Alberti, R. E., & Emmons, M. L. (1982). *Your perfect right*. San Luis Obispo, CA: Impact.

Baldwin, J. (1974). *If Beale Street could talk*. New York: Dial Press.

Bragg, B. (as signed to E. Bergman). (1989). *Lessons in laughter*. Washington, DC: Gallaudet University Press.

Braithwaite, E. R. (1973). *To sir with love*. Moonachie, NJ: Pyramid Publications.

Campbell, B. M. (1989). *Sweet summer: Growing up with and without my dad*. New York: Putman.

Campbell, J. (1972). *Myths to live by*. New York: The Viking Press.

Curtis, N. (Ed.). (1987). *The Indians' book*. New York: Bonanza Books.

Fair, R. L. (1975). *Cornbread, Earl, and me*. New York: Bantam.

Gabor, D. (1983). *How to start a conversation and make friends*. New York: Simon & Schuster.

Grier, W. H., & Cobbs, P. M. (1970). *Why do they act that way?* New York: Basic Books.

Hillerman, T. (1989). *A thief of time*. New York: Harper and Row.

Jung, J. H. (1989). *Genetic syndromes in communication disorders*. Waltham, MA: Little, Brown.

Kingston, M. H. (1989). *The woman warrior*. New York: Random House.

Noyes, J., & MacNeill, N. (1983). *Your child can win.* New York: William Morrow.

Parsons, F. M. (1988). *I didn't hear the dragon roar.* Washington, DC: Gallaudet University Press.

Ritter, B. (1988). *Sometimes God has a kid's face.* Fort Lauderdale, FL: Covenant House.

Rodriguez, R. (1983). *Hunger of memory: The education of Richard Rodriguez.* New York: Bantam.

Washington, M. H. (Ed.). (1975). *Black-eyed Susans: Classic stories by and about Black women.* New York: Bantam.

Wilson, A. N. (1978). *Developmental psychology of the Black child.* New York: Africana Research Publications.

Very Light Reading (not light content)

These stories about children's lives help to understand how they feel during crises and how they learn to deal with conflict and emotion. A brief note following each suggests its focus.

Blue, R. (1976). *Grandma didn't wave back.* New York: Dell. Grandmother's dementia.

Blume, J. (1971). *Freckle juice.* New York: Dell. Peer pressure.

Burnett, F. H. (1971). *The secret garden.* New York: Dell. Self-discovery and friendship.

Byars, B. (1981). *The 18th emergency.* New York: Puffin. Physical fear.

Child of the silent night: The story of Laura Bridgman. (1963). Boston: Houghton Mifflin. Triumph of a deaf, mute, blind child.

Clifton, L. (1979). *The lucky stone.* New York: Delacorte. A myth of hope.

Delton, J., & Tucker, D. (1986). *My Grandma's in a nursing home.* Niles, IL: Albert Whitman. Older adults can have ordinary human characteristics even when in a residential facility.

Dunn, M. L. (1975). *The man in the box.* New York: Dell. Vietnamese youth and a war prisoner.

Estes, E. (1974). *The hundred dresses.* Orlando, FL: Harcourt. Poverty.

Fox, M. (1985). *Wilfred Gordon McDonald Partridge.* Brooklyn, NY: Kane/Miller. Nursing home residents are friendly, ordinary people.

Hassler, J. (1977). *Four miles to Pinecone.* New York: Warne. Risk and responsibility.

Hinton, N. (1979). *Collision course.* New York: Dell. Guilt and anxiety.

Kotzwinkle, W. (1978). *The leopard's tooth*. New York: Avon. Tribal myth, superstition, beliefs.

Lloyd, D. (1985). *Grandma and the pirate*. New York: Crown Publisher. Older people can be active, effective, and full of fun.

Milne, A. A. (1975). *Now we are six*. New York: Dell. Dreams and nonsense.

Moskin, M. (1975). *Waiting for Mama*. Seattle, WA: Coward. Immigrants—hope and fear.

Norris, G. (1969). *A time for watching*. New York: Random House. Hyperactivity.

Patterson, K. (1979). *Bridge to Terabithia*. New York: Avon. Dealing with emotions.

Peck, R. N. (1972). *A day no pigs would die*. New York: Knopf. Life and death, fear and triumph.

Pinkwater, D. M. (1975). *Wingman*. Columbia, SC: Dodd. Racial prejudice.

Sachs, M. (1971). *The bear's house*. Garden City, NY: Doubleday. Classroom teasing.

Smith, D. B. (1976). *A taste of blackberries*. New York: Scholastic. Death.

Smith, G. (1974). *The hayburners*. New York: Delacorte. Mental retardation stereotypes.

Speare, E. G. (1972). *The witch of Blackbird Pond*. New York: Dell. Family and community peer pressure.

Stieg, W. (1973). *The real thief*. New York: Farrar. Guilt and pride.

Tate, J. (1981). *Luke's garden and Gramp*. New York: Harper. Intolerance of differences.

Thiele, C. (1978). *Storm boy*. New York: Harper. Loss of a friend.

Viorst, J. (1975). *The tenth good thing about Barney*. New York: Atheneum. Death of a pet.

The witch of Fourth Street. (1972). Harper. Urban poverty.

APPENDIX D
Selected Characteristics of Aging-Without-Disease

Listed below are some of the recognized characteristics of men and women who live successfully past the age of 75. While a great deal of research still needs to be done, these characteristics reflect a portion of the consensus of current thought. There are strong indications that life review is helpful and settling in the face of current disruptions and to maintaining stability in the presence of unexpected change. The speech-language pathologist and audiologist will want to use these ideas in interacting with aging family members of clients as well as with clients who are themselves members of the gerontological population.

- High variability among individuals in biological, psychological, and sociological interrelationships
- Individual variations in all aspects of life, action, and reaction
- Physiological processes slower than earlier in the same individual's life
- Increased reaction time, causing slower responses to stimuli in the daily environment
- A tendency to conserve strength and resources as necessary to meet perceived needs
- Roles in daily life assumed or discarded to adjust to other changes of aging
- A narrowed scope of social interaction
- Given the time to respond, functions as accurately as when younger
- Activity and involvement highly correlated with life satisfaction
- Expressed attachment to things that surround the individual in daily life
- Review of one's life typically part of self-evaluation in the search to maintain personal integrity
- Self-evaluation based on the self as an integrated whole; self-esteem separated from life style or work role
- Changes in health and body function accepted as part of a natural process while maintaining interest in life
- Tendency to perceive self in the perspective of one's surroundings
- Death considered a part of living, viewed as a step that one can prepare for
- Evaluation of self by others perceived accurately and objectively
- Changed social roles (public or familial) undertaken with adaptation
- An internal locus of control maintained
- An attitude of self held in a tough but flexible manner
- Social influence may replace personal power
- Approval of oneself outweighs regrets
- Acceptance of oneself exceeds recognition of deficits

APPENDIX E
AIDS: Acquired Immune Deficiency Syndrome

INFANTS AND YOUNG CHILDREN
Causative Agents
- Human Immunodeficiency Virus (HIV)
- Transplacental during pregnancy
- Contact with blood and secretions at delivery
- Breast-feeding
Teratogenic Effects
- Microcephaly
- Hypertelorism
- Prominent box-like forehead
- Flattened nasal bridge
- Mild obliquity of eyes
Clinical Manifestations
- Small size
- Failure to thrive
- Respiratory disease
- Delayed psychomotor development

PRE-ADOLESCENTS, ADOLESCENTS, AND ADULTS
Transmission
- Sexual contact with infected partner
- Sharing of contaminated hypodermic needles
- Transfusion with infected blood
Clinical Manifestations
- Loss of immunity (no clear-cut symptoms)
- Fever
- Loss of appetite
- Chronic diarrhea
- Oral candidiasis
- Fatigue
- Weight loss
- Lymphadenopathy
- Yeast infections
- Cytomegalovirus (CMV) infection
- Herpes
- Atypical mucobacterial infection
- Cryptococcal meningitis
- Crytosporidium enteritis
- Toxoplasmosis
- Non-Hodgkin lymphomas
- Kaposi's sarcoma (KS)
- Pneumocystis carinii pneumonia

CLINICAL TECHNIQUE
Follow Institution Protocol
- Use, cleansing, and disposal of instruments
- Protection of clinician from exposure to body fluids that may contain blood, such as saliva in a patient with deteriorating gums
- Protection of patient from infection, for example, a clinician with a cold must wear a facial mask while treating a patient

Note. From Flower & Sooy, 1987; Marlow & Redding, 1988; ASHA Committee on Quality Assurance, 1989.

APPENDIX F
Summary of drugs that are often used for their physical or psychological effect

Substance	Physical Effect	Psychological Effect

ALCOHOL	CNS sedation
	Depressant
	Reduced muscular
	    coordination
		Impaired judgment
		Slowed reaction time
		Slowed emotional
		    control
		Dependency

CAFFEINE	CNS stimulant Increased alertness Reduced fatigue	Insomnia Jitteriness Shallow sleep
NICOTINE	CNS stimulant	Habituation

NARCOTICS
Opium
Heroin
Morphine
Methadone
Dilaudid
Demerol
Codeine
Percodan
Darvon
Cough syrup
    Cheracol
    Hycodan
    Robitussin
    Tussionex
	Decreased blood
	    pressure
	Arrhythmia
	Nausea
	Cramps
	Reduced reflexes
	Convulsions
	Urine retention
	Skin pigmentation
	Swollen nasal mucosa
	Shallow respiration
	Slow breathing
		Euphoria
		Lethargy
		Apathy
		Slow comprehension
		Sedation
		Dependency

STIMULANTS
Amphetamines
Cocaine
    Rock cocaine
Methylphenidate
    Rytalin
	Increased blood
	    pressure
	Tachycardia
	Arrhythmia
	Headache
	Loss of appetite
	Dilated pupils
	Hyperactivity
	Hyperreflexia
	Teeth grinding
	Skin Abscesses
	Dependency
		Euphoria
		Insomnia
		Agitation
		Hallucinations
		Paranoia
		Talkativeness
		Tremors
		Delirium
		Outbursts
		Reduced fatigue
		Dependency

APPENDIX F *(continued)*
Summary of drugs that are often used for their physical or psychological effect

Substance	Physical Effect	Psychological Effect
DEPRESSANTS Barbiturates	Reduced cardiovascular function Dizziness, headache Nystagmus Slurred speech Drunken behavior Decreased reflexes Shallow respiration Dilated pupils Weak, rapid pulse	Drowsiness Confusion Irritability Poor memory Depression Impaired judgment Impaired emotional control Abnormal sleep behavior

HALLUCINOGENS Indolealkylamines
  Delysid, LSD
  Psilocin
  Diethyltryptamine
Phenylethylamine
  mescaline
Phenylisopropylamine
	Elevated cardiovascular function
	Gastrointestinal upset
	Neuromuscular malfunction
	Dizziness
	Dilated pupils
	Muscle aches
	Elevated respiratory rate
		Euphoria
		Delusions
		Hallucinations
		Poor perception
		Excitation
		Psychoses
		Blank stare
		Panic reaction

PHENCYCLIDINES	Elevated cardiovascular function CNS disturbance Hyperreflexia Cholergenic effect Dizziness Loss of coordination Slurred speech Nystagmus Vertigo Nausea Tremor Dry mouth	Illusions Numbness Distorted reality Immobility

APPENDIX F (continued)
Summary of drugs that are often used for their physical or psychological effect

Substance	Physical Effect	Psychological Effect
CANNABINOIDS Hashish Marijuana THC	Cardiovascular depression Tachycardia Red eyes Tremor Poor coordination Headache Increased appetite Dry mouth Increased respiration rate Decreased testosterone production Abnormal sperm Abnormal chromosomes Abnormal menstrual cycle	Euphoria Paranoia Relaxed inhibitions Disturbed short term memory Suspiciousness Confusion Disorientation
INHALANTS Alcohols Alipathic hydrocarbons (adhesives) Anesthetics (nitrous oxide) Aromatic hydrocarbons (gasoline, paint) Esters (paint thinner) Ketones (model cement)	Dizziness Loss of concentration Sudden sniffing death (SSD) Tremor Irritability GI tract disturbance GU tract disturbance Anemia Weight loss Necrosis of liver Nystagmus Cerebellar ataxia Paralysis	Psychological dependence Euphoria Excitement Auditory and visual hallucinations Giddiness Recklessness Impulsive and destructive behavior

Note. From AMA Division on Drugs, 1984; Cole, 1990; Ferry, Banner, & Wolf, 1985; Jones & Smith, 1973; Lippman, 1980; Marlow & Redding, 1988; Merker, Higgins, & Kinnard, 1985; Price & Andrews, 1982; Smith & Deitch, 1987; Sparks, 1984; Trapp & Spatz, 1988.

Index

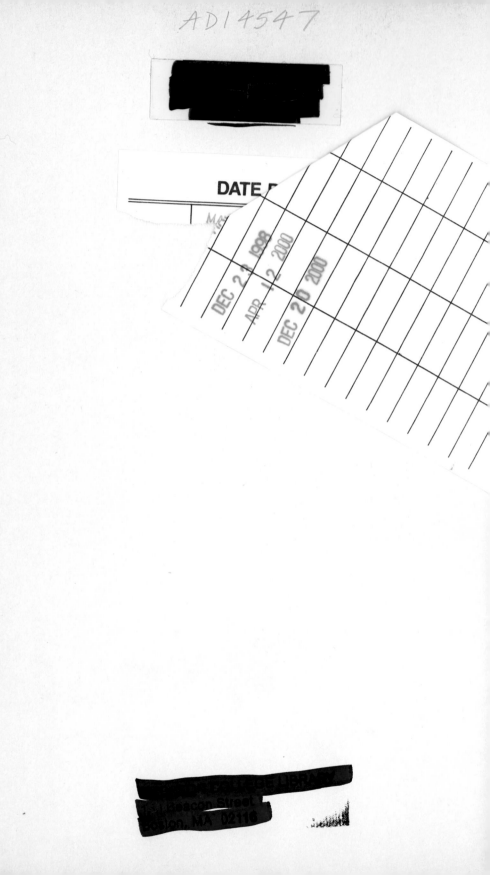